Praise for Lawrence A. Kane...

"I got a chance to read your book *Surviving Armed Assaults* over the weekend. Many thanks for sending it to me. What an excellent contribution to the community! I was particularly impressed by the encyclopedia-like thoroughness and depth of information, tapping into a diverse array of knowledge and experts. WELL done, my friend. This will be an invaluable resource for anyone walking the warrior's path, and anyone who is interested in this vital topic. And you can quote me on that! Hooah! And ALL the best!" – **Lt. Col. Dave Grossman**, US Army Airborne Ranger (ret); Director, Killology Research Group; author of *On Killing: The Psychological Cost of L   Kill in War and Society*, co-author of *On Combat: The Psychology and Physiology of Deadly Co   Board Member of the American Sniper Association, International Law En   ssociation, National Institute of Ethics, and International Confere

"From the very first few pages I could tell that th   would have liked to have written and the sheer vast amount of in   remendous. These days, I can only buy into concepts from people who have worked   conflict and that experience shines through. For me, however, it's how the 'science' of close quarter combat is married with psychology, techniques, and tactics. A really heartfelt 'well done'. It will be on the shelves for years to come." – **Peter Consterdine**, 8th degree black belt, Operations and Training Director of Risk Management and Security Company, Co-Founder and joint Chief Instructor (with Geoff Thompson) of The British Combat Association (BCA), author of *Streetwise: The Complete Manual of Personal Security and Self Defense, The Modern Bodyguard: The Manual of Close Protection Training, Fit to Fight: The Manual of Intense Training for Combat, Travelsafe: The Complete Guide to Travel Security*, and *Powerstrike: The Art of High Impact Punching and Kicking*.

"*Surviving Armed Assaults* is a terrific addition to any serious library of self-defense books. Its emphasis on awareness and avoidance as your most effective survival strategies makes it a worthy companion to works by authors such as Alain Burrese, Loren Christensen, Marc MacYoung, and Peyton Quinn. Kane covers enough aspects of the topic to make the book useful as an encyclopedia, and yet his prose is so readable, and he uses so many real-life anecdotes to illustrate his points, that you'll have trouble putting it down. I'll be drawing on some of the lessons learned from *SAA* in future John Rain books." – **Barry Eisler**, internationally bestselling author of the John Rain series, *shodan* in *Kodokan* Judo.

"As both a private citizen and a security professional, I found this book an outstanding review of self defense tactics and techniques which can be used to save one's life or the life of another. Kane's synthesis of the physical and mental processes of self-defense and counter attack will make this book a must-read for law enforcement, security and self-defense specialists." – **Greg A. Gwash, J.D.**, Chief Security Officer of The Boeing Company, former Deputy Director of the U.S. Defense Investigative Service, decorated Vietnam veteran (5th Special Forces Group).

"Mr. Kane's excellent book covers a broad spectrum of topics associated with surviving armed conflict. It ranges from details about a variety of weapons to philosophical and matters relating to defense and the use of countervailing and potentially lethal force. Tactics, training, and mindset are all discussed; and all of this is presented in a simple and logical format with great anecdotes to illustrate the high points. For a student or teacher of the martial arts, this is a must read." – **Dr. Jeff Cooper, M.D.**, Tactical Medical Director of the Toledo Ohio SWAT; Commander, US Naval Reserve; 4th degree black belt in *Goju Ryu* karate.

"Some two million people in the United States are the victims of a weapon attack each year, and that includes black belts. The de-escalation and survival skills in this book will set your feet on the right path and put your head in the right place so you don't become a shocking headline in your local paper, or lead story on the six o'clock news. Kane gets it: get this book and get it too." – **Kris Wilder**, author of *Lessons from the Dojo Floor*, co   in *Goju Ryu* karate, 2nd degree black belt in Tae Kwon

"*Surviving Armed Assaults* is a far-reaching and superbly informative text that relies on the author's firsthand knowledge of weapons as a martial artist and security officer. His experiences are backed by recent statistics. A crucial part of the self-defense equation is the ability to understand violence, including knowledge of how weapons function and how they can fail, how an armed assailant reasons, and what he (or she) is looking for prior to an attack. Lawrence Kane's knowledge of violence has allowed him to write a very valid and insightful book. I particularly appreciated the color-coded awareness levels, which help the reader classify and quantify the danger in order to understand it better." – **Martina Sprague**, author of *Fighting Science, Strength and Power Training for Martial Arts, Combat Fitness for the Elite Female Martial Artist*, and *Norse Warfare: A History*.

"At long last, a no-nonsense book on armed assaults! Lawrence Kane has written a thorough, well-researched and highly-accessible guide to this vitally important subject. This book should in no way to be confused with those that claim to offer "practical" techniques and advice, but instead perpetuate many dangerous myths and impractical elaborate disarms. This book tells it how it is! *Surviving Armed Assaults* covers all aspects of dealing with armed assailants and gives you all the information you need to keep yourself and your loved ones safe. All serious martial artists should read this superb text." – **Iain Abernethy**, author of *Bunkai Jutsu, Karate's Grappling Methods, Throws for Strikers, Arm-Locks for All Styles*, and *Mental Strength*; British Combat Association Hall of Fame Member, 5th degree black belt in *Wado Ryu* karate.

"Lawrence Kane has done an excellent job of giving very practical and realistic information on how to handle a variety of scenarios that is helpful even for non-karate practitioners. His examples help get the message across. In addition, he includes valid probability statements on the likelihood of an incident occurring or not occurring, based on crime statistics. The book will spark your thinking of what you should or shouldn't do in different scenarios, and gives some practical solutions, weighing different ethical, moral, criminal, and civil principles. Kane's advice on self-defense and moral and legal aspects is right on target and sound advice. This book is highly recommended!" – **Vicky M. Stormo**, Chief of Police, University of Washington Police Department.

"Read this book, it is a very well researched summary of street violence. Kane mixes the right amount of sociological data with well chosen first hand accounts of past events to present a refreshingly clear illustration of what actual street violence is. The book's title can be deceiving, as the book is about much more than weapon involvement in street violence. This book presents street violence from the perspective of a civilian, in a refreshingly non-macho, un-romantic manner. Kane understands that most combative or combative-sport practitioners are filled with numerous fallacies when it comes to actual violence. This book sets forth to offer real perspective without being preachy. Kane has something for everybody in this book. No matter if you are an expert or novice, you will glean something from reading this. Rarely do we find such a good summary of a topic that is so broad, no aspect is ignored, including those aspects, which are not so obvious." – **Aaron Fields**, 4th degree black belt; firefighter.

"I was fortunate enough to receive an advance copy of Mr. Kane's newest book. As with a previous effort of his, *The Way of Kata*, this one was again a researcher's dream. Kane's book is, if nothing else, comprehensive. He goes over far more than just physical self-defense techniques. This book covers the psychology of an assailant as well as what to look for in any situation. Kane peppers his text with a fine mix of statistics as well as quotes from other notables in the field such as Loren Christensen, Marc MacYoung, Massad Ayoob, and others. I would bet that he has lectured on this topic quite a bit as his text is a good mix of conversational English and lecturer. It is an easy read and never gets dull. My favorite section covers the viewpoint of the law regarding a self-defense situation and how you should act when confronted by an investigating officer at the scene. This one section is worth the price of the book alone and this is a small section. I heartily recommend Mr. Kane's book. It certainly has something for everyone from novice to master." – **Dan Anderson**, 8th degree black belt, four-time national karate champion (who has won over 70 Grand Titles), 2002 Master's Division World Champion; author of *American Freestyle Karate: A Guide To Sparring*.

SURVIVING ARMED ASSAULTS

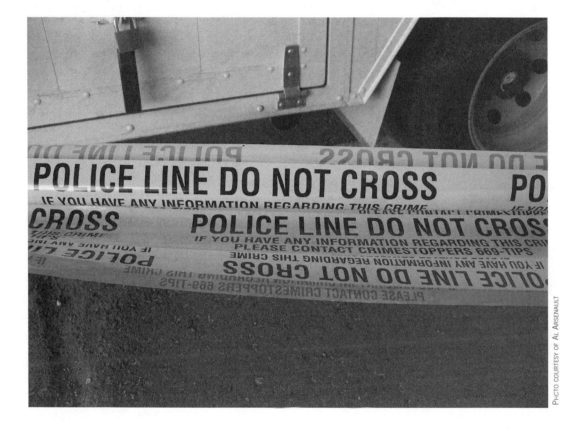

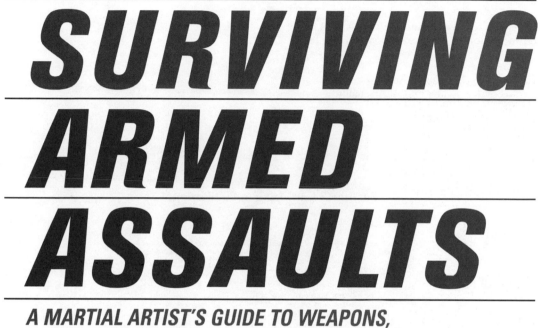

SURVIVING ARMED ASSAULTS

A MARTIAL ARTIST'S GUIDE TO WEAPONS, STREET VIOLENCE, & COUNTERVAILING FORCE

LAWRENCE A. KANE
FOREWORD BY LOREN W. CHRISTENSEN

YMAA Publication Center
Boston, Mass. USA

YMAA Publication Center, Inc.
Main Office
4354 Washington Street
Boston, Massachusetts, 02131
1-800-669-8892 • www.ymaa.com • ymaa@aol.com

Editor: Susan Bullowa
Cover Design: Richard Rossiter
Photos by Jeff Miller and Al Arsenault

ISBN-10: 1-59439-071-1
ISBN-13: 978-1-59439-071-5

10   9   8   7   6   5   4   3   2   1

Publisher's Cataloging in Publication

Kane, Lawrence A.

Surviving armed assaults : a martial artist's guide to weapons, street
violence, & countervailing force / Lawrence A. Kane ; foreword by
Loren W. Christensen. -- 1st ed. -- Boston, MA : YMAA Publication
Center, 2006.

p. ; cm.

ISBN-13: 978-1-59439-071-5
ISBN-10: 1-59439-071-1
Includes bibliographical references and index.

1. Self-defense--Handbooks, manuals, etc. 2. Assault and
battery--Prevention--Handbooks, manuals, etc. 3. Violence--
Prevention--Handbooks, manuals, etc. 4. Assault weapons--
Handbooks, manuals, etc. 5. Martial arts. I. Title.

GV1111 .K56 2006   2006929523
613.6/6--dc22   0609

Warning: No text, no matter how well written, can substitute for professional hands-on instruction. Training with live steel, firearms, and other potentially deadly weapons described in this book should always be undertaken responsibly, ensuring every available precaution for participant safety. Information presented herein inevitably reflects the author's beliefs and experiences under specific circumstances that the reader cannot duplicate exactly. Consequently, these materials should be *used for academic study only.* Readers are encouraged to be aware of all appropriate local and national laws relating to self-defense, reasonable force, and the use of weaponry, and act in accordance with all applicable laws at all times. Neither the author nor the publisher assumes any responsibility for the use or misuse of information contained in this book.

Nothing in this document constitutes a legal opinion nor should any of its contents be treated as such. While the author believes that everything herein is accurate, any questions regarding specific self-defense situations, legal liability, and/or interpretation of federal, state, or local laws should always be addressed by an attorney at law. This text relies on public news sources to gather information on various crimes and criminals described herein. While news reports of such incidences are generally accurate, they are on occasion incomplete or incorrect. Consequently, all suspects should be considered innocent until proven guilty in a court of law.

Printed in Canada.

Dedication

To Todd Beamer, Mark Bingham, Sandra Bradshaw, Tom Burnett, Andrew Garcia, Jeremy Glick, Richard Guadagno, Cee Cee Lyles, and the other passengers and crew who fought back against the hijackers on United Airlines Flight 93. On September 11, 2001 these apparently average people, showed their extraordinary valor by rising to an unexpected and horrific moment. In attempting to regain control of the aircraft by arming themselves with a variety of makeshift weapons and storming the flight deck they showed their gallantry by overcoming terrorists who had already killed innocents and callously intended to kill many more. While their attempt tragically fell short, their actions should be a marker for all readers against which to measure our lives. If faced with the same circumstances, could you? Would you?

These brave souls should not be forgotten.

Table of Contents

Foreword

by Loren Christensen

During my 40 plus years in the martial arts and 29 years in law enforcement, I've learned that we need to tread carefully when using absolutes in our training, teaching and thinking about fighting, no matter if the battle is between two people or ten. Consider the absolutes "always" and "never." These can be dangerous words.

"An assailant with a knife would never attack like that."
"A gunman will always threaten you this way."
"A strong punch here will always drop an attacker."
"Nine out of ten fights always go to the ground."

You have to wonder how the speaker knows these things. Were there studies done? Did someone compile statistics? To my knowledge, there has never been such an impossible study. Even if there were, there is no way to predict future fights.

So, what is so bad about these commonly heard claims? For one, they are not always true. Just because the scuffle you had on the basketball court ended up on the floor, or just because your cousin's friend was attacked by a guy who stabbed at him with a downward slash, doesn't make these characteristics absolutes in the world of fighting. It is dangerous to have these claims ingrained into your mind because they can cause you to train a certain way—a limited way. If you believe that an assailant would never attack in a particular manner, you are not going to train for that possibility. That can come back to bite you big time.

I always get a kick out of this one.

"A trained knife fighter would never attack you that way."

It's been my experience and the experience of every cop I've ever talked to, that being confronted by a trained knife fighter is about as rare as finding a Yellow Page ad for a martial arts school where the teacher isn't a past world champion.

During my decades policing the mean streets of Portland, Oregon and the war-torn streets of Saigon, Vietnam, I went toe-to-toe with assailants armed with shards of glass, boards with nails protruding from an end, a table leg with a screw sticking out, sharpened sticks, screwdrivers, knives of every make and style, and many other cutting instruments. Not one of these wielders of pointy objects was trained in ways of combat with these weapons. Yet they were still dangerous. While I was fortunate enough to never get nicked, people they had attacked before I got to the scene were not so fortunate.

During my first week as a rookie cop, my partner and I responded to a domestic fight, finding the wife sitting in a comfortable living room chair with a kitchen knife protruding obscenely from her throat. Her husband was a railroad man who had never trained with a blade. He resisted arrest long and hard, but we eventually prevailed.

On another occasion, I was in a rough part of town taking a report from a man who was clearly in shock. His girlfriend, he said, had "threatened" him with a knife. After talking with the frightened man for nearly five minutes, he turned his head to the side to look at something. That is when I saw it, or maybe I should say, did not see it. His right ear was gone, sliced neatly from his head by his girlfriend who had clearly done more than just threaten. We looked for it for several minutes, eventually finding it under a parked car. Was the woman a trained knife fighter? No. Just a 50-year-old intoxicated street person.

Most knife assaults are not carried out by trained knife fighters. However, how trained do you have to be to wield a sharp tool and stick it into someone? In the 1998 movie *The Mask of Zorro*, master swordsman Anthony Hopkins's character asks Antonio Banderas, the new Zorro-in-training, "Do you know how to use that thing?" referring to a sword.

"Yes!" he answers. "The pointy end goes into the other man."

That is how simple it is and, consequently, what makes a cutting weapon so dangerous. And why you should never rule out any kind of attack? The next time your training partner or even your teacher tells you that a knife fighter would never hold a knife in such a grip or attack in such a way, say politely, "I'd like to practice it anyway."

British Comedian Eddie Izzard says, "Guns don't kill people; people kill people. And monkeys do too, if they have a gun." For sure, a monkey can shoot a gun, and so can a drunk, your angry buddy, a disgruntled co-worker, and a six-year-old child.

The classic way to practice disarming is for your partner to point a gun at you from your front, side, or back. You train this way because for the most part these are the positions in which you are likely to try to disarm.

I know cops who have successfully disarmed people from this classic position. I've done it once, but it was not against a bad guy. It was against my six-year-old daughter. For years, I drilled and drilled into my kids that they were never to touch my guns. I told them I would not leave them out in the open, but should I make a mistake and do so, they were not to touch it but to come and tell me. This worked all the years they were growing up. Except once.

I had placed my .38 snub-nosed revolver in its holster on top of the camping gear that was to go into the car trunk. I then went into the kitchen to get something and when I turned around my daughter stuck my revolver in my stomach, and said with a smile, "Bang, bang," as she tried to pull the trigger with her too-weak finger. As quick as a wink I bladed my body and snatched the gun away.

After I got out of the bathroom, I talked to my crying child about how daddy had made a mistake and so had she.

My other disarms were not as textbook (if you want to think of your child trying to gun you down as textbook).

There was the guy who after shooting a store clerk ran into the phone booth to make a call. My partner and I spotted him and we jammed him so he couldn't reach for his gun. But that didn't keep him from trying. There isn't a lot of room in a phone booth for one person making a call, let alone three people fighting for a gun. The good guys won, but not without a heart-hammering struggle.

There was the 16-year-old burglary suspect my partner and I were interviewing in his home with his mother. All was going well until he stood up to supposedly stretch, but then lunged for a rifle that was propped against a wall behind a door. I dived for the weapon with one hand and squeezed the front of his throat with the other, while at the same time my partner wrapped his 19-inch biceps around the kid's neck in a choke hold and grabbed the barrel of the gun with his other hand. We had control of the weapon, but it took a few seconds to free my hand that was trapped under my partner's massive arm.

There was the guy I pulled out of his car by his hair as he tried to retrieve his pistol from the floor.

And there was the guy I punched reflexively in the ear as he yanked my partner's gun from its holster.

There were many others, but you get the idea that not all disarm situations are those classic ones typically practiced in class. It makes sense, therefore, to practice in as many ways as your imagination can conjure, and then some. Just don't let anyone ever tell you, "A guy with a gun would never do that." Should you hear that, say to the person, "Just in case, let's practice it anyway." Hey, it's your life you might have to defend.

The book you are about to read takes the same self-defense philosophy I've been discussing. Lawrence Kane has done a marvelous job within these pages drawing upon his own vast experience in martial arts training and in real-world self-defense situations. Just as he has left no possibility unexamined in his own training and teaching, he has done likewise in his research and presentation in this excellent work. If you bought this book thinking you're getting a self-defense manual against weapons, you are. But he goes beyond mere technique to teach you all facets of the subject.

Lawrence begins with a discussion on the critical importance of personal awareness and ways to avoid dangerous situations. Understanding these chapters alone will help keep you out of danger. He then discusses common everyday places where you are likely to come face to face with a violent perpetrator. Should it happen, he teaches you ways to de-escalate an aggressor's intent. A rarity in this type of book,

Lawrence next discusses the ethical, moral, and religious aspects of self-defense, as well as the necessary mindset to use extreme force in your defense.

The next three chapters deal with the down and dirty of fighting for your life against an armed assailant. Lawrence gives you more than just the physical; he also discusses ways to think before, during, and after the confrontation.

The book ends with critical information on a variety of weapons you're likely to run into. A martial arts teacher once said, "I don't want you to fight, but if you have to, it's nice to know how. With this last chapter, I hear Lawrence saying, "I hope you never have to defend against a weapon, but should it happen, here are a number of weapons you might run into and critical information you need to know about them."

You made a good choice getting this book. Read it. Study it. Ingrain it. And train.

Always train.

Loren W. Christensen
www.lwcbooks.com

Loren Christensen began his martial arts training in 1965, earning 10 black belts over the years, 7 in karate, 2 in jujitsu, and 1 in arnis. He is a retired police officer with 29 years experience in military and civilian law enforcement, where he specialized in street gangs, defensive tactics, and dignitary protection. He is the author of 31 books on the martial arts, self-defense, law enforcement, nutrition, prostitution, and post traumatic stress disorder. His book On Combat, *which he co-authored with Lt .Col. Dave Grossman, is mandatory reading at the United States War College in Washington, DC. Loren's web site is www.lwcbooks.com.*

Preface

"Not to be the bearer of bad tidings, but the reason someone uses a weapon on another human being is to stack the deck in their favor. People don't use weapons to fight, they use weapons to win. The absolute last thing any attacker wants to do is to fight you with equal weapons. If he was looking for a fight he wouldn't have attacked you with a weapon in the first place. And if he knows you have a knife, he is going to attack you with a bigger and better weapon to keep you from winning. You pull a knife and he gets a club. You pull a club and he pulls a gun. There is no fighting involved, you use the superior weapon to disable your opponent. And you do it before he does it to you." [1]

– Marc "Animal" MacYoung

Most people intuitively understand that dealing with weapons effectively is far more challenging than surviving unarmed assaults, yet many martial artists are not adequately prepared for such encounters. Unfortunately armed assaults are quite commonplace. The sad fact is that ordinary citizens are victimized an average of 1,773,000 times per year by weapon-wielding thugs in the United States alone. More than 90 percent of all homicides, about half of all robberies, and a quarter of all assaults involve an armed assailant.

Self-defense training that does not consider the very real possibility of an armed attack is dangerously incomplete. Unfortunately, many martial systems, particularly traditional ones, lack a comprehensive weapons familiarity program. There is an awful lot of dangerous stuff out there to be concerned about. About a third of all homicide victims are killed by knives, blunt objects, or similar weapons, while the rest are typically murdered by some type of firearm, more often than not a handgun. Although crimes committed with or without weapons are about equally likely to result in victim injury, armed assaults are 3.5 times more likely to result in serious damage to the victim such as broken bones, internal injuries, loss of consciousness, or similar trauma resulting in extended hospitalization.

No one wants a fair fight, least of all a criminal who is looking to make a quick profit at your expense. It really does not take a whole lot of skill or special training to use many types of weapons effectively. That is why lawbreakers frequently use them to stack the deck in their favor. In the minds of many, the term "fight" implies a rule-based contest between relative equals such as you would find in a martial arts tournament or boxing match. I prefer to use terms like ambush, slaughter, or assassination when describing armed combat on the street. Anyone coming at you with a weapon is planning to win at all costs. There is no fight, at least not in the traditional sense of the word.

If your self-defense training does not consider the very real possibility of an armed attack, you are putting yourself at risk. I do not assert that all martial artists need to be experts in any particular weapons form nor do they even have to demonstrate a particular interest in such techniques, but I sincerely believe that it is remiss to suggest that we do not need to know about weapons at all. Bad guys simply do not hesitate to use them even in public places where you might not naturally expect them to do so. That is part of what classifies such individuals as "bad."

Colonel Jeff Cooper[2] wrote, "Anyone who is aware of his environment knows that the peril of physical assault does exist, and that it exists everywhere and at all times. The police, furthermore, can protect you from it only occasionally." When it comes to defending yourself from armed aggressors, you cannot count on receiving timely assistance, nor any help at all for that matter. You may have to go it alone. Consequently, you must acquire the knowledge, skills, and ability to safeguard yourself.

The evidence is compelling; the danger is quite real. Anyone whose interest in martial arts is driven in part by a desire to remain safe must learn about weapons in order to do so. Every martial practitioner should be both mentally and physically prepared to deal with an armed assault. Exposure must be comprehensive enough to account for the plethora of pointy objects, blunt instruments, and unfriendly projectiles that may someday be used against them.

Acknowledgments

I would like to express my sincere appreciation for the following talented individuals who spent many hours modeling for the photographs included herein: Frank Getty, Tracy Taylor, Laura Vanderpool, and Kris Wilder. Frank is a former U.S. Marine MP who currently works corporate security and practices Krav Maga. Tracy is a former U.S. Army MP who currently works corporate security. A certified firearms instructor, she took responsibility for clearing the weapons and ensuring everyone's safety during the photo session. Laura is a public relations consultant, musician, and songwriter who studies *Goju Ryu* karate. Kris is a martial arts instructor, author, and small business owner who has earned black belts in *Goju Ryu* karate, tae kwon do, and judo. Jeff Miller let us drag copious quantities of guns, knives, swords, pole arms and various and sundry other implements of destruction into his studio and, without flinching (much), took the outstanding photographs included herein. His web site is www.jeffmillerphoto.com.

A gigantic thank you also goes to Dr. Jeff Cooper, Norman Dobin Esq., Rory Miller, David Ripianzi, and Laura Vanderpool who helped me with the production of this book. Using his experience as tactical medical director of Toledo (Ohio) SWAT, Jeff vetted the medical information presented herein and gave me important insight into close-quarters combat and weapons. Norman, an attorney at law, vetted the legal information presented herein. Rory reviewed the draft manuscript and provided outstanding feedback; helping me benefit from the vast experience and insight he has gained as a tactical team leader, close-quarters combat instructor, and Use of Force policy counselor. David came up with some great ideas that helped shape the content and direction of this work. Laura reviewed the draft manuscript, gave me discerning feedback, and helped shore-up my grammatical deficiencies.

Last but certainly not least, I would like to express my heartfelt gratitude to Loren Christensen. Thanks for all the help and inspiration over the years.

Introduction

"There will be no justice as long as man will stand with a knife or with a gun and destroy those who are weaker than he is." [1]

– *Isaac Bashevis Singer*

When dealing with weapons, awareness is the best defense followed immediately by avoidance and strategic withdrawal. Most violent encounters with a blade, for example, begin with a victim who is unaware of the fact that the aggressor is even armed until he or she has already been injured, sometimes fatally. Unfortunate, but all too often true. Even though they must take place at very close range, knife attacks typically occur unexpectedly when assailants can use the element of surprise to ambush a victim.

It really does not matter how fast or strong you are, nor how developed your martial prowess, if you do not detect the presence of a weapon before it is used against you. For example, on April 29, 2001, tae kwon do champion Mark Acaley, 25, was shot to death by gang member Grin "Smurf" Arkanit who was sentenced a year later to 51.4 years in prison for the murder. Acaley, a Minneapolis native, had traveled to Seattle (Washington) to compete in the annual West Coast Tae Kwon Do Championship at Bellevue Community College in the hours prior to the shooting. After winning a silver medal, he and a group of friends went to a nightclub in Seattle's International District to celebrate.

Later in the evening, they were driving from the nightclub to a nearby restaurant when Arkanit opened fire on their rented SUV. Hit in the chest, Acaley died at the scene. His friend James Franklin took two slugs to his right leg and later recovered. The remaining passengers were unharmed. Sadly, Acaley and Franklin never even recognized the threat until Arkanit began firing the first of 13 rounds into their vehicle. The shooter was motivated by a mistaken belief that Acaley and his friends were men with whom he had a confrontation earlier that evening.

Another self-defense expert who recently suffered a similar fate was Alex Blue, a 41-year old Scottish kickboxing champion, who was murdered in Glasgow on June 21, 2004. A few weeks before his murder he demonstrated his martial prowess by successfully fending off an attack by two baseball bat-wielding thugs near his home. Another champion kickboxer James Curran, 42, was shot to death during a karaoke session at the Green Lizard pub in Dublin Ireland on April 3, 2005. A 47-year-old security guard was charged with his murder.

Even trained law enforcement professionals can succumb to sneak attacks. On May 8, 2005 Denver police detective Donald Young, 43, was shot to death and a second detective, John Bishop, was also wounded while the two worked off-duty providing uniformed security at a private party. Young, a decorated 12-year veteran detective, was shot three times in the back, while his partner Bishop was also shot from behind. Bishop was treated and released from the hospital shortly thereafter. Young and Bishop were off-duty but in uniform while providing security outside a rental hall often used for birthday and baptism parties. Two other officers who were nearby rushed to the aid of the fallen detectives and saw a man fleeing with what appeared to be a weapon, early reports said.

On April 17, 2005, detective James Allen, a 27-year veteran of the Providence, Rhode Island police department, was overpowered by a prisoner he was interrogating and killed in the police conference room with his own gun. Esteban Carpio, who was being questioned about the stabbing of an 84-year-old woman (who survived the attack), allegedly grabbed the officer's gun, shot him, broke a third floor window in an adjacent office, and jumped onto a service road to make his escape. He was captured after a brief struggle a few blocks away and subsequently charged with murder. Police said Carpio was injured in his jump from the window and was subsequently treated at a hospital for injuries to his leg, arm, and head.

If you are thinking feet and fists only to discover a knife or other weapon in the middle of a fight you are more than likely doomed. The stark reality is that most victims of weapon attacks do not recognize the severity of the threat in time to react properly. Imi Sde-Or[2], the founder of Krav Maga, wrote,

> *"Victims who survived a violent confrontation against a knife-wielding assailant consistently reported that they were completely unaware of the existence of the weapon until after they had suffered stab or slash wounds. In essence, these survivors of edged weapon attacks state that they believed they were engaged in some sort of fist fight; only later, after sustaining injuries, did they realize that the assailant was armed."*

Many such attacks are made from behind. In order to remain safe you must be vigilant, aware of everything happening around you at all times, at least in places where potential adversaries may be present. Constantly scan your environment, being sure to listen as well as look. Take special care near potential ambush areas such as building corners, doorways, and ornamental foliage. Beware of people acting strangely. Stay out of bad neighborhoods and dangerous locations if at all possible.

If you can, keep sufficient distance between you and a potential assailant to give you time to react. Minimum distance is generally considered to be 21 feet though some experts argue that even that gap is not sufficient. While that may seem a rather lengthy separation, several tests, including the famous Tueller Drill, have been conducted that validate this assertion. This drill, named for Sergeant Dennis Tueller of the Salt Lake City Police Department, was first described in his 1983 *S.W.A.T.* magazine article "How Close Is Too Close."

In his drill, Tueller conducted a series of tests showing that people of various ages, weights, and heights could close a distance of 21 feet in an average time of 1.5 seconds, about as long at it takes for a highly trained officer to draw a handgun and fire one or two aimed shots. Knowing that people who have been shot do not often fall down instantly, or otherwise stop dead in their tracks, Tueller concluded that a person armed with a blade or a blunt instrument at a range of 21 feet was a potentially lethal threat. A defensive handgun instructor whose class I took reiterated this point, stating that it takes a fatally wounded person between 10 and 120 seconds to drop so you must fire then move off-line, expecting your attacker to continue their assault even after your bullets have hit him or her.

In training as well as in real-life encounters, even highly-trained police officers are frequently unable to draw their guns and fire a shot before being cut, sometimes fatally, by a knife-wielding opponent moving toward them from distances as great as 20 to 30 feet. It is reasonable to assert that the average martial artist is somewhat less prepared for such encounters than the typical law enforcement professional. The best response I have found for dealing with these situations is either to run like hell, respond with a bigger weapon, or both.

If you have an avenue of escape, your best course of action is usually to swallow your pride and run away. Unfortunately, that is not always a possibility and you may have to defend yourself or a loved one from armed assault. If you cannot escape but can do something that immediately prevents the attack from getting started that is your second best bet. The third alternative is to create sufficient distance to deploy a better weapon.

If all else fails, you can try to go berserk, hoping to stop your attacker before you are fatally injured yourself. This is the least preferred scenario. In such cases you must be prepared to use any available weapon (e.g., rock, stick, belt, shoe, flashlight, set of car keys, garbage can lid) to even the odds. Unlike a gunfight where a bullet can miss or a fistfight where you can use your martial skills to avoid being hit, you can pretty much count on being injured in a knife attack. Never forget, the term "assassination" more accurately describes such encounters than the word "fight" does. This is a perspective that merits careful consideration.

Footwork is the most important defense fundamental when engaged with a weapon-wielding assailant. Your ability to move quickly in any direction will not only help you avoid being injured, but may also open windows of opportunity for counterattack. These types of encounters are extremely anaerobic and typically brutal. If you have been hurt and are bleeding, you will weaken rapidly and must end the fight as quickly as possible.

There are no absolutes in real-life self-defense encounters. Too many variables exist. Nevertheless, the bottom line for most professionals is that the only way to guarantee survival in an armed encounter is to avoid getting into one in the first place through a combination of awareness, avoidance and, where possible, de-escalation. De-escalation is an essential skill. At times, it is possible to talk, negotiate, or even laugh your way out of a fight. Yes, I have actually been able to laugh my way out of a knife fight:

It was late in the third quarter of a nationally televised football game between two intrastate college rivals. The winner would receive not only bragging rights of a heroic victory in this annual event, but an invitation to the Rose Bowl as Pac 10 champion. Emotions amongst the 78,000+ attendees were naturally running hot, especially in the east end zone where students and alumni from both schools sat in close proximity hurtling insults and the occasional solid object at each other. I was responsible for keeping them in line and, along with my crew, ensuring that no one got hurt.

Though alcohol was prohibited, many of the students applied ingenuity bordering on sheer genius to smuggling in and consuming mass quantities undetected. Anyone we had already caught drinking had previously been ejected from the game, so we were dealing with primarily hard-core fans and hard-core party animals, two of which began a shoving match in the stands.

As I approached the scuffle, I scanned the rest of the crowd. Most were uninterested, intently watching the game so I felt little concern that things would escalate too badly before I got there. After all, it was more pushing, shoving, and expletives than an outright fight. I also spotted two pairs of police officers, the closest 60 or 70 feet away. Like most of the fans, however, their attention was focused on the field yet they were close enough to react if I needed help.

I felt confident that I could handle the situation. Wanting to put a damper on things quickly before someone actually got hurt or other fans got involved I broke my own safety rule and decided not to bother bringing anyone else along to back me up.

As I approached the two rowdies, one saw me coming, had a change of heart, and backed off. The other noticed my approach and turned to face me. As I prepared to speak to him, he reached into his pocket, withdrew a four-inch switchblade knife, flicked open the blade, and took a step toward me.

Now I have had more than a few occasions when irate fans took a poke at me with a fist and/or a foot, but that was the first time anyone had drawn an actual weapon. Not only was the switchblade illegal in its own right, but weapons of any kind were banned from the stadium.* Moreover, there were thousands of witnesses not to mention camera crews all around the incident. I just could not fathom the mentality of anyone who thought they could stab someone in such a public place and not get caught.

---

*Except active duty for law enforcement personnel, of course.

The first thing that flashed through my mind was not fear of being cut, though perhaps it should have been. My first thought was actually trepidation of being spot-lighted on national television beating the tar out of somebody, even if I had a darn good reason for doing so. I should also point out that unlike the vast majority of my time away from the stadium I was not armed myself. Yet even if I had been, there was no way I would discharge a firearm with a 100 percent certainty of hitting an innocent bystander should I miss my opponent or the bullet travel through my attacker.

In the second or two, I had to figure out how to stop this guy from killing or maiming me without being accused of excessive force I was so struck by the absurd-ity of the situation that I broke out laughing. It was not an intentional tactic, but my unexpected reaction froze the guy in his tracks nevertheless. Sometimes laughter real-ly is the best medicine.

When he gave me a puzzled look I cocked my head toward the nearby officers and said, "Put that thing away before they shoot you!" It suddenly dawned on him that he had pulled a blade in front of a huge crowd of witnesses including two cops (who still had not noticed) so he closed the knife, shoved it back into his pocket, and sat back down. I had him arrested a short while later.

To assure our personal safety, we must be prepared to face just about anything on the street. Beyond the obvious knives, swords, chemical spray canisters, stun guns, and good old fashioned firearms, you can potentially find sticks, stones, baseball bats, pool cues, boards, bottles, hammers, tire irons, wrenches, screwdrivers, ice picks, chop sticks, box cutters, belts, chains, rolled coins, canes, attack dogs, chain-saws, hair dryers, furniture, fire extinguishers, and even laptop computers in an adversary's makeshift arsenal. Understanding how such implements work in actual combat is much more useful than one might initially imagine.

"Good guys" can use weapons too. I have blocked a punch with a clipboard and poked an opponent in the ribs with a radio antenna to great effect. I have also defended myself with a ski pole as well as an expandable baton and have even flashed a gun to convince an aggressor to find someone else to pick on. Fortunately, I did not have to withdraw it from the holster and shoot him. Had I not been bet-ter prepared and better armed then he was at the time, however, things could have gotten ugly.

If your goals for learning a martial art include the ability to defend yourself from a real-life attacker, you absolutely, positively must learn how to contend effectively with an armed assault. Experience dictates that if you do not have at least a passing familiarity with how weapons work you are practically begging to get hurt by one.

At a minimum, your tactics must adapt to the longer range and greater lethality of an armed aggressor as opposed to an unarmed one. You should also consider the fact that untrained adversaries, many of whom employ weapons, often act in erratic and unpredictable ways. Even though traditional martial systems contain techniques for dealing with certain types of weapons (e.g., *kobudo*), some empty-hand strategies are simply incompatible with armed attacks.

When facing the prospect of an armed opponent you must understand where, how, and when you would need to adapt if you wish to survive. Many grappling techniques, for example, require you to get a bit too close to a knife for my comfort. Kelly Worden[3] agrees. He wrote, "In reality, whether in the streets of our inner cities or on the battlefield in a war zone, it takes nothing more than a simple boot knife or folding pocketknife to kill or maim a grappling strategist during a physical engagement." That is not to say that there

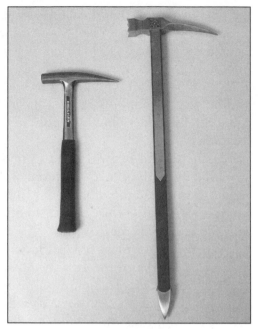

MODERN ROCK PICK AND MEDIEVAL WAR HAMMER. THE ROCK PICK IS ON THE LEFT. NOTE THAT THEY ARE SIMILARLY CONSTRUCTED.

is absolutely no place for traps, locks, and disarms when dealing with knives, assuming you are a true master of such techniques. No matter what martial style you practice, controlling an opponent's arms (or elbows) and disrupting his or her balance is a sound strategy, one best executed at close range. For the lesser-trained practitioners, however, many grappling applications are risky indeed. No matter how well trained you are, against a blade many types of takedowns are a recipe for murder—your own.

Even if you do study a weapon-based form that does not automatically mean that you are prepared to deal with an armed assault on the street. *Kobudo* practitioners, for example, learn how to turn common farm implements such as the *bo* (staff), *tonfa* (gristmill handle), *kama* (sickle), *kuwa* (hoe), and *ueku* (oar) into effective weapons yet they do not always consider other improvised devices they might confront on the street or how to respond when the practitioner him or herself is unarmed. Furthermore, these forms frequently assume specified lines of attack and often do not deal with scenarios where an opponent has taken the practitioner by surprise.

One of my favorite weapons for home defense is a rock pick,* a short-hafted tool with a hammer on one side and a slightly curved spike on the other. This weapon is not only effective in close quarters, but it also eliminates the worry of stray bullets

*Other than a gun which is my first choice.

traveling through sheetrock into an innocent victim. Used by rock hounds and lapidaries, it costs around $35 at most hardware stores. Little to no training is required to deliver crushing blows with the hammerhead, while the tempered steel pick can punch through heavy clothing or even high-tech body armor much like a medieval war hammer could break through a knight's protective plate.

An important advantage of this tool is that should an opponent only block your arm or the haft of the rock pick they will be hit by the point anyway. I have seen training knives and guns in many *dojos*, but never a rubber ax, rock pick, or war hammer. Do you know how you would defend yourself against extrusion weapons? If so, have you practiced the appropriate techniques recently? This type of attack is not as far-fetched as it seems. On March 9, 2005, a 36-year-old Lynnwood (Washington) man murdered his father with an ax just a few miles north of where I live in Seattle. He then turned himself in at a nearby mental services center in Edmonds and confessed his crime. Axes and other extrusion weapons are used to commit numerous murders throughout the world each year.

Training must be holistic, realistic, and adaptable. Any mistake you make when dealing with an armed opponent may well be your last. It is critical to think about how to adapt your martial arts techniques to unexpected movements by your assailant.

Several years ago, I had a confrontation with an aggressive teenager who was breaking car headlights in my neighborhood using an aluminum baseball bat. Although I probably had a legal right to draw my gun and respond with countervailing force when he attacked me, he was much younger than I was and I felt that such a response would literally be overkill. For a martial arts instructor and firearms expert, I am a really a very non-violent guy. Besides, I had enough experience with weapons that I thought I had a pretty good idea of what to do.

In my sword training, there is a tandem drill that teaches practitioners how to use range and angle to avoid a strike. As the blow comes toward us, we shift slightly out of range to keep from being hit, then follow the weapon back in to counterattack before it can be redirected. Although it is a sword-to-sword drill, I figured that the same principles would apply to an unarmed confrontation against a bat as well.

Assuming I could use the same technique to disarm this kid without either of us getting seriously hurt I prepared to do so. Unfortunately, he was not on the same lesson plan. As I shifted out of range, he simply let go of the bat, something I had never seen done with a sword. It flew a short distance through the air and rapped me across the head and shoulder with stunning force.

Before I realized what had happened I was on the ground in dire straits. I still do not actually remember falling, yet once I hit the ground, I had the presence of mind to scissor his legs, knocking him down before he could do anything worse. I followed up by grabbing a hold of one of his feet, pulling him in, and simultaneously kicking him in the family jewels to end the fight. Not quite what I had planned, yet effective nevertheless.

Some martial styles begin with empty-hand techniques then progress to weapons while others begin with weapons forms and work the other way around. Unfortunately, not all styles cross-pollinate. If I had a less varied background, I doubt I would have survived my close encounter with a baseball bat and come away with only a few bruises.*

If you do not regularly train with weapons yet have an opportunity to participate in a seminar or visit an instructor of such arts I highly encourage you to do so. After all, you simply cannot learn everything you need to know from any book, not even this one. Knowledge must be applied; techniques must be practiced. Regardless, the broader your understanding of weapons, the greater your odds of reacting appropriately when you run into one on the street. Such encounters are, unfortunately, quite commonplace.

This book includes nine chapters that can be briefly summarized as follows:

Chapter 1 (Awareness) helps you develop the skills necessary to identify a potential threat and prepare for an assault before it is too late to react. This section covers crime statistics, the types of weapons you might encounter on the street, common concealment strategies, situational awareness, and fighting ranges/danger zones.

Chapter 2 (Avoidance) demonstrates that, ego notwithstanding, it is far better to withdraw than it is to face the consequences of causing or allowing an argument to escalate to the point of physical confrontation. This section covers fundamental principles of personal safety, the escalation process, evasion, escape, concealment, and cover.

Chapter 3 (Scenarios) delves in-depth into various self-defense situations you could encounter in your everyday life to help you better prepare for any eventuality. Scenarios discussed include carjacking, cash machine safety, hostage situations, intimate (domestic) violence, public transportation, sexual assault, and workplace violence.

Chapter 4 (De-Escalation) covers strategies you can employ to help keep confrontations from boiling over into violent encounters.

Chapter 5 (Countervailing Force) covers important aspects of physical confrontations including the legal aspects of self-defense, ethical/moral considerations, psychological effects of violence, combat mindset, triggers, and the unpredictability of bystanders.

Chapter 6 (Armed Conflict) delves into what happens when real-life confrontations get ugly. This section covers levels of force that you might employ to defend yourself, principles that can help you defeat an armed attacker, angles of attack, empty hand vs. weapon combat, footwork, and range considerations.

---

*Yes, I'm not ashamed to admit that my ego was one of them.

Chapter 7 (**Nine Rules to Live By**) summarizes essential principles from the rest of the book that can help keep you safe on the street, collecting them all in one place for added emphasis. If you remember nothing else from this book, Chapter 7 hits the highlights.

Chapter 8 (**Aftermath of Violence**) covers what happens after your survive a violent encounter, focusing on medical triage, legal concerns, and associated issues such as dealing with law enforcement personnel, attorneys, and the press.

Chapter 9 (**Weapon Features/Functions**) describes how various types of weapons are used so that you can be more familiar with the strengths and limitations of the various items you might use for self-defense or that might be used against you during an attack.

How to Use this Book

As you can no doubt tell from the chapter summaries above, there is a lot of material in this book, perhaps more than most people can absorb in one pass. It may be useful, therefore, to read this work from cover to cover, and then go back and focus on the sections most applicable to your situation to help you internalize the materials most pertinent for you. Everything in here is important and necessary to provide a comprehensive picture of weapons, street violence, and countervailing force yet select areas may be more or less urgent for each individual reader.

The majority of readers will fall into one of three broad categories. Aligning yourself in this manner will help you individualize the contents to meet your needs.

Category 1. Little or no martial arts background combined with little or no street experience. The majority of people fall into this category, including those with a year or two of boxing, wrestling, or martial arts training who have managed to avoid serious violent encounters and wish to continue to do so.

Category 2. Advanced martial arts skills but little or no street experience. This includes professional or semi-pro boxers, wrestlers, and higher ranking martial artists (e.g., black belts) as well as individuals with concealed weapons permits who have received a high degree of training yet have not had to use that training on the street.

Category 3. Significant martial arts experience and a great deal of street savvy. This can include law enforcement officers, security personnel, and other professionals who have a high degree of training as well as experience with weapons and violence.

xxviii · SURVIVING ARMED ASSAULTS

If you fall into Category 1, you will likely want to focus on awareness, avoidance, and de-escalation, the things that precede violent encounters. Without the knowledge, skill, and ability to fight back successfully, your greatest urgency is avoiding harm in the first place. Situational awareness and de-escalation skills are paramount. The various scenarios in chapter 3 may be especially useful.

If you fall into Category 2, you will probably want to focus on countervailing force, armed conflict, and the aftermath of violence. Without actual street experience it is easy to underestimate the seriousness of a violent encounter, particularly if you have never faced a weapon before. It is easy to develop a cavalier attitude, perhaps even subconsciously looking for conflicts in order to prove your martial prowess. You will want to understand the emotional, legal, and medical cost of such actions to assure that you will act in a prudent and well thought out manner should you be confronted by an adversary on the street. You will also benefit from a thorough understanding of the weapons features and functions to help plan your response in an unavoidable encounter.

If you fall into Category 3, you will probably want to focus on de-escalation, armed conflict, and aftermath of violence. Many people who fit this category have a high probability of experiencing a violent encounter because of their chosen profession. With both skill and experience comes a higher level of responsibility than most. You will want to refine your ability to resolve bad situations peacefully as well as to survive if de-escalation does not work. You will also benefit from a thorough understanding of the weapons features and functions to help plan your response.

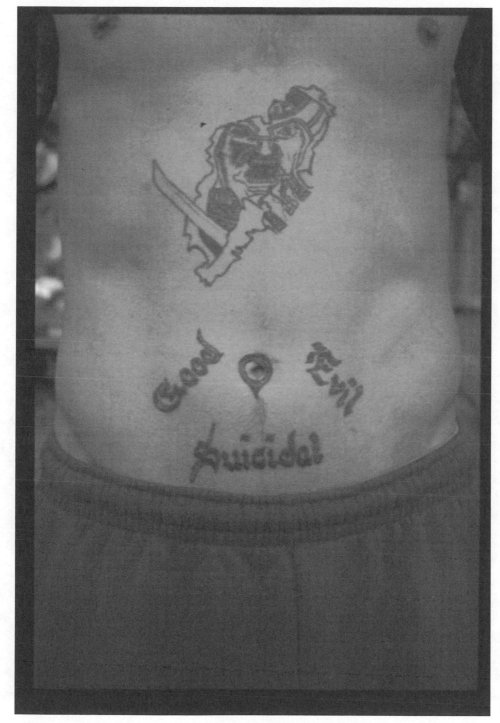

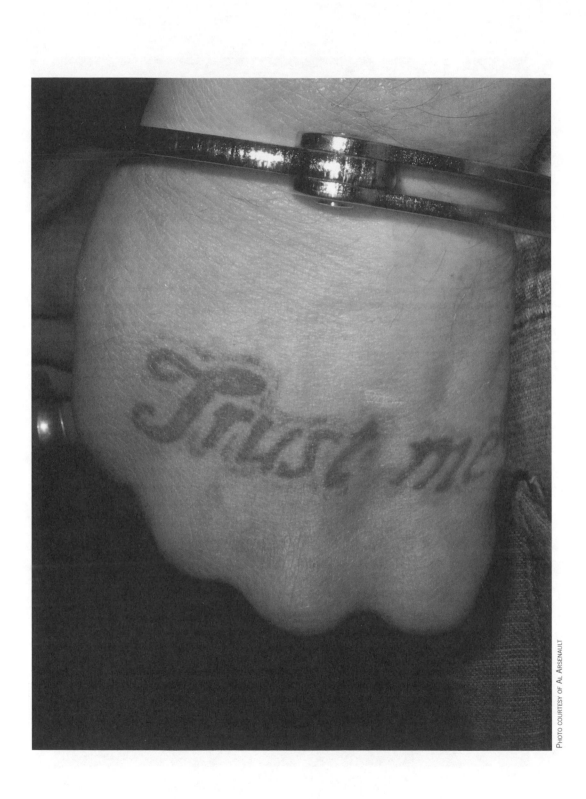

CHAPTER 1

Awareness

"Any tool is a weapon if you hold it right."[1]

– Ani DiFranco

Weapons can be found practically anywhere, even in public places where you might not expect to find them. A few years back I was beginning to enter my PIN into a cash machine located inside a crowded QFC store when I caught movement in my peripheral vision. A young man of perhaps 18 to 20 had sidled up alongside me in direct viewing range of my keypunching. This behavior was certainly rude, though not initially alarming. As I pivoted slightly to get a better look at him, I began to feel uncomfortable about the way in which he was standing. Not exactly knowing why, but reacting to my intuition, I carefully and evenly said, "Son, you're going to have to step back a little. You're crowding me."

When he shifted back a couple of feet, I turned to continue my banking transaction then suddenly realized what had been bothering me. I became conscious of the fact that I could not see his right hand that he held along his side hidden from my view. Reacting to this realization I abruptly hit the cancel button while turning back to face him, blindly grabbing my card out of the slot as I did so. His expression went from carefully neutral to clearly exasperated as I continued to keep an eye on him.

Not wanting to provoke a confrontation, I slowly angled away, maintaining eye contact the entire time. I kept my hands free, but did not do anything overtly aggressive. As I passed him, he quickly shoved something metallic into his pants pocket. I moved on another ten or twelve feet behind a bakery display and stood there watching him until he left the store. If he was ever planning to use the cash machine in the first place, he had clearly changed his mind and left without doing so. I strongly suspect, however, that he had much more nefarious intentions.

Had I just foiled the plans of a would-be robber or murder? Though the local newspapers had reported a few stories of victims who were robbed while using ATM machines near my neighborhood during that time period, I'm actually not quite certain and undoubtedly never will be. None of the reported crimes took place inside a store, but always at parking lot or bank-front kiosk. Nevertheless, had I not been paying attention to my surroundings I am certain that I would have uncovered whatever that young man's plans were the hard way.

Did he shove a weapon like a knife into his pocket or something innocuous like a cell phone? I will never know. Could I have completely misinterpreted that chain of events, embarrassing myself in public? You bet I could.

Barry Eisler's fictional character John Rain once said, "If I have to err, it's on the side of assuming the worst. This way, if I am wrong, I can always apologize. Or send flowers. You err on the other side; the flowers will be coming to you." Likewise, I am more than happy to err on the side of caution. Embarrassment? I can live with that.

Violent Crime by the Numbers

"Estimates from the National Crime Victimization Survey indicate that between 1993 and 2001 approximately 25% of the average annual 8.9 million violent victimizations were committed by offenders armed with a weapon. Males, American Indians, and Hispanics, the young, and those with the lowest annual household income were more vulnerable to weapon violence in general and firearm violence in particular than their respective counterparts." [2]

– Craig Perkins

While violent crime rates in the United States have been trending steadily downward over the last decade or so, the threat of armed assault is still quite real. Between 1993 and 2001 there was an average of 847,000 firearm attacks, 570,000 edged weapon victimizations, and 356,000 violent crimes perpetrated with blunt objects every year. Every single violent assault is one too many, especially if it happens to you or someone you love.

Although all violence is bad, armed assaults are far more dangerous to the victim than unarmed ones. While crimes of non-lethal violence committed with or without weapons were about equally likely to result in victim injury (~ 25 percent), armed assaults are 3.5 times as likely as unarmed encounters to result in serious injuries. In fact, during this same period, 96 percent of all homicides involved some type of weapon.* If you are concerned about your personal safety and well-being, you simply cannot overlook the fact that armed aggressors frequently injure or kill their victims.

Let's briefly explore some more recent examples to reinforce how dangerous weapons can be. Odd as it may seem, sword attacks are truly not limited to the moldy dustbin of history. Even in modern times, thousands people are hacked to death each year by swords, machetes, and similarly pointy objects in countries like Rwanda, Sudan, Israel, Philippines, Ivory Coast, and even here in the United States.

---

*Not counting terrorism-related deaths on 9/11 which would raise this percent even higher.

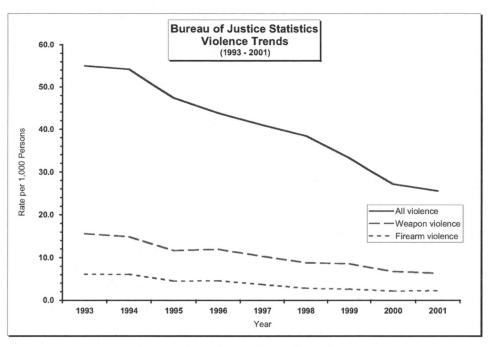

BUREAU OF JUSTICE STATISTICS VIOLENCE TRENDS CHART.

In fact, dozens of sword incidents take place in the United States almost every week. Here is a brief sample that occurred over a four day period:

- On October 30, 2004, James Flemons allegedly used a sword that he fabricated at the Detroit metals plant where he worked to kill a co-worker. The victim, Anthony Williams, was struck in the neck and nearly decapitated by the sword the suspect had apparently been working on for several days without his coworkers or plant security doing anything to stop him.
- On November 1, 2004, police arrested Benjamin Pulliam, a 22-year-old central Florida man, for allegedly stabbing his roommate 35 times with a sword. The 20-year old victim, Richard Owens, was pronounced dead at the scene.
- On November 2, 2004, Richard Taylor was arrested for entering a Wal-Mart store in Cape Girardeau Missouri and allegedly threatening employees and customers with a sword.

Interestingly enough, it is not just the bad guys who bring swords to a fight. The following incident occurred in Snohomish County, Washington—about a 30-minute drive (in light traffic) from where I live. On November 7, 2004 a man used a machete to defend himself against three gun-wielding intruders who allegedly tried to rob him. Neighbors armed with a baseball bat and a gun helped him fight off the perpetrators, two of which were later arrested at the hospital. Police were still looking for the third attacker a day later.

Knife attacks are far more common than assaults with swords or any other type of pointy object, at least in the United States. While statistically speaking an encounter with a sword-wielding assailant is not terribly likely, knives are frequently a villain's best friend. In fact, armed assaults perpetrated with edged weapons are becoming increasingly common since they are much easier to obtain and conceal then handguns, and are carried by far more people. Their relatively low cost, near silent application, and comparative ease of disposal are definite bonuses for the criminally minded.

For example, even though knives are prohibited in the stadium where I work and all fans must pass through a security checkpoint upon entry, only bags and backpacks are thoroughly inspected. In the last few years, I have had to confiscate a half dozen or more knives at almost every game. Imagine how many you will find where they are actually legal to carry, something that an estimated 70 percent of adult males do in the United States.* A few recent examples of where knives are misused:

- High school student Joshua Goldman, 18, pled guilty on September 2004 to first-degree murder for killing John Jasmer with a kitchen knife in Marysville (Washington) the previous year. He also agreed to testify against co-defendant Jenson Hankins who was convicted on November 6, 2004. The two killed Jasmer by hitting him on the head five times with a hammer then, when that did not work, stabbing him 29 times in the neck, arms, back, and abdomen because they believed he had raped one of their girlfriends, a claim she later recanted.
- On October 22, 2004, Tony Sukto allegedly murdered his wife, Pranee, and attempted to kill his 8-year-old son Anthony with a knife. Anthony's heroic 9-1-1 call made headlines nationwide. Tony Sukto was charged with murder and held on a $1,000,000 bond. Sukto reportedly told Lakewood (Washington) police he used a knife in each hand to attack his wife and son, stating that he was on drugs at the time of the murder and that he attacked because, "the spirits made me do it."
- On October 25, 2004, Man Hong Chung used a knife to kill his wife Kwang Ja Chung and then himself at the Happy Sushi and Teriyaki restaurant they owned in North Bend, Washington. Earlier in the week he was accused of domestic violence, arrested, and subsequently released from the Issaquah jail on his own recognizance. Violating a court issued no-contact order; he entered the restaurant the day after his release and perpetrated the murder/suicide.

---

*Though that statistic includes multi-tools such as the Leatherman, which I'd argue has only limited value as weapon, so it may be a bit misleading.

Furthermore, uninvited guests who crashed two different Halloween parties in the University District (of Seattle, WA) recently attacked the homeowners who tried to turn them away. During the scuffles, one victim was stabbed in the thigh while the other was wounded in his lower back. Knife assaults are so common, in fact, that many never even make it into the newspapers at all. To get a feeling for the magnitude of those that do, a recent Yahoo.com search of the key words "stabbed to death" turned up 4,749 news stories within 30 days of my query.

According to the Bureau of Justice Statistics, between 1993 and 2001 most victims of armed violence were attacked somewhere other than in their home by someone they did not already know. A majority of such attacks took place at night. Consequently, you are probably more at risk from armed attacks from strangers than spouses, intimate relations, or even non-intimate relatives or acquaintances. More specifically, the offender was armed in a third of all violence committed by strangers and in a sixth of all violence committed by a known individual. Locations of armed, violent victimizations occurred as follows:

Leisure away from home	*26.9%*
Traveling to or from work	*22.9%*
In the home	*20.5%*
At work	*14.5%*
Other (e.g., open areas, public transportation)	*7.7%*
Out shopping	*4.7%*
At school	*2.8%*
Total of all attacks	*100.0%*

Violent crimes at night were more likely than crimes occurring during the day to involve a weapon (30 percent versus 21 percent) or a firearm (12 percent versus 6 percent, respectively). Three of every five crimes committed by an offender with a firearm occurred at night, something to consider when traveling after hours.

Interestingly enough, non-firearm violence actually accounted for more injuries though fewer deaths than crimes with firearms. Of all violence with a weapon, crimes committed with blunt objects and other weapons (e.g., ropes, chains) were most often associated with victim injury (36 percent), followed closely by knives and sharp objects (28 percent), and finally firearms (15 percent). Offenders armed with knives, for example, accounted for six percent of all violence but 24 percent of all serious injuries—those involving broken bones, internal injuries, loss of consciousness, or injuries requiring two or more days of hospitalization.

Armed robbery is theft of property or cash directly from a victim by force or threat of force.* About half of armed robbery victims were injured when blunt objects were used to commit the crime compared to a third of those held up by

---

*As opposed to burglary where the victim is not present during the theft.

knives or similar pointy objects. In fact, robbery victims are much more likely to be attacked without prior threat by perpetrators who use these types of weapons than they are by criminals who carry firearms, a situation that bodes well for the prepared martial artist and poorly for the untrained.

In most jurisdictions aggravated assault is an attack or threatened attack with a weapon regardless of whether or not an injury occurred as well as attack without a weapon when serious injury results. Simple assault is attack without a weapon that resulted in either no injury or minor injury to the victim such as bruises, black eyes, cuts, scratches, swelling, or other injuries requiring less than two days of hospitalization.

Although there are relatively few armed rapists, about half of all victims of rape/sexual assault by an unarmed attacker were injured compared with three quarters of such cases when the crime was committed by an armed assailant. This statistic, while alarming may actually be a bit misleading. Since pathogens such as HIV/AIDS and hepatitis can be transmitted during forced intercourse, such crimes might ultimately be fatal for the victim years after the initial molestation, something to consider when deciding how to respond to such attacks. Other STDs, while not fatal, can cause lasting or permanent harm. Furthermore, the psychological trauma from such incidents can last for years or even a lifetime as well.

Overall vulnerability to victimization by an armed offender varied with the age, gender, ethnicity, and income of the victim. Younger persons, particularly those aged 18 to 20, had the most encounters with armed opponents. About a third of males and a fifth of females who were attacked faced an armed aggressor. Victimization rates for Caucasians (22.7 percent) were lower than those of African Americans (36.1 percent), Hispanics (33.0 percent), Asians (31.2 percent), or American Indians (26.1 percent). Persons with annual household income of less than $7,500 experienced both armed victimization and firearm violence rates at about three times the rates of persons with annual household incomes of $50,000 or more.

About 703,800 violent crimes against persons aged 12 to 17 occurred at school or on school property each year during the survey period. About eight percent of those crimes were committed with a weapon while one percent involved a firearm. About a third of all armed assaults in schools resulted in injury to the victim. Between 1994 and 1999, the most recent data available at this writing, 172 homicides of students and non-students took place on school property, 69 percent of which were committed with a firearm. Eighteen percent were committed with a knife or other sharp object. Of the firearm homicides, three-quarters were committed with a handgun.

Between 1993 and 2001, 61 percent of all victims of violent crime reported taking some sort of self-defensive measure during the incident. Most used non-aggressive means, such as trying to escape, getting help, or attempting to scare off or warn the offender. About 13 percent of victims tried to attack or threaten the offender, while only two percent used some sort of weapon with which to defend themselves. Half of those brandished a firearm.

Again, these statistics may be a bit misleading. According to countervailing force expert Massad Ayoob,[3] for every one criminal that gets shot in self defense, another 13 to 15 are driven off merely by the sight of a firearm in the hands of someone who is willing and able to use it. Such incidents are rarely reported. This seems consistent with my own personal experience. While I have been forced to display a gun in self-defense, a few times I have fortunately never had to pull the trigger.

A 2004 study by Professor Gary Kleck published in the November issue of the journal *Criminology* supports this perspective. He found that, "Self-protection in general, both forceful and non forceful, reduced the likelihood of property loss and injury, compared to non-resistance. A variety of mostly forceful tactics, including resistance with a gun, appeared to have the strongest effects in reducing the risk of injury… Combined with the fact that injuries following resistance are almost always relatively minor, victim resistance appears to be generally a wise course of action." The bottom line is that taking a proactive measure of self-defense is often necessary and prudent, though certainly not in all cases.

Despite the fact that they get a lot of news play, terrorist attacks are actually quite rare in most parts of the world. Terrorism is defined as violence, or the threat of violence, calculated to create an atmosphere of fear and alarm. These acts are designed to coerce others into actions they would not otherwise undertake, or refrain from actions they desired to take. All terrorist acts are crimes. Many would also be violation of the rules of war if a state of war existed. This violence or threat of violence is generally directed against civilian targets.

The motives of all terrorists are political, and terrorist actions are generally carried out in a way that will achieve maximum publicity. Unlike other criminal acts, terrorists often claim credit for their acts. These acts are intended to produce effects beyond the immediate physical damage they cause, having long-term psychological repercussions on a particular target audience. The fear created by terrorists may be intended to cause people to exaggerate the strengths of the terrorist and the importance of the cause, to provoke governmental overreaction, to discourage dissent, or simply to intimidate and thereby enforce compliance with their demands.

According to the National Counterterrorism Center (NCTC), there were 3,192 terrorist attacks worldwide in 2004, with 6,060 people killed, 16,091 wounded, and 6,282 taken hostage for a total of 28,433 victims. Every death is one too many and 2004 was a particularly brutal year for terrorism, well above the historical average. Despite this appallingly high number of victims, it is important to point out that we average 41,962 automobile accident related fatalities in the United States alone every year, roughly seven times number of people murdered by terrorists worldwide.

None of the major incidents took place in the United States. The single bloodiest incident of 2004 was the September 1 armed takeover of a school in Beslan, Russia, perpetrated by 32 members of the Riyad us-Saliheyn Martyrs' Brigade.[4] A two-day standoff ended in a horrific firefight with police. By the time it was over, 331 people (including 172 children) were killed, and 727 people were injured. The second worst attack, in terms of casualties, was the bombing spree in Madrid (Spain) perpetrated by the Abu Hafs al-Masri Brigade, an al-Qaeda offshoot, that killed 191 riders on the city's commuter train system and injured more than 1,800 others. The third-worst incident was a bombing aboard Superferry Number 14 in the Philippines' Manila Bay by members of Abu Sayyaf Group, another radical Islamist group, which killed 132 people.

The NCTC estimated that Islamic extremists were responsible for 2,623 deaths in 2004, followed by 1,030 people killed for "secular political" reasons.[5] Officials remain uncertain about the motives (and in some cases the perpetrators) in the remaining 2,407 terrorist-related deaths. Regardless, suicide bombers and other terrorists do represent a threat, albeit less of one than common, everyday criminal thugs.

Weapon Awareness

"In my time I have been clobbered by or attacked with hairbrushes, a pot, rope, scissors, beer bottles, pens, a cat, tables and chairs, pool cues, shuriken, playing cards, keys, razor blades, rocks, a candleholder, shoes, a cup of Coke, and, of course, chains. I have used leaves, dirt, the water from a dog dish, a shirt, a belt, trash cans, paint scrapers, beer, orange juice, spit, and many of the things previously listed, to open conversations. Many of these serve to knock you off balance or mildly hurt you so you'll choke and your attacker can get in there with something more serious. Others are more serious by themselves."[6]

– Marc "Animal" MacYoung

Not all weapons are inherently deadly, yet many dangerous objects are not even recognized as such by the average martial artist. Before reading the quote above, how many of you have seriously considered a hairbrush a weapon? What about orange juice? After that tragedy of 9/11 several of my martial arts buddies and I got together to discuss how one might defend oneself during an airplane hijacking attempt. Frankly that is a pretty unlikely occurrence now that cockpit doors are hardened[7] and there is limited access to the pilots. Nevertheless, it was an interesting discussion.

In narrow airplane aisles, there is little room to maneuver if confronted by a knife or box-cutter-wielding assailant. We mutually agreed that this lack of maneuverability pretty much necessitates some type of counter-weapon to have the best chance at successfully disabling an armed hijacker. After all, running is simply not an option in such situations. We ultimately decided that a laptop PC would be our ideal weapon of choice. It is permitted aboard every flight, heavy enough to deflect a knife thrust, yet maneuverable enough to be used as a cudgel on its own. The cord and power brick can be used offensively or defensively as well. They are certainly not cheap but I would rather replace a computer than eat a knife. Regardless of whether or not you agree with our conclusion, have you seriously thought of using your computer as a weapon before reading this?

Bad guys do not come with giant neon signs announcing nefarious intent; they look much the same as anyone else. While completing his undergraduate studies at the University of Washington, my sister's orthodontist lived in the same fraternity house as infamous serial killer Ted Bundy.[8] While he did not know him well, he indicated that he had thought Bundy an affable guy with a good sense of humor and was totally shocked to discover that his fraternity brother was a mass murderer.

Other famous killers looked perfectly normal to their friends, relatives, and victims as well:

- John Wayne Gacy, a once respected businessman who strangled more than 30 boys and buried them under his house.
- Ian Brady who along with his girlfriend Myra Hindley tortured and killed several children committing England's infamous "moors murders."
- Albert Fentress, a former schoolteacher who killed and ate a teenager.
- Jeffrey Dahmer, cannibal serial murderer.
- Lyle and Erik Menendez, convicted of murdering their parents.

Another recent addition to this is list is 60-year old Dennis Rader, the Cub Scout leader, Lutheran church member, and family man who pled guilty on June 27, 2005 to the infamous BTK serial murders[9] in the Wichita area of Kansas. Since you simply cannot tell by appearance alone whether or not that gentle-looking man or woman walking down the street next to you is a harmless accountant, a violent rapist, or even a mass murderer, you must always be on your guard, vigilantly identifying and avoiding hazardous circumstances and knowledgeably detecting and steering away from the precursors of potential violence.

It has been said that the first step to recovery from alcoholism is to admit that you have a problem. Similarly, the first step to keeping yourself safe from armed assault is to admit that it can happen to you. No matter what the facts and figures say, far too many people feel that the statistics simply do not apply to them.

Lt. Col. Dave Grossman[10] popularized the theory that there are three kinds of people in the world: sheep, wolves, and sheepdogs. Sheep are regular, productive, law abiding citizens with little or no capacity for violence. For the most part, they would rather not even know that such dangers exist. Paradoxically some even get violent about their beliefs.* Wolves are, of course, the dregs of society who prey upon the ignorant sheep. They are robbers, rapists, murderers, muggers, and such. If you do not believe that they exist, the odds are good that sooner or later a wolf will get you.

Sheepdogs protect the sheep as well as themselves from the wolves. They are prepared to use countervailing force as necessary to defend themselves and others. They would rather not have to resort to force, of course, but clearly feel a need to know how and when it is appropriate to do so. Since there is not a police officer on every corner, you must proactively take responsibility for your own safety. Be a sheepdog rather than a sheep. Once you begin to take the possibility of armed assault seriously, the second step is to develop sufficient awareness to identify potential weapons before they can be deployed against you.

Types of Weapons

Since just about anything can be used as a weapon, it is simply not practicable to list them all. I find it useful to classify the plethora of pointy objects and deadly devices one might encounter into the following general categories, each of which will be discussed in greater detail in Chapter 9 (weapon features/functions):

- Hand weapons
- Knives
- Swords
- Mass weapons
- Pole arms
- Multi-element weapons
- Projectile weapons
- Unusual weapons

(1) Hand weapons

Hand weapons fall into two main sub-categories: strike enhancers and control devices. Together these types of devices augment empty-hand (unarmed) applications generally taught to martial practitioners by increasing the effectiveness of punches, blocks, locks, takedowns, and similar techniques. Strike enhancers include such things as keys, *neko te* (cat claws), *shuko* (tiger claws), fighting rings, rolled coins, brass knuckles, and sap gloves that add impetus to your punches and hand strikes. Control devices include *kubaton, yawara* sticks, *karambit* trainers, flashlights, certain pens, and other objects that enhance the efficiency of control techniques and pressure point applications.

---

*Such as riots at peace rallies, death threats against law enforcement officers, and assaults on soldiers.

(2) Knives

Knives include single edge, double edge, fixed blades, folders and specialty devices such as ice picks, *karambits*, switchblades, and *balisongs*. Just about any pointy object (e.g., pen, chopstick, box cutter, and scissors) can be used like a knife. Knives are the most common type of street weapon used by criminals other than a gun. In court, they are often considered "thug" weapons, potentially increasing the likelihood of legal consequences from their use, even in legitimate self-defense scenarios. An estimated 70 percent of adult males in the United States carry a knife or multi-tool on a regular basis.

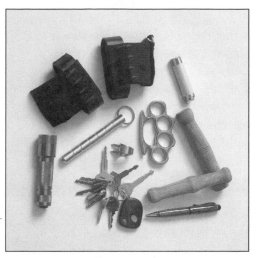

HAND WEAPONS.

(3) Swords

In the ancient world, swords evolved from daggers as metallurgical sciences advanced. In Pre-Colombian South America and Mesoamerica, several cultures made use of sword-like weapons without developing metallurgy by mounting obsidian teeth along the edges of a wooden blade. Swords eventually became a symbol of authority. In feudal Japan, for example, only members of the *buke* (nobility) such as the *samurai* (elite warrior class) were allowed to carry *daisho* (set of two swords, *katana* and *wakizashi*). Even today in most service branches, military officers' dress uniforms in nearly every country throughout the world include swords.

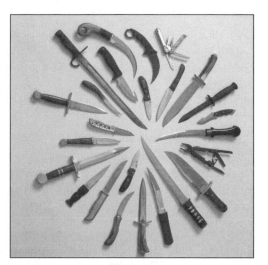

KNIVES.

Swords include single-edge and double-edge varieties. They can be designed for use primarily by one hand (e.g., *gladius*, short sword, *wakizashi*) or predominantly by two hands (e.g., claymore, *grosse messer*, and *katana*). Even though two-handed weapons can be wielded with one hand, their weight and balance are best suited to double-hand techniques. For example, although the initial draw and strike with a *katana* is performed one-handed,* the coup d'grace is almost always a double-hand swing.

Some varieties are balanced to facilitate use with either one or both hands like a "bastard" sword. This hand-and-a-half sword earned its name after the propensity for its usage by medieval knights born out of wedlock who could not display their heraldic arms on a shield, thus often entering tournaments

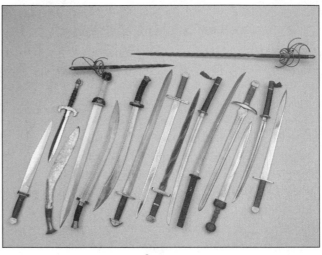

SWORDS.

with just a sword. That is not to say that one cannot use a primarily two-handed weapon effectively with only one arm, it is just not generally the most effective or commonly taught approach.

Another important distinction is whether the sword is primarily designed for thrusting (e.g., *gladius*, rapier) or slashing (e.g., broadsword, claymore). The weight, balance, and even blade thickness are affected by the weapon's intended use. While you can thrust with a slashing weapon or vice versa, it is often unwieldy and generally less effective to do so.

(4) Mass weapons

Mass weapons include blunt instruments, extrusion weapons, and specialty devices. These devices generally cause crushing damage upon impact as opposed to swords or knives, which primarily cut or impale a victim. Some mass weapons such as axes can cut as well as crush, yet the weight of the weapon adds significantly to the force of the blow.

Blunt instruments are simply heavy objects you can hit someone with such as a cane, club, tactical baton, *jutte*, tire iron, pipe wrench, flashlight, laptop computer, bottle, mug, blackjack,[11] or chair. Extrusion weapons have an extruding head that extends beyond the haft. They are extremely dangerous because even if you block the opponent's arm or the haft of their weapon, the business end can still hit you. Examples include *kama* (sickle), hammers, hand axes, rock picks, war hammers, and ice axes. Specialty weapons include martial arts devices like *sai* and *tonfa* that can also be used to capture other weapons or are simply employed a bit differently than your basic heavy object.

---

*Since the other usually holds the *saya* (scabbard) to optimally position it for the draw.

(5) Pole arms

Pole arms include basic pole weapons, pointed pole weapons, and bladed pole weapons. Basic pole weapons include long wooden poles such as pool cues, *ueku* (oars), and *bo* staffs. Pointed pole weapons include spears, *nunti bo* (hooked spear), bayonets,[12] lances, and pitchforks. While they can be used similarly, the primary difference between pointed and non-pointed pole weapons is a predilection for using the sharp end to impale

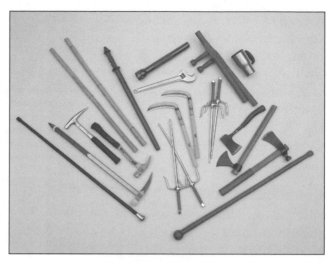

MASS WEAPONS.

rather than the haft to crush an opponent. Some, like certain spears, can also be thrown. This category also includes long-hafted blade weapons such as *kuwa* (hoe), halberds, glaives, boar spears, and *naginata*, which can be used to slice an opponent at long distances.

These devices have been around for a long, long time. Until the twentieth century, more people throughout history were killed by spears than any other type of weapon. In the ancient world, spears were also a symbol of power and authority long before creation of the sword.

(6) Multi-element weapons

Multi-element weapons include pliable weapons and composite weapons. Pliable weapons are such things as chains, whips, *suruchin* (weighted chains), *kusarigama* (weighted chain and sickle), and belts among other things. Composite weapons can include *nunchaku, sansetsu kon bo* (three-sectional staff), and flails. These types of weapons are especially challenging to defend against, but also difficult to use, requiring extensive training for best effect. *Sansetsu kon bo*, for example, were effective at striking around a soldier's shield yet could also clobber the wielder if deployed improperly.

Assuming it is used properly, it is virtually impossible to block a flexible weapon unless you have some sort of weapon yourself. Consequently, you will need to employ other tactics to avoid being hit by them if you are unarmed. In the hands of an untrained individual, on the other hand, these types of weapons can be more dangerous to the wielder than they are to the potential victim. For example, if you miss the target on your first strike you are likely to lose control of the weapon making it very challenging to launch a second blow, and/or hit yourself with it.

(7) Projectile weapons

Projectile weapons include liquids, thrown objects, arrows, darts, javelins, *fuki-dake* (blowguns), firearms, and non-lethal projectiles. Liquids such as hot coffee, chemical sprays and flammable fluids can be used offensively to distract, incapacitate, or damage an opponent. While just about any weapon can be thrown, certain varieties are more or less designed to be projectiles (e.g., rocks, baseballs, certain knives, *shuriken*, spikes, and darts). Bows include traditional, compound, and crossbow varieties. Firearms fall into the broad categories of handguns, rifles, and shotguns.

Non-lethal projectiles, those intended to subdue without always killing, can

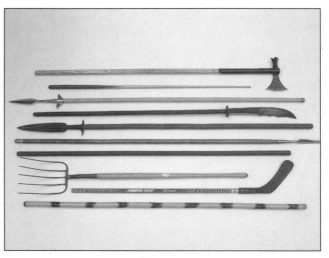

POLE ARMS.

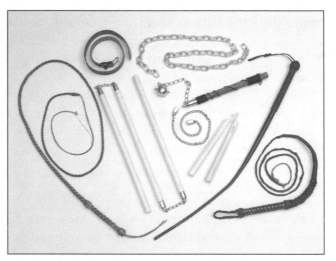

MULTI-ELEMENT WEAPONS.

include gas canisters, Tasers, rubber bullets, nets, water cannon, and bean bag rounds. This does not necessarily mean that they never cause grave injury or death, only that killing is not their primary purpose. Some non-lethal projectiles can affect a group of people (e.g., chemical spray, water cannon), while others are designed to stop a single target (e.g., Taser, beanbag round).

(8) Unusual weapons

Unusual weapons is a catchall category for anything that does not fit neatly into some other bucket such as bodily fluids which can be used to deliver pathogens such as HIV/AIDS or Hepatitis C, including syringes, spittle, blood, and semen. Other unusual weapons can include attack animals, vehicles, chainsaws, bombs, hand grenades, and other improvised explosive devices (IEDs).[13]

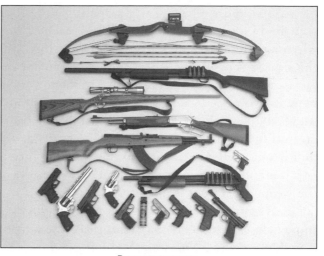

PROJECTILE WEAPONS.

Common Concealment Strategies

With few exceptions, civilians who carry a weapon need to do so in a manner where it cannot be seen by those around them yet can be drawn in very big hurry should the need arise. If you are legally carrying a weapon for self-defense purposes, you will not want to be stopped every twenty feet by a police officer summoned by some frightened bystander who spotted and reported your weapon. Further, you will not want to forewarn possible aggressors of the fact that you are armed. Bad guys also conceal their weapons not only for the reasons list above but also to increase the chances of a successful ambush when they attack you or whomever they have chosen as their victim.

It is paramount to be able to identify anyone around you who may be carrying a weapon since they can be found almost anywhere, even in locations where they are legally prohibited such as schools, courthouses, and bars.* Certain weapons such as those made of wood, Zytel (nylon), Grivory (fiberglass-reinforced plastic), Lexan (polycarbonate resin), plastic, or other non-ferrous materials can even be smuggled past metal detectors.

Since you will not generally see a weapon carried openly, it is really important to know how to spot when someone is armed with a concealed device. The vast majority of weapon concealment strategies have one thing in common: accessibility. After all, a weapon does no good if you cannot get to it rapidly when you need it.

Blades, handguns, batons, and just about anything else concealable can be hidden in similar ways, most of which are centered on or around the waist. There are varieties of holsters that can be attached to one's belt either inside or outside of the

---

*In most jurisdictions.

pants. The most reliable carry systems rigidly fix the weapon to a specific spot on your body so that you can always find it when you need it under stress. That is also why many folding knives come with belt clips designed to hold them firmly against the side of your pocket where they are easily located by touch.

Pants or jacket pockets are always a handy choice yet not as reliable or easy to get to when you need rapid access since the weapon may become repositioned as you move about during the day. For example, a pistol slid into your pocket may flip around such that the handle cannot be grasped without moving the gun first. If you pull it out by the barrel, it will not do you much good until you change your grip. In a fast and furious encounter, you may not have enough time to do that and deploy the weapon before it is too late.

Every type of concealed carry has strengths as well as weaknesses. For example, some belt-attached holster systems make the weapon nearly impossible to draw while seated, especially if you are belted into a vehicle's restraint system. Ankle systems that are easy to access when seated, on the other hand, require stooping and moving a pant leg before you can access to the weapon while you are standing. If you spend most of your day sitting down (e.g., taxi driver, air marshal) you might make a different choice than if you spend most of your day standing up (e.g., construction worker, store clerk).

Shoulder holsters, which gained popularity on TV's Miami Vice, are a reasonably popular method of carrying guns, knives, and even tactical batons. Unlike most hip or small-of-the-back holsters, they have the benefit of ready access while sitting, yet require reaching across the body to retrieve the weapon. Not only may this extra reach take a certain amount of time to perform, but also an opponent could press against your arm to keep you from being able to retrieve your weapon. Fanny pack and purse holsters offer excellent concealment as well as accessibility when seated but typically require both hands to free the weapon, something that not only takes time to perform but may also be stopped by an attentive opponent.

Some concealment strategies require no holster or sheath at all. Weapons can be palmed, hidden behind an arm or leg, or held out of sight beneath a covering object such as a folded jacket or newspaper. These systems facilitate rapid access but can be easier to spot than other methods and preclude the use of the hand that carries the weapon for anything other than deploying the device in combat. Weapons can also be "hidden" in plain sight. Heavy keys on a lanyard can work much like a flail or *manriki kusari* (weighted chain). A solidly built pen can operate like a *kubaton* or stiletto. A cane or walking stick can be used as a bludgeon.

You will frequently rely on your eyes to spot a concealed weapon, though you can use your ears too, listening for the sound of a weapon being drawn or readied for action. This will be described in more detail in the next section (weapons delivery systems). Pay particular attention to a person's hands and midsection, looking for unusual bumps, bulges, out-of-place items of clothing, or odd movements. Look for clips that indicate a knife, heavy belts that may indicate a holster, and other visible signs of something hidden from plain view. Don't worry about being confused by cell phones, pagers, PDAs or other harmless devices. It is far better to be overly cautious than injured or dead through ignoring warning signs. Just because you believe that someone is armed does not necessarily imply that you will take immediate action but you should be prepared to do so as necessary. Trust your instincts.

To summarize, there are a ton of different ways to hide a knife or a gun including through the use of weapon retention devices such as holsters (e.g., belt slide, high rise hip, belly band, inside-the-pants, shoulder, and ankle), pouches (e.g., fanny pack, purse), pockets, and clips such as those built into many folding pocketknives. Furthermore, weapons can also be disguised by hiding them under jackets, in bags, beneath towels, or simply holding them behind one's back. The following are detailed descriptions of some common concealment methods to help you become more familiar with how they work.

Weapon retention devices (e.g., holsters, sheaths):

Fanny pack holster – A hip bag with two to three pockets that can be used to carry a wallet, keys, or other small items that can also conceal a firearm within. It is typically worn bag-forward on the front hip or below the stomach and looks much like a normal fanny pack save for a small loop, tab, or string between the zippers that facilitates rapid deployment of the weapon.

Purse holster – Similar to a fanny pack holster, a secret pocket, typically in the center of the bag, holds a weapon. A snap is usually released to free the weapon.

High-rise hip holster – Worn on a heavy belt, this type of holster conceals the weapon firmly against the wearer's kidneys, just above the hip. It is typically covered by a loose shirt, sweater, or jacket to facilitate concealment and rapid access.

Belly band holster – Holds the weapon snug against the wearer's mid section. It is typically covered by a loose fitting shirt to facilitate concealment and rapid access.

Inside-the-pants holster – Similar to a hip holster save that it is worn under the pants with only the pistol grip and securing strap/snap visible around the belt. Offers slightly better concealment than a high-rise hip holster but also requires looser trousers (or a relatively small gun) in order to fit properly. It is typically covered by a loose shirt, sweater, vest, or jacket to facilitate concealment and rapid access.

Shoulder holster – There are two major varieties of shoulder holsters: vertical and horizontal. Either way, the weapon is held snug against the side of the chest and concealed beneath a loose-fitting shirt, vest, or jacket. Unlike a hip holster, the concealing garment must be moved relatively far in order to free the weapon unless it splits down the middle so buttoned shirts or zippered jackets are the most common type of cover.

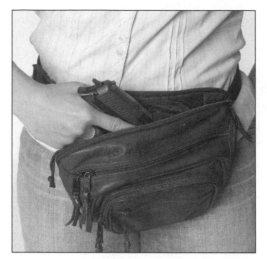

Fanny pack holster.

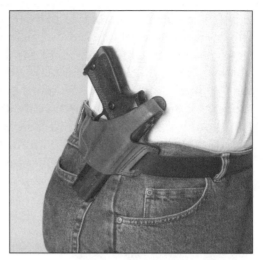

High-rise hip holster.

Ankle holster – Holds the weapon at the base of the shin just above the ankle, covered by the pants leg. The weapon is frequently placed on the inside of the weak-side leg (e.g., left leg if right-handed).

Belt slide holster – Similar to a high-rise hip holster, another method of securing a weapon to your waist. It is typically covered by a loose shirt, sweater, or jacket.

Pocket pistol – Small handguns can simply be dropped into a pocket. This is quick and easy to do but somewhat dangerous as the trigger is not properly covered and the weapon can shift around, repositioning as you move. Further, the trigger can become entangled with keys or other items in your pocket leading to

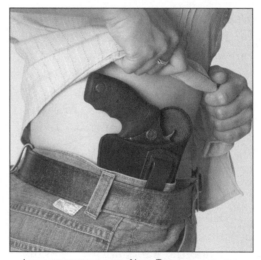

Inside the pants holster. Note: This is usually worn lower but was pulled up a bit so that it would be easier to see in the picture.

inadvertent discharge of a bullet. Many manufacturers make wallet-like pocket holsters that can hold these weapons more safely and securely while reducing the obvious gun-like outline that can be seen when the weapon is pocketed without one.

Waist band – Weapons can be placed into your waist band without using a holster. This is quick and easy to do but somewhat dangerous as the trigger is not properly covered and the weapon can move around or fall out easier than when an actual holster is used. If the weapon falls to the ground it may inadvertently discharge a bullet. Some

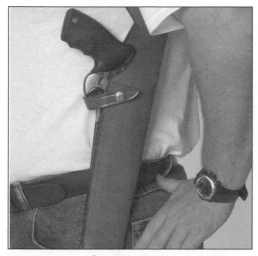

SHOULDER HOLSTER.

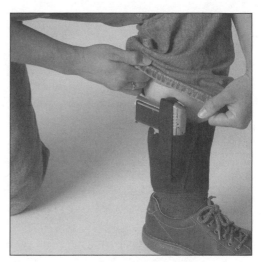

ANKLE HOLSTER.

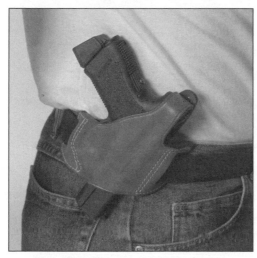

BELT SLIDE HOLSTER.

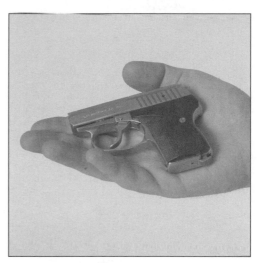

POCKET PISTOL.

firearms have optional belt clips that can help secure the weapon without a holster. The trigger is still not protected with these devices however. The weapon is typically covered by a loose shirt, sweater, or jacket.

Knife clip – Many folding knives come with built in clips to secure them in your pocket.

Knife sheath – Like a firearm, knives may be holstered on your belt. Knife sheaths can also be strapped to your forearm, hung around your neck, or clipped onto your boot.

Pocket knife – Many folding knives are carried loose in the pocket.

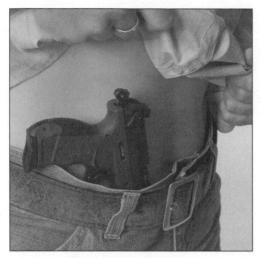

PISTOL IN WAIST BAND – FRONT.

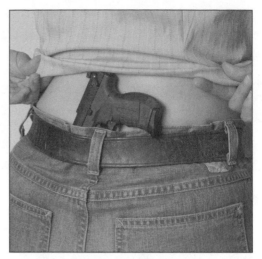

PISTOL IN WAIST BAND –BACK.

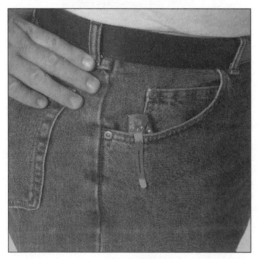

KNIFE CLIP.

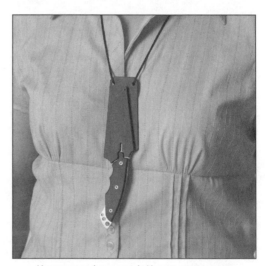

KNIFE SHEATH (NECK KNIFE). KNIFE SHEATHS CAN BE
STRAPPED TO YOUR FOREARM, CLIPPED ONTO YOUR BOOT,
AFFIXED TO YOUR BELT, OR HUNG AROUND YOUR NECK.

Concealment clothing - Common articles of clothing like jackets, vests, and even underwear have been designed specifically to conceal firearms within built-in holsters. Companies like 5.11 Tactical, Coronado Leather, Roma, and Thunderwear manufacture these items.

Weapon Disguises (e.g., stealthy deployment):

Trailing leg – A gun or knife can be held out of sight tucked in behind a person's trailing leg until it is about to be deployed.

Behind the back – Another method of keeping a gun or knife out of sight until it can be deployed is to hide it behind your back. The front hand is often used to distract an adversary, placing their attention on the moving limb rather than on what is hidden.

Palmed knife – A knife can be held concealed in the palm. Stiffened fingers often give away the fact that something is held therein.

Reverse grip along arm – A knife held in reverse grip can be hidden alongside the arm. A bent wrist may indicate something held in concealment.

Arms crossed – Another way to hide a knife alongside one's arms. The weapon is typically held in the hand closest to the body beneath the arm farthest out. This keeps the weapon invisible from most angles.

Covered – A knife or gun (or just about any weapon for that matter) can be concealed beneath a towel, jacket, newspaper, or similar covering until it is deployed.

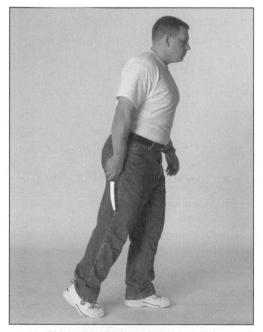

KNIFE HIDDEN ALONGSIDE THE TRAILING LEG.

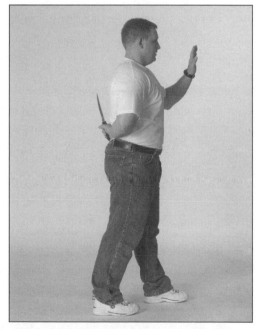

KNIFE BEHIND BACK, FRONT HAND DISTRACTING. NOTICE HOW THE FRONT HAND IS USED TO DISTRACT AN ADVERSARY, PLACING THEIR ATTENTION ON THE MOVING LIMB.

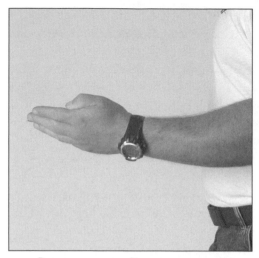

PALMED KNIFE – FRONT. NOTE THE STIFF FINGERS
INDICATING THAT SOMETHING MAY BE HIDDEN WITHIN.

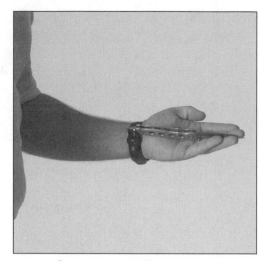

PALMED KNIFE – BACK. YOU CAN SEE THE
WEAPON MORE CLEARLY FROM THIS ANGLE.

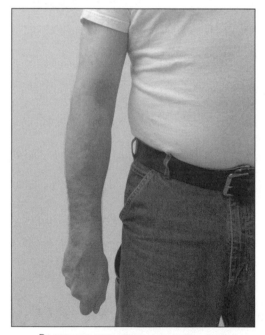

REVERSE GRIP KNIFE HIDDEN ALONG ARM – FRONT.
NOTE THE BENT WRIST WHICH INDICATES SOMETHING HELD
IN CONCEALMENT.

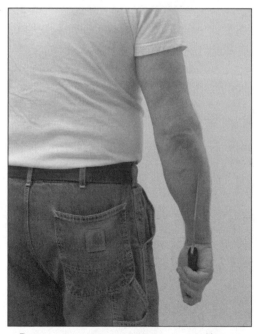

REVERSE GRIP KNIFE HIDDEN ALONG ARM – BACK. YOU CAN
SEE THE WEAPON MORE CLEARLY FROM THIS ANGLE.

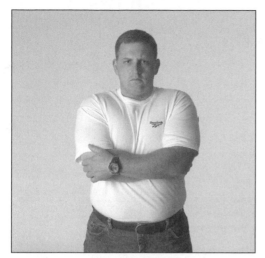

ARMS CROSSED HIDING KNIFE — FRONT. THIS IS SOMETIMES CALLED THE "PISSED OFF" STANCE.

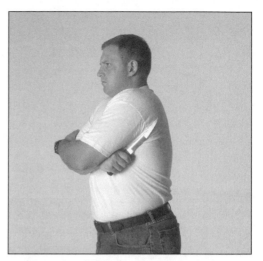

ARMS CROSSED HIDING KNIFE — BACK. YOU CAN SEE THE WEAPON MORE CLEARLY FROM THIS ANGLE.

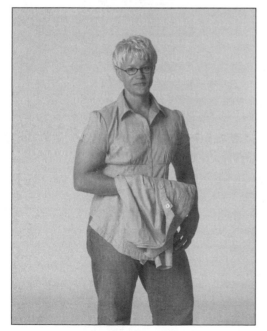

JACKET COVERED KNIFE.

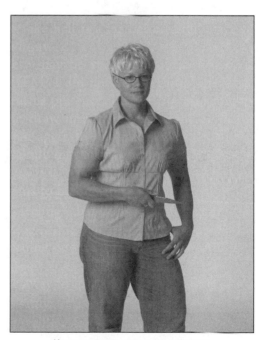

KNIFE UNCOVERED, SHOWING HOW IT WAS HELD BENEATH THE JACKET.

Now that you have a little experience, can you spot the weapons in this picture? While I am carrying more objects than one might reasonably expect, I am not so overloaded that I cannot walk around naturally or move swiftly. Here are two views:

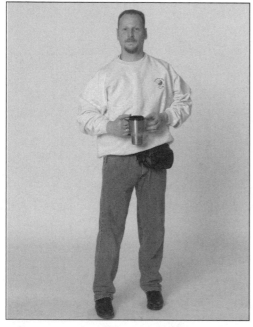

FRONT VIEW.

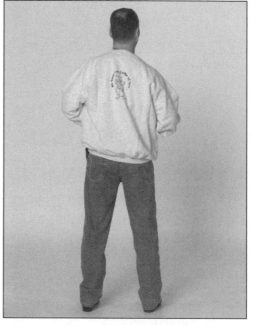

BACK VIEW.

Here are all the nasty objects I am carrying. Let's begin with the coffee. Both the hot liquid and the cup holding can be practical, improvised weapons:

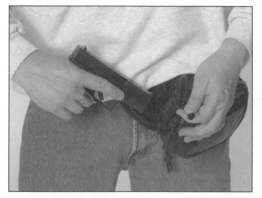

GLOCK 30 .45 CALIBER PISTOL IN BELT POUCH HOLSTER.

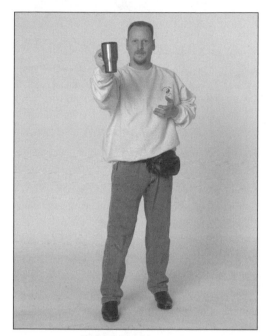

FIGURE 1.32 – HOT COFFEE.

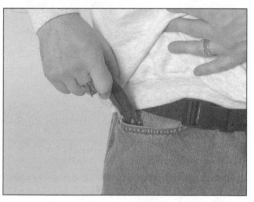

FOLDING KNIFE IN RIGHT FRONT POCKET.

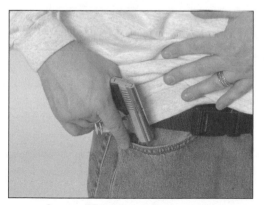

SEACAMP .32 PISTOL IN RIGHT FRONT POCKET.

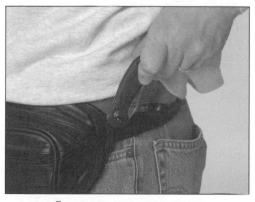

FOLDING KNIFE IN LEFT FRONT POCKET

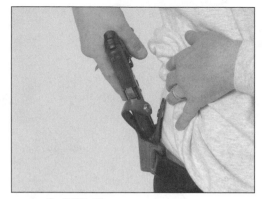

SIG P220 .45 PISTOL IN RIGHT HIP HOLSTER.

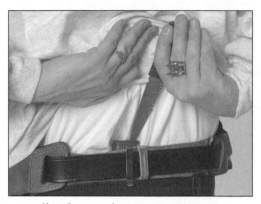

KNIFE (*SKEAN DHU*) IN SMALL OF BACK SHEATH.

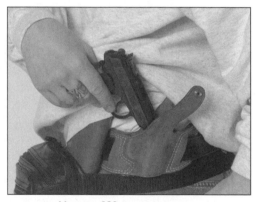

MAKAROV .380 IN LEFT HIP HOLSTER.

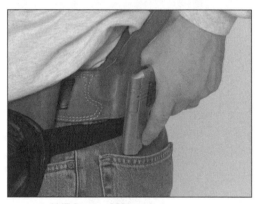

AMT BACKUP .380 IN LEFT REAR POCKET.

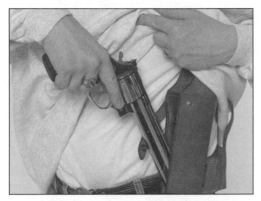

.44 MAGNUM TAURUS IN SHOULDER HOLSTER.

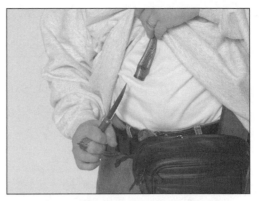

KNIFE IN NECK SHEATH.

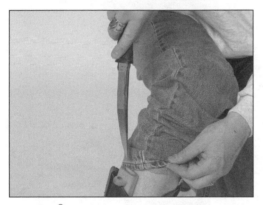

COMBAT *TANTO* IN RIGHT BOOT SHEATH.

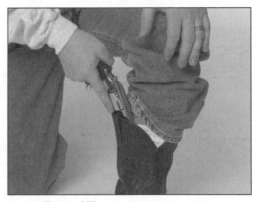

TAURUS .357 IN LEFT BOOT ANKLE HOLSTER.

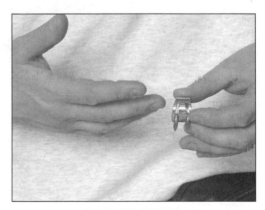

FIGHTING RING ON FINGER.

It is important to understand that just about anyone can carry a knife, gun, or other hand weapon concealed under just about anything. Just because you cannot see a weapon does not mean that a person is not armed. In fact, I have successfully concealed a firearm wearing only a pair of shorts at the beach, for example. Here is a look at all the lethal objects I had hidden around my body in the first picture. Scary, ain't it?

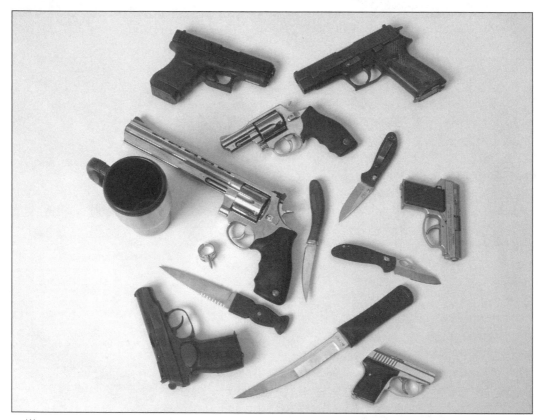

WHILE THIS PILE OF WEAPONS MAY SEEM EXAGGERATED, I WAS ABLE TO WALK AROUND EASILY AND MOVE QUICKLY WHILE CARRYING ALL THESE OBJECTS. ADDITIONALLY, I HAD NO WEAPONS STRAPPED TO EITHER ARM SO I COULD EASILY HAVE HELD A COUPLE MORE KNIVES THERE. FURTHERMORE, MY RIGHT BACK POCKET WAS EMPTY AND COULD EASILY HAVE HELD ANOTHER GUN. IT IS INTERESTING TO NOTE THAT DETECTIVES RECOVERED 14 GUNS, 107 KNIVES, TWO HAMMERS, TWO WRENCHES, AND NINE LARGE FLASHLIGHTS IN AND AROUND HARRAH'S CASINO AFTER AN APRIL 27, 2002 FIGHT BETWEEN HELL'S ANGELS AND MONGOLS MOTORCYCLE GANG MEMBERS IN LOS VEGAS NEVADA. DOZENS OF SHOTS WERE FIRED IN THE CROWDED CASINO, SEVERAL PEOPLE WERE BRUTALLY BEATEN AND STABBED, AND WHEN THE DUST CLEARED THREE BIKERS WERE DEAD. FOURTEEN MEMBERS OF BOTH GANGS WERE CHARGED WITH MORE THAN 70 CRIMES FROM THE MELEE. ASSUMING THAT THOSE CHARGED CARRIED A MAJORITY OF THE CONFISCATED WEAPONS THAT IS ROUGHLY NINE DEADLY OBJECTS PER PERSON. I WAS CARRYING TWELVE (PLUS THE COFFEE AND COFFEE CUP).

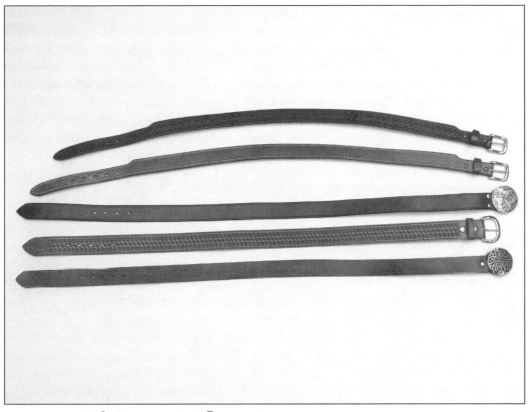

SELECTION OF PISTOL BELTS. THE TOP TWO ARE TAPERED, BOTH TO DISGUISE THEIR GIRTH
AS WELL AS TO BETTER DISTRIBUTE A WEAPON'S WEIGHT, WHILE THE LOWER ONES ARE STRAIGHT.

Here is another way to tell that someone might be armed. Most concealment strategies involve a holster of one type or another. Holsters only work well on heavy belts that can support both the weapon's weight and simultaneously hold it solidly in place. Another possible way to tell whether or not someone is armed is to look at his or her belt. A businessperson in a suit with an overly heavy belt, no matter how dressy, may well be carrying a holstered weapon that you cannot detect underneath his or her jacket. While some pistol belts are wider in the back and narrower in the front to disguise their girth, it is useful nevertheless to look for heavy leather belts from roughly 1–2 inches wide. This is no guarantee, of course, simply another indicator to be aware of.

Also, look for concealing clothing that may be covering a weapon. Examples include a jacket worn in hot weather, a vest that covers the waistline (especially the hips/lower back), or a loose shirt that is buttoned high but not low. Anyone who wears his or her outdoor wear (e.g., jacket) indoors may well be concealing a weapon under it.

Weapon Delivery System Identification

As you can see from the previous photos, just about anyone can be carrying a weapon in a manner that you cannot with certainty detect until it is deployed. It is essential, therefore to look, listen, and even feel for the presence of such devices. If you cannot see someone's hands and ascertain that they are empty, be very, very cautious around them. The hands are, after all, the primary delivery system for most lethal devices, at least those you are likely to encounter. To paraphrase the National Rifle Association, weapons do not kill people, people kill people. In addition, they almost always do so using their hands to deploy the weapon.

Hands buried in pockets, hidden under a jacket or shirt, or simply out of sight may be deploying a weapon. Or the person could simply have cold fingers. It never hurts to be prudent yet can hurt an awful lot if you are not cautious. This is somewhat situational, of course. If you cannot see a waiter's hands because he or she is serving your meal, the chances are great that you need not be concerned. Same thing goes for a close friend or relative in most cases. In public places and situations where danger may be real, you will definitely want to scrutinize people's hands. Be wary of stiff fingers, clenched fists, and other odd hand movements as they could be used to conceal a lethal device or indicate a general precursor of violence.

Also, watch for the upward or sideways motion of withdrawing a weapon from its sheath/holster. I once bluffed my way out of a fight by reaching for an imaginary handgun under my jacket. When my would-be adversary saw me shift my weight to the balls of my feet and reach toward my right hip he naturally assumed that something bad was about to happen to him. With one hand facing him in a warding gesture and the other hidden behind me, I politely stated that I did not want any trouble and asked him to stand there while I walked away. He complied.

Be sure to listen for the sounds of deployment, especially when you cannot clearly see a potential adversary such as when you are in a crowd, where someone is behind you, or when it is very dark. Audible indicators can include:

- Click (e.g., releasing mechanical safety on a handgun locking open a knife blade).
- Snap (e.g., unlocking a retention device such as a holster safety strap).
- Rustle (e.g., moving clothing aside to facilitate drawing the weapon).
- Velcro* (e.g., opening a pouch, removing a retention device such as a holster safety strap).

Feeling is important too, both psychologically and physiologically. When the kid at the QFC encroached on my personal space, I became more uncomfortable than would normally be warranted simply by his proximity. While I could not tell why at first, upon further scrutiny he was hiding something along his side. Pay attention to

---

*Is Velcro a noise? I'm referring to the ripping sound that Velcro makes when unfastened.

your intuition. Though we are often conditioned to ignore it, everyone has a biologically built-in danger sense. Use it.

Furthermore, many martial artists train to react to unexpected physical contact, especially from behind. This is valuable training. With the proper practice, you can become adept at thwarting pickpockets as well as minimizing damage from a surprise knife or weapon attack by reacting immediately to the contact without conscious thought. You will need to temper your reaction to the circumstances, of course, but the unconscious reaction training is important.

Recognizing Available Counter-Weapons

If an armed aggressor attacks, you may find yourself needing to deploy an improvised weapon with which to respond. Imi Sde-Or wrote, "You must become accustomed to quickly scanning your immediate environment for objects that can be used as improvised weapons should the need arise. When you come to a new place, survey the area thoroughly, noting any objects nearby that could prove useful. Similar to an expert chef who is capable of preparing a gourmet meal from various ingredients that he finds in his refrigerator, you should be ready to 'cook' for an occasional assailant from an impressive and effective 'menu' of your own, using standard, everyday objects that you can find within reach."

There are techniques you know, techniques you can do, techniques you use, and techniques you would stake your life on.[14] It is important to know the difference. I may be a black belt in karate, but I am really hesitant to go up against an armed attacker empty-handed. If given a choice, I would prefer to have my gun in a legitimate self-defense situation. The challenge is that a gun is a tool designed for a very narrow purpose. In some situations, it is literally overkill. In others, such as when I travel to other countries or other states on vacation or for business, my gun is legally unavailable. Without access to a firearm (or whatever instrument you prefer), improvised weapons can fill the void.

When your life is on the line, you will want every advantage to protect yourself. Look for rocks, pipes, hand tools, boards, bricks, sticks, mugs, beer bottles, belts, chairs, chains, pool cues, car keys, pens, books, briefcases, and other devices that you may already have on your person or can readily pick up and deploy to protect yourself. In some locations, you may find household or commercial chemicals, fire extinguishers, and other items that you can use to thwart an attacker as well.

Almost anything can become a weapon if you know how to use it. Some items are better used as simple distractions to help you maneuver or escape while others can become legitimate offensive or defensive weapons. A belt, for example, is not a particularly dangerous tool in most people's hands yet victims have been killed by them nevertheless. Even a common umbrella can be deadly. Eighteen year-old

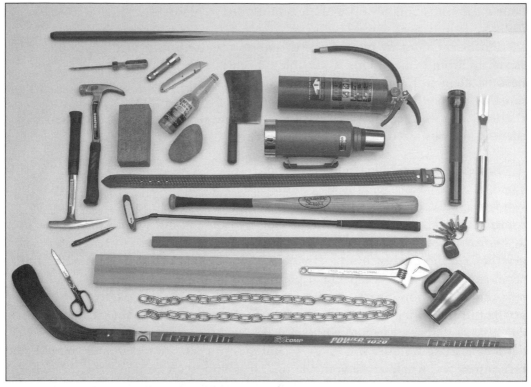

IMPROVISED WEAPONS. IN THE RIGHT HANDS, ALMOST ANYTHING CAN BE USED AS A WEAPON.

Christopher Williams was murdered on October 21, 2003 by a golf umbrella following an argument with a 16-year-old youth at a suburban Essendon (Australia) tram stop. On July 11, 2005, a 23-year-old college student, Tombol Malik, was beaten to death near the University of Illinois campus by two thugs armed with a bicycle lock. Improvised weapons in the hands of criminals are a concern yet they are also an important component of your self-defense toolbox as well.

Situational Awareness

"The ordinary person concerned with self-defense has a job that is easier than the professional's in some ways and harder in others. It is easier because, except in truly dire circumstances people are not required to seek out danger, or carry out missions regardless of danger. It is more difficult because, when danger is present, their knowledge is less accessible, their skills are likely to be less practiced, and (at least compared to police, military,

and firefighters) their allowable actions are more restricted. Being mindful of one's surroundings takes additional effort and skill, beyond that required in one's daily life. For the professional, that is one's daily life." [15]

– *Jack M. Feldman, Ph.D.*

Situational awareness means a solid understanding of time and place and how they relate to you, your family, friends, and others around you at any given moment. Any time you are near others, especially strangers, you must be vigilant, striking a good balance between obliviousness and paranoia. If you can sense danger before stumbling across it, you have a much better chance of escaping unscathed. Most self-defense experts agree that nine out of ten dangers can be identified and avoided simply by learning to look out for them.

By constantly surveying and evaluating your environment, you achieve more control over what ultimately happens to you. Tom Givens[16] wrote, "You can be stupid, inattentive, and oblivious in your work environment day in and day out and get away with it until one day the odds catch up with you and you are injured. The same applies on the street. You can be stupid, inattentive, and oblivious and get away with it until your path happens to cross the path of a criminal. The vast majority of criminals are opportunists, who only strike when presented with a viable opportunity. Remove the opportunity and you remove the risk to you!" This is absolutely correct. You can make yourself a hard target by eliminating easy opportunities for those who would do you harm to take advantage of.

Once you understand the basic concepts, situational awareness can be developed and improved through practice. There are two potentially dangerous errors that must be avoided to have truly good situational awareness, however. The first is improperly identifying danger, where none exists. The second is failing to perceive true jeopardy when confronted with it. With the former, you pose a danger to others while in the latter others pose a danger to you.

About two decades ago, I was walking through Northgate Mall, a shopping center just north of Seattle (Washington), when I noticed movement out of the corner of my eye. I glanced back to spot a metallic gun barrel pointing up at me. Adrenaline surging, I pivoted, smacked the pistol off-line with the palm of my left hand, and smoothly started to draw my gun with my right. As it cleared the holster, I suddenly realized that I was staring down at a frightened eight-year-old kid.

This was before the days when the government mandated orange safety tips and toy firearms were all made of plastic, so his metal cap gun looked pretty realistic. Nevertheless, I was so focused on the perceived threat that I had completely failed to realize how short and young my "attacker" actually was. Having not drawn it completely and pointed it at anyone, I managed to return my gun to its holster without causing too much of a scene but it could easily have turned out otherwise.*

---

*Several preoccupied bystanders noticed nothing amiss. That says something about their level of awareness too, doesn't it?

After venting my spleen about suitable toys and gun safety on the kid's mother, I fled to the parking lot where I sat in my car shaking uncontrollably for several minutes, knowing that I had nearly shot a little kid with a cap gun in the middle of a shopping mall. I was incredibly lucky to have neither killed an innocent kid nor been arrested for flashing a gun in public. I learned a very important lesson that day: improperly perceiving a threat can have dire consequences.

Not noticing a real threat can be just as bad if not worse than misperceiving an illegitimate one. About six months after the incident at the mall, I was out driving on a Saturday afternoon. The sun was shining, the traffic was light, and I was rocking out to my favorite music on a stereo system that was worth almost as much as my car. As I came upon an intersection between the four-lane arterial on which I was driving and a two-lane side street that crossed it, the light turned red. Waiting for the light to change, I became aware that something was wrong when the driver on my left suddenly burned rubber, pulling an illegal left turn through the red light and speeding away down the side street.

I look around for what seemed like a minute but was probably only a second or two before noticing half a dozen police cars in my rear view mirror as they came barreling toward me in hot pursuit of another vehicle that was suddenly looming far too close for comfort. Following the other guy's example, I drop-shifted, slammed the accelerator and ran the red light, turning right onto the side street to get out of the way. Using this maneuver, I managed to avoid a collision at the very last second. Had I not noticed the other guy's movement and reacted accordingly, I almost certainly would have ended up with another car in my back seat.

This incident was a near thing yet completely unnecessary. If I had kept the music at a reasonable level, I most certainly would have been able to hear the police sirens in plenty of time to move toward safety as the other guy did. It is important to be capable of situational awareness at all times whenever you are out in public places. At a minimum, that means looking and listening for danger. That is one of the reasons why many jurisdictions ban the use of headphones while driving. If you cannot hear an approaching siren, you may become a hazard to emergency personnel, yourself, or both.

Good situational awareness can let you predict and avoid most any potentially difficult situation. It is something all of us instinctively have yet few really pay attention to. In most cases, we should be able to spot a developing situation, turn around, and walk (or drive) away before anything bad happens.

Remember a time you were driving along the highway, suddenly "knew" the car beside you was going to swerve into your lane, and took evasive action to avoid an accident? Almost everyone who drives has done that on numerous occasions. The ability to predict what other drivers are going to do is an example of good situational awareness. Sometimes, however, try as you might to avoid it, trouble finds you and you will have to react accordingly.

Threat Level Color Codes

> *"By learning to observe your environment, constantly evaluate it, and react appropriately to what you see, you can achieve a large degree of control over your fate. This requires you to learn to shift up and down a scale of readiness, just like shifting gears in a car, so that you can match your level of awareness / readiness with the current requirements of your situation… The colors simply let us conceptualize and discuss the basic mental states. You must learn to go up and down this scale as the situation and circumstances around you change, as they invariably do as you go through your daily routine."* [17]

— *Tom Givens*

Many self-defense experts use a color code system to help define and communicate appropriate levels of situational awareness. The most commonly used approach, codified by Colonel Jeff Cooper, was based in large part on the color alert system developed by the United States Marine Corps during World War II then later modified for civilian use.* These color code conditions include White (oblivious), Yellow (aware), Orange (alert), Red (concerned), and Black (under attack). This should not be confused with the similar U.S. Department of Homeland Security threat level alerts that use similar colors. The mindset and attitude of each condition are described below:

Condition White (Oblivious)

As I was when rocking out in my car, people in this state people are pretty much oblivious to their surroundings, completely unprepared for trouble if it arrives. They are distracted or unaware, not only perceiving no danger in their immediate area, but also not alert for any that may be presented to them. Drivers carrying on conversations with passengers or talking on cell phones, joggers wearing headphones and grooving to the music, and other generally preoccupied individuals fall into this category. Their head is commonly tilted downward toward the ground in front of them or fixed on a spot in the distance such as one might do when looking at a tourist map, reading a book, or searching for a distant address or landmark.

In Condition White, you become an easy mark for just about any pickpocket, mugger, rapist, or deviant you come across. If you are attacked, you are likely going to be hurt. If armed, you can easily become a danger to yourself or others. Even police officers, who have access to much better training than the average civilian,

---

*While the highest level of situational awareness required that soldiers would shoot an enemy on sight, most law enforcement agencies tend frown on that sort of behavior among civilians.

have been killed by their own weapons when they relaxed their vigilance.

Street criminals may be strong, fast, and mean, but in general, they are neither particularly bright nor hardworking. I am stereotyping here, but seriously, how many rocket scientists or Mensa members are there on death row? Further, many crimes are quick fix substitutes for earning a living the old fashioned way via hard work. Why then would a street thug go out of his/her way to tangle with a tough, prepared target when easier prey is readily available? In Condition White, you are that easy prey.

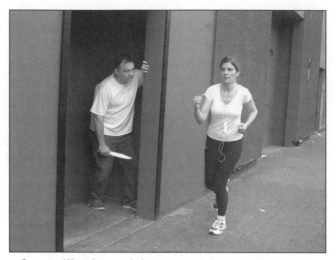

Condition White (oblivious). Joggers wearing headphones cannot hear threats. When listening carefully to the music, overly focused on the exercise, or tired after a long run they will likely not see approaching dangers either. When distracted (Condition White) in this fashion, you become an easy target for predators.

The only acceptable spot for Condition White is within the confines of your own home and then only if you are safely behind layered security appropriate for your situation. For example, motion sensor lights in the yard that warn of intruders, doors and windows secured against unauthorized entry, alarm set to sound a audible warning, an alert police dog curled at your feet, and gun safely stowed in a quick release safe within easy reach should someone get through all the other layers of protection.

Condition Yellow (Aware)

Although you are not looking for or expecting trouble in Condition Yellow, if it comes up you will have a good chance to know about it in time to react. People in this condition are at ease, not immediately perceiving any danger, but generally aware of their surroundings. They can identify, without re-looking, generally who and what is around them—vehicles, people, building entrances, street corners, and areas that might provide concealment and/or cover should something untoward happen. To clarify the difference between these two concepts, concealment (e.g., a bush) keeps bad guys from seeing you but does not provide much physical protection, while cover (e.g., a stone wall) can keep the bad guy and/or his weapon from getting to you should he wish to attack.

Body language is important. People in Condition Yellow should be self-assured and appear confident in everything they do, yet not present an overt challenge or threat to others. Predators typically stalk those they consider weaker prey, rarely victimizing the strong. People in this state look confident, walking with their heads up and casually scanning their immediate area as well as what is just beyond. They see who and what is ahead of them, are aware of their environment to each side, and occasionally turn to scan behind them.

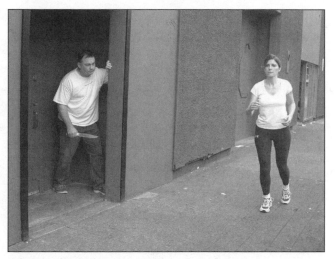

CONDITION YELLOW (AWARE). IN THIS CONDITION, YOU ARE GENERALLY AWARE OF WHAT IS HAPPENING AROUND YOU.

Condition Yellow is appropriate any time a person is in public. If you are armed in any way, it is essential. You should notice anything out of place, anyone looking or acting in an unusual manner, or anything that is simply out of context and further evaluate for potential threat. Examples might include a crowd gathered for no apparent reason, someone wearing heavy clothing on a summer day, a person studiously avoiding eye contact, anyone whose hands are hidden from view, a person moving awkwardly or with an unusual gait, or someone who simply stares at you for no apparent reason. Anything that stimulates your intuitive survival sense, suspicion, or curiosity should be studied more closely.

Condition Orange (Alert)

People in this condition have become aware of some non-specific danger (via Condition Yellow) and need to ascertain whether or not there is a legitimate threat to their safety. The difference between conditions Yellow and Orange is the identification of a specific target for further attention. You may have heard a nearby shout, the sound of glass breaking, or an unidentified sudden noise where you would not have expected one. You might also have seen another person or a group of people acting abnormally, someone whose demeanor makes you feel uncomfortable, or somebody whose appearance stands out as unusual.

In this state, you should focus on the nebulous danger, but not to the exclusion of a broader awareness of your surroundings. Trouble may be starting in other places in addition to the one that has drawn your attention (e.g., ambush situation). It is wise to look for escape routes and nearby areas of cover or concealment. If unarmed you should also try to spot objects that can be used as makeshift weapons or distractions. It may be prudent to reposition yourself to take advantage of cover, escape routes, or impromptu weapons should it become necessary to use them. It is usually premature to make any aggressive moves at this point.

If the trouble is immediate, but not directed at you, de-escalation may be appropriate, but assess the situation before you intervene. If you have not honed your communication skills and/or you have no legal or hierarchical authority to get involved,[19] your interference

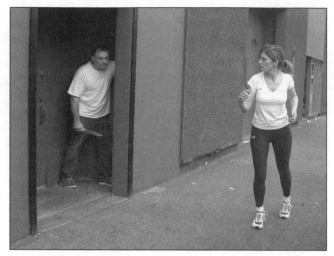

CONDITION ORANGE (ALERT). IN THIS CONDITION, YOU HAVE BECOME AWARE OF A POTENTIAL THREAT THAT WARRANTS FURTHER EXAMINATION.

may shift the violence toward you or spark a confrontation that you could have otherwise avoided. Even though I have more than 20 years of experience defusing volatile situations at the stadium, unless I am near 100 percent certain that my involvement will help a situation I am unlikely to directly intervene in everyday encounters outside of my work. I am much more likely to get out of the way, pull out my cell phone, and dial 9-1-1. Similarly, you may also wish to move to safety and call for help as precaution in such situations. (The de-escalation process and methods will be covered in-depth in Chapter 4.)

If armed, it is a good idea to be sure that your weapon is accessible, though it is probably not prudent to call attention to it at this point. If in a lonely area like a parking garage or alley, it is usually wise to move into a better-lit or populated area like a store. Denying privacy for criminal acts to occur or escalate once started is one of the most fundamental principles of self-defense.

This is also a good time to prepare a plan of action; shortening the OODA (Observation, Orientation, Decision, and Action) loop to hopefully take a would-be adversary by surprise should it become necessary to do so. The OODA loop, oftentimes referred to as Boyd's law for military strategist Colonel John R. Boyd who codified it, is a way of quantifying reaction times in combat.

Here is how the OODA loop works. Each party to a confrontation begins by observing themselves, their physical surroundings, and their adversary. This takes a quantifiable amount of time which delays immediate action, even if only by milliseconds. Next each combatant must orient themselves by making a mental image of the tactical situation, building on past experiences to interpolate the current environment before deciding how best to respond. Because it is impossible to process information as quickly as we perceive it, there is also an orientation delay that precedes any action a person chooses to take. This decision ultimately takes into account the various factors present at the time of the orientation. Once deciding upon an appropriate response, there is another delay between thought and action.

A person who can consistently cycle through Boyd's OODA loop faster than his or her opponent can gains a tremendous advantage. By the time the slower person reacts, the faster one may already be doing something different so the defensive action is less effective than anticipated. With each cycle, the effectiveness of the slower party's action becomes more and more diminished. Boyd's law dictates that the aggregate resolution of these cyclic episodes will eventually determine the outcome of a conflict.

Whether you prepare ahead of time or not, the more comprehensive your martial arts training and the more experience you have with various weapons, the faster you can move through this cycle. Preparing a plan of action ahead of time can significantly reduce your OODA loop cycle-time giving you a significant advantage in defending yourself should the need arise.

If it turns out that trouble is not brewing, you simply return to Condition Yellow, abandoning the plan unimplemented. Consider your effort good practice, be thankful that nothing untoward happened, and go on with your day. Conceivably a potential adversary may even sense your preparation and choose not to act. If, on the other hand, you become convinced that trouble truly is likely forthcoming, you will need to escalate to Condition Red.

Condition Red (Concerned)

People in this condition have been confronted by a potential adversary or are in close proximity to someone who is becoming aggressive and is near enough to confront them quickly. Condition Red means that you have every reason to believe that someone poses a clear and present danger to you or someone with you.

You must be prepared to fight, hopefully taking advantage of the plan you visualized in Condition Orange. At this point it is prudent to begin moving away toward escape routes, locations with strategic cover, or areas of concealment if you can do so. If the confrontation is immediate, it is often a good idea to try to move away from any weapons being brandished or distractions being made, while at the same time keeping well aware of them.

If you are armed, this may be the point where you draw and ready your weapon or at least make its presence known.* A verbal challenge at this point may prove useful if time permits. De-escalation may still be an option but it can also backfire so you must be prepared in case it does not work. Every reasonable attempt should still be made to avoid a fight yet you must resign yourself to the very real possibility that it will be unsuccessful.

---

*Such as by reaching under your jacket to grab a hold of your pistol and thumbing your holster's safety release.

For example, a show of ability and readiness to resist with countervailing force may stop the confrontation yet it could also elevate it to the next level, open conflict. Either way, your intent should be to stop the potential assault that is forthcoming, escape to safety, or stay safe until help arrives, doing so without harming anyone including those threatening you. You must not want to kill or hurt anyone nor teach them a lesson. Such attitudes can make you the aggressor in the eyes

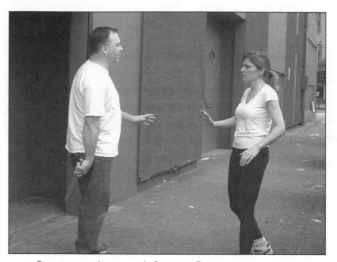

CONDITION RED (CONCERNED). CONDITION RED MEANS THAT YOU HAVE EVERY REASON TO BELIEVE THAT SOMEONE POSES A CLEAR AND PRESENT DANGER TO YOU.

of the law. In addition, even if you are never charged with a crime you will still have to live with yourself afterward.

Many fights are over before the loser fully comprehends what has happened. This is because of the OODA loop we discussed previously. Although it is possible to skip nearly instantly from Condition Yellow all the way up to Condition Black (under attack), you can still more or less align Boyd's law with the various alert conditions. In Condition Yellow, you observe something amiss. In Condition Orange, you ascertain that it may be a threat, building on past experiences to orient and interpolate this new information. In Condition Red, you pre-determine a response and decide what to do. This merely leaves the decision to take action unfulfilled. You act in Condition Black. By pre-cycling through the OODA loop your reaction time may be faster than that of your opponent. Without doing so, it most assuredly will not be.

Reaction being slower than action, mental preparation gives you an essential edge before combat. You must be both mentally and physically prepared to fight, merely waiting for a mental trigger to up the ante to Condition Black. This trigger is a typically a pre-determined action on the part of a potential adversary (e.g., closing distance, pulling their arm back in preparation for a punch, flashing a knife, attempting to draw a gun), that will clarify in your mind the imperative to act. Do not be too locked in on something specific yet try not to overreact either. After all, Condition Red is still not open conflict that, at this point, you are still trying not to initiate. Condition Red is only a precursor to violence. See Chapter 5 for more information on triggers.

Condition Black (Under Attack)

People in this condition are actively being attacked. Verbal challenges and de-escalation attempts are no longer useful. You must flee or fight back, using any appropriate distractions and/or weapons at your disposal. If armed and confronted by an armed attacker or multiple unarmed assailants, you may decide to use your weapon in self-defense. Be sure that you are legally, ethically, and morally entitled to do so before employing lethal counter-vailing force. (See Chapter 5 for information on the legal, moral, ethical, religious, and psychological considerations of coun-tervailing force.) Once again, your intent must be to stop the assault that is in progress so that you can escape to safety or otherwise remain safe until help arrives. Your goal is to be safe, not to kill your attacker or teach him/her a lesson.

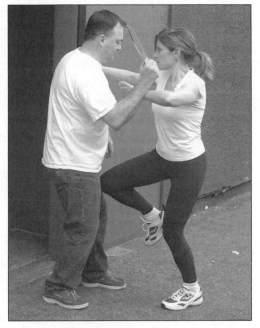

CONDITION BLACK (UNDER ATTACK). IN THIS CONDITION, VERBAL CHALLENGES AND DE-ESCALATION ATTEMPTS ARE NO LONGER USEFUL. YOU MUST FLEE OR FIGHT BACK, USING ANY APPROPRIATE DISTRACTIONS AND/OR WEAPONS AT YOUR DISPOSAL.

Each encounter is different; its unique characteristics will determine an appropriate response. It is important to use suffi-cient force to effectively control the situation and keep yourself safe without overre-acting. You will, no doubt, want to treat a drunken relative at a family reunion quite differently than a homicidal street punk coming at you in a drug-induced rage.

Indicators of Impending Attack

Violence rarely happens in a vacuum. There is always some escalation process—even a really short one—that precedes it. There are physiological, behavioral, and ver-bal indicators that you can spot to warn you of imminent conflict. Some are subtle and may indicate nothing of an alarming nature. Others are overtly hostile and should cause immediate action. Most fall in between and require judgment to be applied before taking action. As a general rule, you should error on the side of caution, trying to avoid or evade problem situations before they spin out of control. It is important to trust your instincts in such situations. Whether you see it or not, there will often be some indicator that can warn you of a person's intent just before they attack.

This indicator is often called the "tell." Poker players coined this term, which refers to some movement or gesture that lets them ascertain that an opponent is bluffing. In the martial arts, the tell has been called many things such as the adrenal dump or the twitch. If you do not see the tell you are bound to lose. Even if you are really, really fast, action is always faster than reaction. In other words, missing the tell is what gets you sucker punched. Recovery after the first strike is challenging, though not impossible.

The sign you are looking for could be a slight drop of the shoulder, a tensing of the neck, a puckering of the lips, or any other small movement that precedes an attack. Because it is small, it is really hard to see. Consequently, the best way to find the tell is to look for a change, the physical manifestation of an adrenal response that implies a person is about to attack. Looking for the tell is a little different than looking for a change in the person, however. You actually look for a change in a person's energy.

Here are some examples of where changes of energy constitutes a tell:

- A person who was standing still moves slightly. A weight shift is far subtler than a step, but the change is possibly preparation for attack.
- You notice a sudden pallor or sudden flushing of the person's face (e.g., adrenaline-induced vasoconstriction).
- A person who was looking at you suddenly looks away or, conversely, a person who was looking away suddenly makes eye contact.
- You notice a change in the rate, tone, pitch, or volume of a person's voice. An overt example is when someone who is shouting becomes suddenly quiet or, conversely, one who has been quiet begins raising his or her voice.
- You notice a sudden change in the person's breathing (i.e., shallow, fast for untrained adversaries; slow, deep for trained opponents).

While the tell immediately precedes violence, other behaviors can be part of the escalation process that may eventually lead to violence. Possible trouble indicators to be concerned about include:

- Glaring, staring, or otherwise "sizing you up."
- Attempts to follow, herd (control your direction), flank, or mirror your movements.
- Making unprovoked accusations, threats, aggressive requests, demands, or using foul language for no apparent reason.
- Baiting or attempting to provoke an aggressive response from you (e.g., "What's your problem?" or "What are you looking at?").
- Unusual or out of place body movements, aggressive gestures, agitated pacing, clenched fists, forward weight shift, or adaptation of a fighting stance.
- Clearing space to move or draw a weapon.

- Hands and/or teeth clenched, neck taut, or other stiff or shaking body movements.
- Shouting to startle or paralyze you as an attack begins.

Fighting Ranges and Danger Zones

"Once a criminal selects a victim, he must move into a position from which an attack is possible. Always remember that to assault, rob, or rape you, he must be close enough to talk to you. He will attempt to maneuver into this position by stealth (which is defeated by being alert), or by ruse… Positioning prior to the assault is vital to him, as he relies almost totally on surprise for success. If you avoid his attempts to properly position himself, you forestall the attack." [20]

— Tom Givens

There are no absolutes in self-defense. Every situation will be different and unique. The closest thing to an absolute, however, is that it is critical to maintain sufficient distance between yourself and a potential assailant to give yourself time to react. You may be in imminent danger from an unarmed attacker within about 10 feet. For an armed attacker this range is extended to a bare minimum of 21 feet. As stated previously, the Tueller Drill established a minimum distance of about 21 feet for armed attackers since most adversaries could close that gap and fatally assault you with a knife, sword, or blunt instrument in about 1.5 seconds, as fast as most trained practitioners can react. [21] One and a half seconds seems like an awfully long time until you try it for yourself.

At a handgun retention [22] class I took several years ago we tried a modified version of this drill. Everyone wore white t-shirts and protective eyewear. The attackers carried Sharpie markers to simulate knives while the defenders used paintball guns to simulate firearms. The rules were that the defenders had to hold their guns by their sides* and could not move until the attackers had already moved first. If an attacker got hit in a vital area with a paintball pellet, he or she would to take one more step, and then fall forward. It was permissible to strike while falling.

Admittedly, it is harder to aim and fire a paintball gun than a real firearm, but it sure seemed like an easy "win" scenario for the shooters until we actually got started. The results were interesting. Between fifteen and twenty feet, many of the defenders ultimately missed hitting their fast-moving attacker on their first shot, frequently not getting off a second without being "cut." The old adage that action is faster than reaction was very apparent. Even though we did not have to withdraw the paintball guns from a holster, we had to wait for the attackers to make the first move. Because a

---

*Since there weren't any holsters available for them.

"critically wounded" attacker got one step after being hit, almost every defender was cut regardless of whether or not they shot their attacker first. Furthermore, attackers only had to stop after suffering vital area hits (e.g., torso, head). The room was not big enough to try this at even longer distances but the instructor noted that most people can close thirty feet in about 2 to 2.5 seconds so the results would likely be similar even at slightly longer ranges.

I suspect that since the paintball splats really hurt at close range through a light t-shirt, the knife-wielders were motivated to move with realistic combat speed. I know I was when I took that role! I further suspect that is why we did not use squirt guns for this drill. At ten to fifteen feet, all the defenders received "fatal" wounds every single time, even when the defenders attempted to move off the line of their opponent's attack.* I am not sure this was a completely realistic scenario; nevertheless, it was illuminating. Although I came home covered with bruises, paint, and ink, this drill really drove home how fast a motivated aggressor can move under stress conditions and how difficult it is to aim at and hit a fast-moving target when you are adrenalized yourself.

A distance of 21 feet is not necessarily great enough to keep you safe from a determined attacker. You need to pay attention not only to how far away from you a potential attacker is, but also to whether or not he or she is armed or in close proximity of a makeshift weapon. It is important to point out that while an armed attacker at 21 feet is a potentially deadly foe, this does not automatically imply that you should kill him or her out of hand. If, for example, you are armed with a firearm and already have a bead on your knife-wielding attacker, there may still be sufficient time to request his surrender or otherwise warn him off before you have to fire. If he charges, you obviously have to shoot, yet until you get to that point you may still have other non-lethal options available. Regardless, distance is critical for safety.

Now that we know distance is important, I find it useful to break weapon-defense fighting down into ranges, as certain instruments deploy better at some distances than they do at others. In general, the closer you are to an opponent, the more danger you are in simply due to reaction time, yet this is not always the case. Each weapon will have an optimal range wherein it is most effective.

With certain devices such as pole weapons, you may be better off fighting close up so that you can work inside their most effective range. With other devices such as knives, you may be better off further away so that you have a chance to run. Given the chance to do so, you would be better off running from a pole weapon too, of course, but that applies to all types of weapons and goes without saying. Other weapons, such as firearms, are less effective up close where you can grapple with them as well as far away where it is easier to miss. In every case, a good understanding of the optimal fighting range for whatever weapon you are facing can help you ascertain how much danger you are truly in and help plan the best way to keep yourself safe.

---

*There were numerous "double kills," however, where both the attacker and defender were struck simultaneously.

This will be further discussed on a weapon by weapon basis in Chapter 9.

Since fights are dynamic, ranges will vary throughout an encounter. For the most part, rather than describing distances in feet or inches I prefer to use body or weapon lengths so that descriptions can be applicable for practitioners and weapons of any size. Try not to be too hung up on exact distances; the important message is ensuring that you understand enough about your proximity to danger to make wise decisions. I like to use the following general range categories:

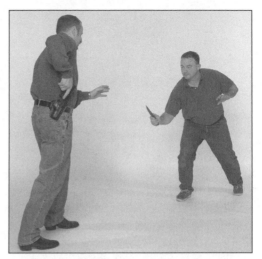

EVEN A DISTANCE OF 21 FEET IS NOT NECESSARILY SUFFICIENT TO KEEP YOU SAFE FROM A DETERMINED ATTACKER.

- Grappling range (touching)
- Close range (arm length)
- Short range (leg length/short weapon distance)
- Mid range (long weapon length)
- Long range (pole weapon length)
- Extreme range (projectile weapon length)

Grappling Range

Grappling range requires body-to-body contact. This is the range at which martial artists can effectively perform locks, throws, sweeps, and takedowns. At this range, you may have the best chance of defeating an armed opponent when you are unarmed since you will have leverage to control the opponent's weapon and attack his body with your arms and legs simultaneously. Longer weapons such as swords, staffs, and baseball bats are at a disadvantage in this range as you can get inside their most effective reach. Even guns can be defeated from this distance if you know how to do so and have a little luck on your side. Shorter weapons such as certain knives, and control devices such as *kubatons* and *yawara* sticks can be highly effective and very dangerous at this distance.

Close Range

Close range, an arm's length away, is the optimal distance for most *Goju Ryu* karate applications. If you are in a fighting stance where one leg is in front of the other such as you would be in *sanchin dachi* (hourglass stance), this distance would be measured by

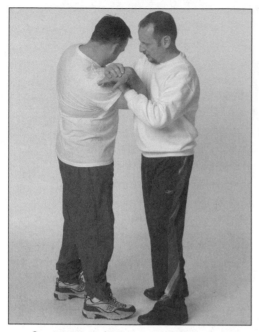

GRAPPLING RANGE (TOUCHING DISTANCE). YOU MUST HAVE GOOD BODY-TO-BODY CONTACT TO APPLY GRAPPLING TECHNIQUES EFFECTIVELY SUCH AS THIS ARM LOCK.

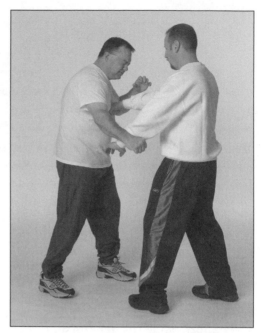

CLOSE RANGE (PUNCHING DISTANCE). THIS IS THE RANGE FROM WHICH YOU CAN LAND A *GYAKU TSUKI* (REVERSE PUNCH) EFFECTIVELY.

what you can touch from your back (trailing) fist.* From this range, practitioners can throw effective punches, elbow strikes, or knee strikes from either side of their body.

It is too close to effectively launch certain kicks yet not so close as to optimally perform many control techniques and takedowns. You might begin a takedown from this distance but will have to move in closer to grappling range to complete the application. This is an especially effective range for strike enhancers (e.g., fighting rings/brass knuckles), certain control devices (e.g., *tonfa*), most knives, and even some swords (e.g., *wakizashi*, *gladius*) and certain mass weapons (e.g., flashlight).

Short Range

Short range is kicking distance, a preference of many Korean martial styles. Again, you should measure from your trailing leg if in a fighting stance since you will want to be able to connect with either leg. At this range, the effectiveness of hand techniques begins to diminish while the effectiveness of many weapons increases. Certain swords, clubs, tactical batons, large wrenches, hammers, hand axes, and a host of other weapons can be highly effective at this distance.

*This is a *gyaku tsuki* (reverse punch) for those who recognize the Japanese term.

Mid Range

Mid range is slightly beyond kicking distance, approximately the length of an extended sword. Longer weapons such as swords, bats, and *bo* staffs, become exceedingly effective at this range, as they are hard to counter. *Bo* staffs, when held near the middle (e.g., traditional *kobudo* grip with hands at even thirds along the shaft), are effective here as well. Chemical sprays and hand-launched projectiles such as rocks, bottles, knives, darts, as well as liquids like hot coffee can be effective at this distance as well.

This is also a decent range from which to shoot someone—most gunfights take place at a distance of less than ten feet. In fact, according to FBI statistics, 95 percent of officer involved shootings occur at less than 21 feet, with approximately 75 percent taking place at less than 10 feet

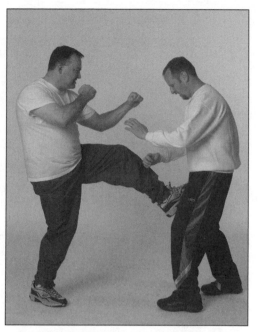

SHORT RANGE (KICKING/SHORT WEAPON DISTANCE). THIS IS THE RANGE FROM WHICH YOU CAN LAND A SOLID KICK SUCH AS THIS *MAE GERI* (FRONT KICK).

and a little over half at closer than five feet. It is also about as close as you can reasonable use a Taser to assure that you get the minimum appropriate spread between the probes.[23]

Long Range

Long range is the length of an extended *bo* staff, the purview of pole[24] and projectile weapons. It is far beyond where you can land a punch or a kick without taking a long step or two to close the gap. Pole weapons include pool cues, spears, pitchforks, *bo* staffs, halberds, pole axes, and *naginata*, to name a few. Projectile weapons such as guns, bows, Tasers, and thrown knives, tend to be especially effective here as well, since they can frequently be used to attack more than once before someone can close the gap to counter or clear enough distance to find cover or get away.

Extreme Range

Extreme range derives its name because it is impractical to engage an opponent at this distance with anything other than a projectile weapon. From this distance, you are almost always better off running away than pursuing any type of countervailing force, even if you are carrying a gun, unless there is no available cover or your path of escape

has been blocked. It is challenging for even highly trained
combatants to hit a moving
target at distances beyond 10
to 15 feet, especially if they
themselves are moving too.

Identifying Escape Paths

Since the best way of avoiding injury in a fight is not getting into one in the first place,
our prime strategy is to become
aware of and steer clear of the
danger before it is too late. On
occasion, however, either we
miss the cues or the situation
spins out of control too fast to
avoid. In these cases, we need to
protect ourselves from immediate threat then find a way to
escape safely. The next chapter
will go into more details about
escape and evasion techniques,
but before you begin to run, it
is very important to have an
escape path figured out ahead of
time. This is where awareness
comes into play.

Pay attention to available
escape paths wherever you go.
On an airplane, for example,
know not only where the exit

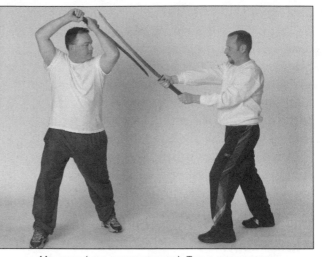

MID RANGE (LONG WEAPON DISTANCE). THIS IS APPROXIMATELY
THE RANGE OF AN EXTENDED SWORD.

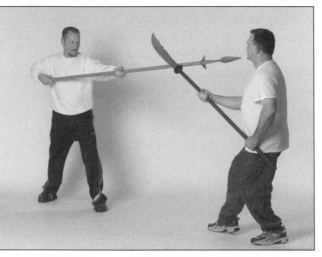

LONG RANGE (POLE WEAPON DISTANCE). THIS IS APPROXIMATELY
THE RANGE OF AN EXTENDED SPEAR THRUST.

doors are located but also how many seats you must pass before you get there. That
way if you need to navigate in smoke, darkness, or other adverse conditions you will
know what to do. Similarly, in public places such as restaurants, bars, schools, and
office buildings note the locations of all available exits. If a gunman enters from one
side of the building, you will want to know how to escape out the other.

Be sure to note the location of any improvised weapons or obstacles you will have
to pass along your route. These items could be employed for countervailing force,

used for cover or concealment, or simply get in your way, barring escape. In addition to your physical location (e.g., building layout, street map, terrain), pay attention to any bystanders in your proximity. They may be a source of aid, additional threat, and/or witnesses to corroborate your claim of self-defense should things get ugly.

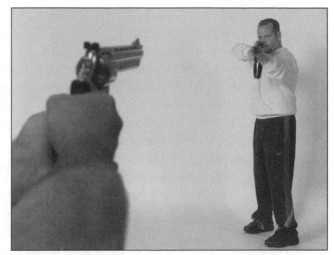

EXTREME RANGE (PROJECTILE WEAPON DISTANCE). THIS RANGE IS THE PURVIEW OF PROJECTILE WEAPONS SUCH AS BOWS (E.G., ARROWS, BOLTS), THROWN OBJECTS, AND FIREARMS (E.G., BULLETS, SHOT SHELLS)

This information can help keep you safe not only during an armed confrontation but also during a fire, earthquake, or other emergency as well. In areas you frequent such as your workplace or school, it is imperative that you know where fire extinguishers, first aid kits, AEDs,[25] and other safety resources are located. Some of these items can be used as improvised weapons during armed attacks while others are lifesaving devices for more mundane emergencies.

Summary

"To be safe you need first an awareness of the danger and a healthy level of common sense." [26]

– *Massad Ayoob*

If your goals for learning a martial art include the ability to defend yourself from a real-life attacker, you absolutely, positively must learn how to contend effectively with an armed assault. In the United States alone, there are nearly two million violent crimes perpetrated with weapons every year. Not only are they fairly common, but armed assaults are far more dangerous to the victim than unarmed ones, about 3.5 times as likely as unarmed encounters to result in serious injuries. More than 90 percent of all homicides involve some type of weapon.

Since just about anything can be used as a weapon, it is simply not practicable to list them all. I find it useful to classify the plethora of pointy objects and deadly devices one might encounter into the following general categories: hand weapons, knives, swords, mass weapons, pole arms, multi-element weapons, projectile weapons, and unusual weapons. Each has unique characteristics.

It is paramount to be able to identify anyone around you who may be carrying a weapon. The vast majority of weapon concealment strategies have one thing in common: accessibility. A weapon does no good if you cannot get to it rapidly when you need it. You will frequently rely on your eyes to spot a concealed weapon, though you can use your ears too, listening for the sound of a weapon being drawn or readied for action.

Pay particular attention to a person's hands. If you cannot see them or cannot tell that they are empty, be extra cautious. Hands buried in pockets, hidden under a jacket or shirt, or simply out of sight may be deploying a weapon. Look for stiff fingers, clenched fists, and other odd hand movements as they could be used conceal a lethal device or indicate a general precursor of violence. Also, watch for the upward or sideways motion of withdrawing a weapon from a sheath, holster, or pocket.

Violence almost never happens in a vacuum. There is some escalation process—even a really short one—that precedes it. There are physiological, behavioral, and verbal indicators that you can spot to warn you of imminent conflict. Situational awareness means having a solid understanding of time and place and how they relate to you, your family, friends, and others around you at any given moment.

Any time you are near others, especially strangers, you must be vigilant, striking a good balance between obliviousness and paranoia. Many self-defense experts use a color code system to help define and communicate appropriate levels of situational awareness. The most commonly used approach describes conditions as White (oblivious), Yellow (aware), Orange (alert), Red (concerned), and Black (under attack).

It is critical to maintain sufficient distance between yourself and a potential assailant to give yourself time to react. For an armed attacker this range is about 21 feet, since most adversaries can close that gap and fatally assault you with a weapon in about 1.5 seconds, as fast as most trained practitioners can draw and fire a weapon. While fights are dynamic, it is important to understand ranges and how they play to the strengths and weaknesses of whatever weapon you might face: grappling range (touching), close range (arm length), short range (leg length/short weapon distance), mid range (long weapon length), long range (pole weapon length), and extreme range (projectile weapon length).

Since the best way of avoiding injury in a fight is not getting into one in the first place, our prime strategy is to become aware of and steer clear of the danger before it is too late. On occasion, however, either we miss the cues or the situation spins out of control too fast to avoid. In these cases, we need to protect ourselves from immediate threat then find a way to escape safely. Pay attention to available escape paths wherever you go.

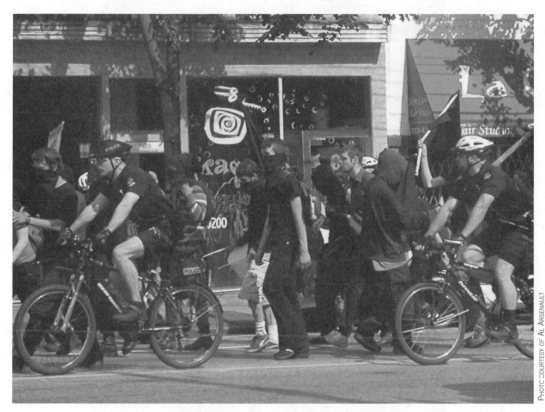

ANARCHY DEMONSTRATION MARCH WITH POLICE ESCORT.

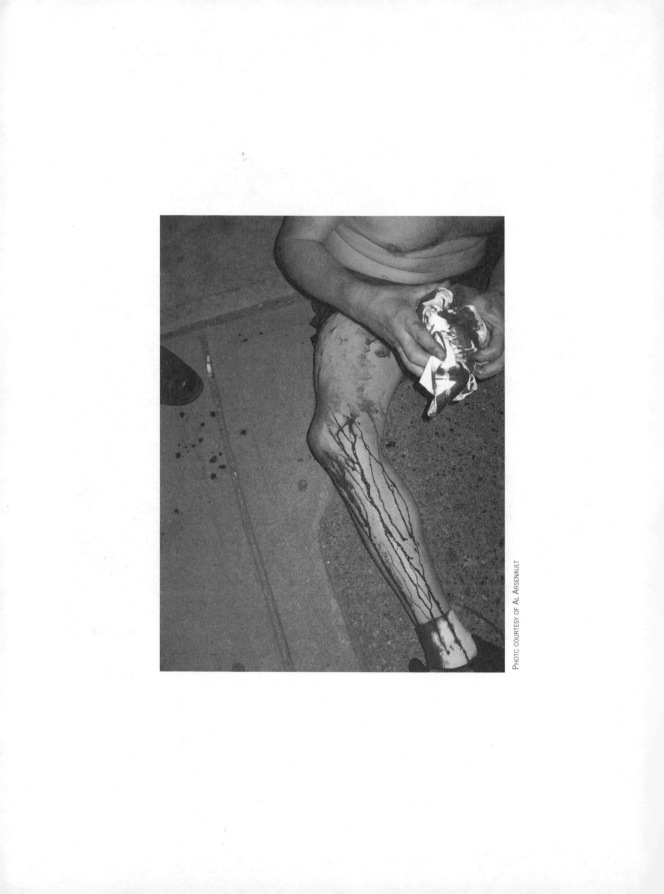

CHAPTER 2

Avoidance

"People should learn to see and so avoid all danger. Just as a wise man keeps away from mad dogs, so one should not make friends with evil men." [1]

– *Buddha*

In a review of Marc MacYoung's book *Street E & E: Evading, Escaping, And Other Ways To Save Your Ass When Things Get Ugly* posted on Amazon.com, one customer wrote, "I guess it was pretty good, and I'm sure that a lotta folks will be able to get something out of it, but I could never run away. Maybe I'm stupid or something, but I just can't do it. Of course, for all of you folks running away is probably really good advice—especially if you're facing three attackers and they've all got knives. Valhalla, here I come!"

I hope this person was not serious, but I have met all too many martial artists for whom his/her perspective would resonate. There is absolutely nothing wrong with running away, especially if you wish to enjoy life beyond an extended stay in a jail cell or a one-way trip to the morgue. Will it kill you to swallow your ego and back down from a confrontation even if you are in the right? Probably not. Failing to do so, on the other hand, can have lasting repercussions including, but not limited to, your untimely demise.

In fact, the only way to guarantee victory in a physical confrontation is to walk away before the first blow is thrown. Although martial artists train to survive (or even triumph) in a fight, we should do everything we can to avoid violence in the first place. We can use humor, deception, bribery, or any other plausible tactic that might work. Even if a person legitimately uses force in order to escape an imminent and unavoidable danger, he or she will still have to live with the physiological and psychological results of doing so. Further, he or she must be prepared to face the prospect of subsequent litigation by the defeated opponent and/or a government prosecutor.

Avoidance is your best strategy for safety and survival. The more dangerous you are, the less you should need to prove it. Ego notwithstanding, it is far better to withdraw than it is to face the consequences of causing or allowing an argument to escalate to the point of physical confrontation.

Avoiding Risky Behavior

"The average citizen makes one terrible, frightening mistake when he buys a gun for self-defense. He sees the weapon as a talisman that magically wards off evil. In fact, it is nothing of the kind." [2]

– *Massad Ayoob*

Martial artists and people who carry weapons for self-defense frequently develop a feeling of invulnerability and begin to court danger in ways they never would have prior to beginning their training. Sauntering through a dark alley in a bad neighborhood after midnight, leering at a professional ballplayer's girlfriend at a nightclub, and antagonizing protesters at a political rally are all bad ideas no matter how well trained or armed you happen to be. If you really need to prove how tough you are, there are plenty of relatively safe and thoroughly legal venues to consider such as Ultimate Fighting and similar "no-holds-barred" style tournaments.[3] Do not court trouble on the streets.

We talked about awareness conditions and danger zones in the previous chapter. Being prepared and alert for trouble can stave off most attacks before they even begin.

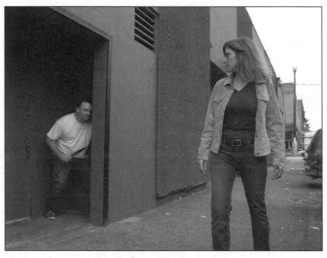

AVOIDING AMBUSHES. SWING WIDE OF DOORWAYS, ALLEYS, AND POTENTIAL AMBUSH LOCATIONS TO GIVE YOUR SELF TIME TO REACT.

Put yourself in a potential attacker's shoes, taking note of locations where you might lurk if you wanted to get the jump on someone. A few extra precautions near these potential ambush sites can add an extra layer of safety.

For example, when approaching alleyways, doorways, and likely ambush locations swing wide to increase your odds of spotting an attacker before he or she can surprise you. Keep your hands free to the extent possible so that you are ready to use them at a moment's notice. The sooner you spot a potential attacker the more time you will have to react.

Do your best to avoid perilous locations, dangerous times, and hazardous people. For example, if you need money from a cash machine during a night out, choose one in a well lit, populated store rather than using a freestanding parking lot kiosk or bank side ATM. Better still, use a credit card and avoid carrying large amounts of cash altogether. There is more information about cash machines and other hazardous situations in Chapter 3.

Principles of Personal Safety

"No one program can train you for every situation you encounter on the street because there are always surprises in a fight, things you never thought would happen. It's important, therefore, that you are aware of your training's strengths and weaknesses. Do all that you can to eliminate or at least minimize those weaknesses, but understand that you can't get rid of them all. Assess the many possible situations you might get into where those weak points could raise their ugly heads and then take every precaution you can to avoid getting into them." [4]

– Loren Christensen

You can avoid risky behavior relatively easily simply by controlling your own actions yet you cannot forestall all danger no matter what you do. To keep yourself as safe as possible you must always be prepared to respond to confrontations, pre-planning what you might do should things go wrong. Purchasing this book is an excellent first step in the process.*

Detective (ret) J. J. Bittenbinder suggests four principles for personal safety that I think are pragmatic, practical, and easy to remember. These include (1) making yourself a hard target, (2) denying privacy, (3) attracting attention, and (4) taking action as appropriate to your circumstances. The following is not a direct quote from his work, but uses his premises as foundational material.

Never Make Yourself an Easy Target

Tough, alert individuals are typically not selected by criminals. Predators are excellent at identifying body language, mental state, and awareness, automatically sorting the metaphorical sheep from the sheepdogs (and fellow wolves). The more alert and prepared you are, the less likely you are to be attacked.

Develop and hone your awareness, listening to your intuition to discern and avoid danger before you stumble upon it. Operate in Condition Yellow or higher in all public places. Train hard and realistically, preparing for the unlikely occurrence that you should need to utilize your martial skills to defend yourself.

I cannot remember who said it, but the phrase "somewhere, every day, someone is training to kick your ass" sums things up brilliantly. You can assume that anyone

*Shameless self-promotion alert.

who attacks you will consider him or herself bigger, tougher, meaner, and more experienced than you are. Either that or he will deploy a weapon to win, likely from an ambush. Either way, you must always be prepared and ready to defend yourself and/or your loved ones.

The first step in being prepared to fight is being able to move freely. Pay attention to your wardrobe. If you train exclusively in a loose-fitting *gi*, you may be in for a big shock the first time you have to defend yourself wearing restrictive clothing (e.g., jeans, dress) or heavy footwear (e.g., boots). If you have a choice about what you wear, select clothing that facilitates your ability to defend yourself or at least does not limit your options in a confrontation by making it difficult or impossible to kick, run, or otherwise move around.

If you carry a concealed weapon, be sure that your clothing choices facilitate your ability to deploy it quickly. Consider what you will be doing as well as what the weather is likely to be in determining your clothing choice. For example, if you drive for a living, a hip holster will not only be hard to draw from when sitting, but may also become very uncomfortable as the butt of your gun or the handle of your knife is jammed into your kidney day after day. A shoulder or cross-draw holster may be a better bet. On a winter day, however, it is nearly impossible to draw a weapon from a shoulder holster that is buried under several layers of heavy clothing. The style and fit of gloves that you wear can affect weapon handling as well. The bottom line is to ensure that your clothing allows you to both conceal your weapon effectively and to deploy it rapidly.

It is challenging to fight when you cannot see. If you wear prescription eyeglasses, you should consider keeping a spare pair in your vehicle in case they get broken during a confrontation, especially if you cannot drive without them. Further, in inclement weather take steps to keep your glasses dry, clean, and fog free such as wearing a brimmed hat and/or applying an anti-fog spray. Be sure to have polarized lenses available in sunny weather as well. In this manner, you can facilitate your ability to apply countervailing force should you be required to do so.

Deny Privacy

Most crimes start in public or semi-public places. Since a robber can take your money when you first encounter him/her, anyone who tries to move you to a secondary crime scene has something more nefarious in mind. Never let someone take you to another location where they will have privacy to commit murder, rape, or other heinous acts upon you. Applying countervailing force at first contact is almost always your best bet for survival should fighting be required due to a criminal encounter.

Do your best to avoid isolated areas like parks, trails, alleys, elevators, and empty buildings, especially at night, unless you have someone else you trust with you. As a general rule, the more public the situation the safer you will be insomuch as violent crime is concerned. Certainly, riots run counter to this principle and certain crimes such as pick-pocketing are facilitated by the anonymity that crowds provide. Terrorist bombers also target populated areas at peak traffic times. Nevertheless, the vast majority of violent acts are perpetrated by one attacker against one victim or among small groups. Relatively few violent acts occur in front of large numbers of witnesses unless the perpetrator is mentally deficient and/or under the influence of drugs which limit his or her inhibitions.

There are no absolutes in self-defense. Every situation will be different. Overall, however, you can expect to be much safer in locations where criminals do not have the privacy necessary to get away with their crimes.

Attract Attention

If you are attacked, yell something that stands out from a generic cry of "help." A request for help is easy for bystanders to ignore since it does not affect them personally. We will talk more about bystanders in Chapter 5 and creating witnesses in Chapter 8, but for the moment, it is important to point out that what you say or do during a violent encounter may ultimately be retold before a jury. A method that not only attracts attention but also highlights your peril in a way that may both clarify who the victim is and justify your use of countervailing force simultaneously is to point out the attacker's weapon.

"Oh my god, don't kill me with that knife!" is a pretty cogent statement. Not only may this tactic have a better chance of attracting attention of a prospective rescuer than a generic shout for help, but it also demonstrates for potential witnesses that you are in legitimate fear for your life should you have to kill your attacker in self-defense. Further, the mere presence of other attentive individuals may make many criminals stop trying to hurt you and become more concerned about out how to escape successfully before authorities arrive to arrest them.

Similarly, children should be taught to scream, "That's not my dad," or similar phrases when approached or grabbed by strangers to draw attention to their plight. It is relatively easy to ignore a cry for help by a kid who may be acting out but much harder to stand by and watch a child be abducted by someone you "know" is really a bad guy. Pleas for assistance must be meaningful to the bystander to get their attention. Even then it does not always work. See bystanders in Chapter 5 for more information.

If you witness a violent act in progress a good intervention strategy is often simply to yell, "Hey, someone just called the cops" whether you or another person has actually done so or not. The mere knowledge that his or her actions have been observed by another person and that police assistance may be on its way is often enough to cause a perpetrator to flee. In this fashion, you can stop a violent assault without getting physically involved. Of course, if you choose this approach, you should consider shouting from far enough away that you can flee to safety should the thug(s) decide to turn attention toward you.

Take Action

A criminal offender has the least amount of control at initial contact with his or her intended victim. The faster you act the better your chances of getting away unharmed. Use your martial arts training to avoid being injured by the initial attack, apply countervailing force as necessary to prevent pursuit, then high tail it away from your attacker. As mentioned previously, the faster you can cycle through the OODA loop the better your chances of winning a violent confrontation.

Repetition in training is not always all that fun but it is important. In a real fight, martial arts training can take over automatically. *Budoka* (martial artists) can literally watch their bodies perform what they have been trained to do, with fists and feet or makeshift weapons, without having to think about it that much. That is why we practice repetitively and realistically. When real danger arises, pre-programmed responses can take over. The better prepared you are the better your odds of survival.

Escalation to Violence

"Most amateur violence comes about because of this stupid game of escalato (upward spiral of one-upmanship). People have no clear-cut idea of what winning means, but by God they know they gotta do it. Think about how many times you have seen things escalate out of control. This simple pattern is behind nearly 90 percent of all conflicts you'll encounter. People get 'locked in' and begin raising the stakes. Each round is more intense. It's a basic human pattern no matter where you go. Escalato is the most dangerous game in the world... Anytime you step in to the arena of physical violence, you have to accept that it may not end until either you or your opponent, maybe both, are dead." [5]

– Marc MacYoung

Glaring, staring, shoving, arguing, threatening, yelling, or other clear signs of escalation precede the vast majority of violent encounters. Insults and other forms of verbal abuse are common precursors to a fight. As a trained martial artist, you simply cannot afford to play that game. As MacYoung indicates in the quote above, escalato is perilous. It only happens, however, when both parties are willing to engage in it. Do not be stupid enough to fall into that trap. Swallow your pride and walk away. As stated previously, the more dangerous you are, the less you should feel a need to prove it.

There are no absolutes in self-defense so walking away will not always work. There are more or less two types of aggressors: dominance attackers and predators. Dominance attackers want to feel superior to their victim. If you walk away, he/she will generally be happy to let you go. Predatory attackers, on the other hand, want a victim who will not put up a fight. If you walk away from one of these individuals, you may trigger the very attack you were trying to avoid. Nevertheless, trying to leave puts you on better legal and ethical ground if you ultimately have to fight back.

While it is common to experience an obvious escalation, ambushes do occasionally occur. In such situations, the escalation has already occurred yet the victim is unaware of it since it took place solely within the mind of the attacker. He or she has already looked you over, conducted a mental interview to ascertain that you are an easy target, and decided upon a course of action against you. This can cause a situation where you have no choice but to fight.

Sneak attackers may ask for the time, directions, a cigarette, or use any other dirty trick to get close enough to launch their assault. It is exceedingly rare, however, for the victim to be caught totally unaware. For example, even if he or she was sucker punched, most assault victims say that they saw the blow coming but did not have time to react. Even when long-range weapons are involved (e.g., firearms) fights typically begin close up. Unarmed confrontations always take place at close range. If a trained martial artist can see his/her attacker, he or she should not be surprised by an attack.

Regrettably, many practitioners are simply not mentally prepared to react to sudden violence, needlessly being hurt or killed despite the fact that they saw it coming. Dave Lowry[6] wrote, "You don't want to live in a state of combat readiness 24 hours a day. It is not practical, and it is not healthy. What you can do is train to eliminate your internal rules that say all aggressive acts must 'make sense.' Insisting that an attack make sense before you respond can get you seriously injured or killed." This is sound advice.

Martial training can help practitioners automatically respond to attacks without much, if any, conscious thought, though it takes years of diligent practice to reach that level. Given enough repetitions, however, the physical movements of *kata* (forms) and *bunkai* (applications) can become "hard wired" into your subconscious. When the unexpected blow comes screaming toward your head you can take advantage of your natural flinch reaction to instinctively intercept it and counterstrike. Only after you have safely dispatched your attacker do you need to wonder about his or her motivation.

Responding vs. Reacting

The escalato follies are a supremely dangerous game—one you really, really do not want to play. It is supremely important that you respond to an aggressor's actions rather than reacting to them. Responding is a planned course of action, one that leaves you in control of your emotions and actions. Reacting, on the other hand, cedes control to the opponent. If you become angry, defensive, or otherwise emotionally involved it is easy to be caught up in the one-upmanship cycle that will inevitably lead to physical violence. It is far better to be alive and free than right, especially if it requires your death or imprisonment to prove your point. See Chapter 5 for more about the legal aspects of countervailing force.

Anger should be used strategically as a tool, never as an unchecked emotion. If you really are upset about something, you generally cannot afford to show it. On the job, you can be perceived as a "loose cannon" by your manager and/or co-workers, facing disciplinary action or possible termination. At home or amongst friends, you can irreparably harm your interpersonal relationships.

If you need to prove a point and you are not actually furious, on the other hand, feigned anger can sometimes be an effective tool. Consider disciplining children—if you yell at them too often they become desensitized. If you do it judiciously, they may learn important life lessons and grow up to become better people. The same thing applies to venting feigned rage. I suggest that you can get away with it only rarely since the vast majority of people remember negative emotions longer than positive ones; hence a long memory of your actions. That means that you really need to save this tactic for the time at which you need it the most.

In his best-selling book, *The 7 Habits of Highly Effective People*, business guru Steven Covey described a concept called idiosyncratic credit. You can think of it as an emotional bank account. Whenever you do good things for the people you are close to and treat them with dignity and respect, you build up credit in your account. Whenever you become abrasive or insensitive, you make withdrawals. So long as the balance remains positive, you remain on their "good" side. Blowing up at someone uses up a huge amount of idiosyncratic credit so make your withdrawals wisely.

Avoid the escalato follies at all costs. Keep your ego in check. In addition, do your best to verbally de-escalate a confrontation before it becomes violent. We'll talk about de-escalation in depth in Chapter 4.

Force Continuum

During the escalation process there are several force options available to help stave off violence: (1) presence, (2) voice, (3) empty-hand restraint, (4) non-lethal force, and, ultimately, (5) lethal force (if required). This continuum is similar to the approach codified by many police departments. The first two levels can prevent violence before it begins, the third may be used proactively as an opponent prepares to strike, and the last two take place after you have already been attacked. We will talk more about levels of force and the concept of "reasonable force" in Chapter 6.

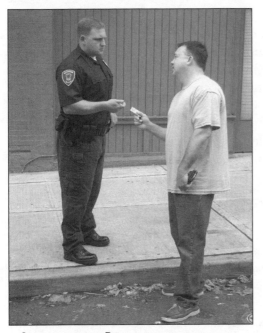 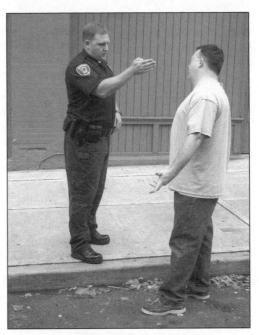

COMMAND PRESENCE. BECAUSE PREDATORS LOOK FOR EASY VICTIMS, BODY LANGUAGE CAN HELP STAVE OFF AN ATTACK. TACTICS TO ENHANCE YOUR PRESENCE INCLUDE UTILIZING GOOD POSTURE AND STANDING TALL ON A CURB OR ELEVATED AREA TO ADD EXTRA HEIGHT.

VERBAL SKILLS. TALKING WITH THE AGGRESSOR MAY ALLOW YOU TO RESOLVE A CONFRONTATION WITHOUT RESORTING TO VIOLENCE.

(1) Presence

If you are a trained martial artist or just a well-conditioned athlete your presence alone can frequently de-escalate a dangerous situation. Carry yourself with confidence and be prepared to act. Criminals who are very good at sensing body language may back off simply because they can tell that you are prepared to act.

(2) Voice

Use you verbal skills and tone of voice to talk an aggressor out of attacking you or otherwise get them to back down. A variety of techniques for doing this are described in Chapter 4 about de-escalation.

(3) Empty-hand restraint

Restraint, disarm, and control techniques can be employed to keep an aggressor from hurting you and/or themselves until law enforcement professionals arrive. You will generally want to respond with a slightly greater degree of force than is used against you. Pulling a weapon on an unarmed attacker almost always makes you the bad guy.

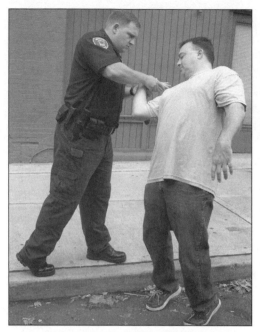

EMPTY-HAND RESTRAINT. THIS WRISTLOCK IS AN EXAMPLE OF EMPTY-HAND RESTRAINT.

Beware of chokes and other violent-looking responses. Pins, locks, arm bars, and similar control techniques are preferable if you can apply them safely and effectively. Be very cautious of going to the ground unless you are absolutely sure that your attacker acted alone and does not have friends who might take advantage of your vulnerability to attack.

4) Non-lethal force

Non-lethal force is the next step up on the force continuum. This includes striking, kicking, and a plethora of other martial techniques that cause damage to your opponent. Certain weapons (e.g., *kubaton*, pepper spray, Taser) can also be used for non-lethal force or restraint applications. If restraint techniques do not work or will put you in danger because your assailant is armed you may have to escalate directly to this level should other options fail.

(5) Lethal force

The final level is lethal force. This includes both martial applications applied to vital areas of the body as well as deployment of various lethal weapons (e.g., gun, knife). This level should be avoided unless there is no other way to escape a violent encounter unscathed. See Countervailing Force in Chapter 5 for more information.

Evasion and Escape

"Brave Sir Robin ran away. Bravely ran away, away! When danger reared its ugly head, he bravely turned his tail and fled. Yes, brave Sir Robin turned about and gallantly he chickened out. Bravely taking to his feet, he beat a very brave retreat, bravest of the brave, Sir Robin!" [7]

— *Monty Python*

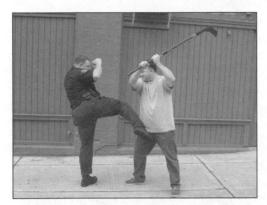

NON-LETHAL FORCE. A SOLID KICK TO THE GROIN IS A NON-LETHAL WAY OF ENDING A CONFRONTATION QUICKLY (THIS KIND OF ATTACK CAN CAUSE PERMANENT INJURY, HOWEVER).

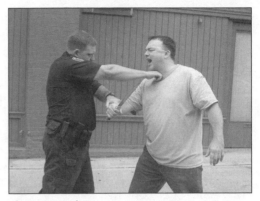

LETHAL FORCE. A WEAPON IS NOT ALWAYS REQUIRED TO DELIVER LETHAL FORCE. A BLOW TO THE THROAT IS A GOOD EXAMPLE OF POTENTIALLY LETHAL FORCE DELIVERED FROM A FIST.

Amusing as the *Ballad of Brave Sir Robin* (above) may be, the tactic of running from danger is a very real and ultimately practical way of saving your hide when things get ugly. I consider the "Brave Sir Robin defense" my first, best option in violent encounters. I hope that I will sense trouble before it catches up with me and thereby avoid any threat altogether, of course. At times, it just does not work out that way. Sometimes you do have to fight, at least long enough to deal with the immediate threat, but as soon as practicable running like hell is a far better alternative to sticking around and slugging it out with a bad guy.

When you sense trouble brewing, subtlety may be your best initial reaction. Remember how I confronted the guy at the ATM? I did not do anything offensive; merely made sure he knew that I had detected his presence. Fast or big movements are generally not recommended as they might draw unwanted attention to you or ignite a smoldering situation. Running from an aggressive dog, for example, might cause him to chase you, while moving away calmly may allow you to escape.

- Be aware and leave an area if trouble seems to be brewing.
- Walk away normally if you only have a "feeling" that things are not right.
- Evade potential or developing threats by crossing the street, turning and walking back the way you came from, turning down another street, or otherwise moving toward a safer location.
- If actual trouble becomes apparent, move away from it quickly but calmly.
- If the trouble starts after you, run away swiftly.
- Call attention to your predicament by yelling for help as appropriate. Remember that pointing out the attacker's weapon or shouting "fire" or other attention getting phrases works better than a generic cry for help.*

*Though shouting "fire" around a gun-wielding assailant is probably not the best way to call attention to your predicament. Words like gun, knife, or rape are good attention-getters too.

It is important to always be prepared and able to escape, evade, or fight for your life. This preparation includes not only the obvious stuff like awareness but also things many people do not think about like using the restroom in a timely manner before you really need to go, for example. At the stadium where I work, there are several Starbucks espresso carts to support our indigenous fanaticism for and addiction to coffee. Like many Seattleites, I typically consume at least two or three lattes game-day mornings. Coffee, in case you do not already know, is a potent diuretic.

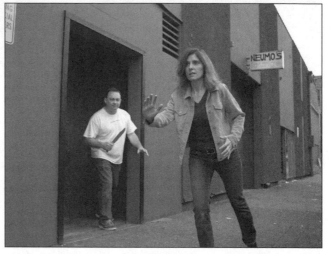

RUN LIKE HELL. STRATEGIC WITHDRAWAL IS OFTEN YOUR BEST DEFENSE AGAINST AN ARMED AGGRESSOR.

Many years ago, I got an emergency call on the radio right after my third cup of coffee and rushed over to where one of my captains needed help breaking up a fight. Long story short: between dealing with a whole bunch of fisticuffs, dragging two drunken fans off each other, interviewing witnesses, interfacing with the police, and writing out a whole mountain of paperwork I became acutely, uncomfortably aware of just how much coffee I had consumed that morning. By the time I was able to do anything about it, I was in no condition to run anywhere let alone fight. I managed to make it to the restroom in time, but that whole incident got me thinking that it could be quite embarrassing to wet oneself in battle due to failing to make a pit stop before you really, really needed one.

Once you are prepared to react to a potentially violent encounter it is important to plan what you will do. Simply running is not good enough. It must be done strategically. To facilitate understanding, I like to break getting away into two pieces: evasion and escape. Evasion is avoiding or dealing with the immediate threat, while escape gets you away to safety.

Evasion

Evasion deals with the immediate threat—be it a weapon, a person, or a situation. Here is an example: When I was twelve years old, I was walking to the bus stop after judo practice one night when four older boys stopped me. They quickly began to hassle me about the *gi* I was wearing, spitting on me, calling me names, and threatening to "kill" me. Verbal threats soon escalated to pushing and shoving, which was clearly evolving toward more serious blows. Although I probably stood a good chance of badly injuring one or two of them, I felt that there was no way I could win a fight against four kids, all of whom were bigger, older, and most likely stronger than I was.

Swallowing my pride, I did my best to ignore their expectorating and taunting while I tried to figure out a way to escape. As soon as I saw a car approaching, I shoved the nearest antagonist out of the way, shoulder-rolled over the hood of the vehicle, and darted across the street. The driver slammed on his brakes, stopping between where I had just run and where the bullies on sidewalk had started to follow. While they were distracted by the irate driver, I hopped over a fence, ducked down another side street, and ran away as fast as I could.

By shoving the nearest attacker out of the way, I dealt with the immediate threat, created an opening, and was able to make further use of the distraction that the passing car provided to make my escape. In a situation where I was outnumbered and could not win, running was clearly the best thing to do. Because I was surrounded by four antagonists, I could not successfully flee until I had dealt with the immediate threat, making a hole in their perimeter through which I could escape.

In fact, that is exactly what you must do in any violent encounter. Marc MacYoung wrote, "Before you consider doing anything else, your first priority is to neutralize the threat! You do what you need to keep from getting hurt by the particular attack. This does not mean you immediately start pounding on someone until he is flat. Nor does it mean you immediately run like hell. It means, before you even consider anything else, you make sure your ass is safe from the specific attack!"

Evasion deals with the immediate threat strategically. If there is a weapon or multiple attackers involved you need to both move and counterattack in a way that both puts you in a stronger position and neutralizes the threat. (We will discuss this topic in more detail in Chapter 6.) Once the immediate threat is neutralized, you have the choice of sticking around and continuing the fight or running away and escaping. If multiple opponents or weapons are involved, escape may be your only viable option. Regardless, it is almost always your most prudent option.

Dealing with multiple attackers is very challenging. Avoidance is obviously the best and most preferable alternative. If you are forced to fight, you can realistically only engage one opponent at a time. Once the first adversary has been defeated, you may have a chance to flee successfully or you may have to move on to defeat the next attacker and then get away. Defense against a large group is generally handled by strategically engaging one person at a time in a manner that confounds the other's ability to reach you.

Your response is a form of triage, striking for the greatest impact or taking on the most dangerous threat first. When I took an advanced defensive handgun course a few years back, the instructor emphasized taking cover, assessing the threat, and killing the most dangerous person such as a shotgun-wielding* assailant first. If all are equally dangerous, take out the easiest target first.[†] The same concept holds true in a fistfight.

Several psychological factors can help you survive. In any large group of attackers, someone will be the primary instigator or leader of the pack. If you can instantaneously and dramatically disable that individual (or pretty much anyone else for that matter), blowing out a knee, shattering a nose, gouging out an eye, or otherwise leaving him huddled in a pool of his own blood, the psychological advantage will be enormous. I am not exaggerating here—the only way to survive assault from a large, determined group of thugs is to be more ruthless and violent than they are is a good reason for avoiding such conflicts in the first place. Further, if you show no fear in the face of overwhelming odds your attackers may hesitate giving you the few seconds you need to disengage and escape.

Even as a 12-year-old, I discovered that knocking the ringleader aside disorients a gang of toughs. Once you have dealt with the immediate threat, you may be able to disengage and escape.

Escape

Once the immediate threat is dealt with you not only need to get away, but you also need to find a way to keep the bad guys from deciding to chase you.[‡] If possible, you further want to discourage them from coming after you again. The primary ways this is accomplished is by either disabling your opponents or by distracting them long enough that you can get out of their line of sight or develop an insurmountable lead. The passing car in my aforementioned confrontation was the vehicle I used to distract my opponents. There are plenty of other ways to do that as well.

For example, several years ago I was accosted in the Pioneer Square area of Seattle (Washington) by two street thugs who demanded that I give them money. Both had large belt knives clearly visible, but not yet drawn. Both were large, muscular, and outweighed me by more than forty pounds. If it came to a fight, however, there was no way that the bad guys could win.

Although they did not know it, these muggers were not the only ones who were armed. I have a concealed pistol license and was carrying a gun hidden beneath my jacket. More specifically, I had a Sig Sauer P220 .45-caliber semi-automatic pistol loaded with MagSafe, +P+ rounds. For readers who are unfamiliar with firearms, MagSafe arguably makes the most effective handgun ammunition in the world.

---

*All things being equal (e.g., everyone has a gun, is equally skilled, and is approximately equal distance away), a shotgun-wielding assailant is the most dangerous (e.g., most likely both to hit you as well as most likely to kill you with his shot).
†Such as nearest aggressor, smallest person, the guy with no cover, etc.
‡Or at least keep them from catching you if they start to follow.

Their pre-fragmented self-defense rounds pretty much guarantee* that one torso hit equals one kill because they "explode" upon entry† causing maximum damage without the danger of over-penetration, which could hit an innocent bystander. The +P+ rounds are so powerful that they require special springs to control the recoil.

At that time, I shot competitively on a regular basis, firing approximately 7,500 rounds down range per year and had extremely good aim. I routinely practiced close-quarter drawing, handgun retention, and stress-fire techniques as well. I had to make a choice between swallowing my pride and handing over some money or escalating a conflict toward an undoubtedly lethal ending.

Legally I had a pretty good case for forcefully defending myself, as I was confronted by two larger, obviously armed individuals and in reasonable fear for my life. Morally and ethically, however, I knew that there was a better choice. Pulling a small wad of bills from my pocket, I threw the money to one side then immediately ran to the other. I generally carry a small amount of cash in my pocket as both a convenience and precautionary measure.‡ Because my cash was held together with a money clip, I was able to throw the stack of bills a pretty fair distance before running in the opposite direction to escape. The only down side is that the money clip was a present§ from my parents, which was never recovered. Sure beats having to shoot someone though…

Had these thugs decided to chase me and I could not get away, I would have had no choice but to meet their attack with countervailing force. Fortunately, however, they took long enough picking up the $27 I had left behind that I was able to escape. I consider that a small price to pay to avoid having to kill or maim two people even if they clearly were bad guys.

Getting away requires that you figure out some way to get the bad guys to stop chasing you. In the example above, I was able to distract them with a few dollars, which gave me sufficient time to get out of their line of sight. I do not know whether they actually tried to pursue me or not, yet I cut across a couple of random streets to make it harder for them to find me again if they did decide to follow and, fortunately, never saw them again.

Physically disabling your attacker works too although it is somewhat less ideal. If you do need to fight your way to safety, a good strategy is to attack the feet, ankles, or knees of your assailant. Not only do you temporarily disable them, but also you make it nearly impossible for them to follow you when you run away. No matter what you do, always use your highest percentage techniques—those things you are truly skilled at performing—which are most likely to disable the attacker so that you can get away. Your number one goal has to be not getting hurt. If there is more than one opponent you must do your best to avoid becoming entangled with any single attacker long enough that his/her buddies can join in the fray.

---

*To the extent that any bullet manufacturer can.
†A lot like being hit by a shotgun from inside your body.
‡Rather than simply keeping everything in my wallet.
§Turquoise inlaid sterling silver.

The way in which you escape is dependant upon how many attackers there are, how badly they want to catch you, and the tactical situation you encounter (e.g., terrain, bystanders). If you encounter a couple of thugs looking to make a quick buck, they should be relatively easy to distract and escape from, especially if you throw a few dollars their way before you run. Similarly, if you wander through some gang's territory and they are more interested in scaring than killing you, your odds of escape are very good.[8]

Most folks that you will encounter on the street will not be motivated to chase you beyond a certain distance. The longer you keep out of their hands, the more likely they will be to give up.* Dragging stuff into pursuer's way, dodging around obstacles, over fences, or through hedges, or otherwise slowing them down is a good way to string your pursuers out, facilitating your ability to escape successfully. Your goal is to get enough of a lead that can lose your pursuers completely, find somewhere safe to hide, convince your opponents to give up, or otherwise gain safety. In the meantime, however, you need to ensure that as few opponents as possible are in striking distance to engage you. After all, if one opponent can tie you up by engaging in combat, the others may have time to join in before you can end the battle.

As you run, look for shops you can duck through, fences you can climb over, gaps in hedges you can worm through, and other bottlenecks where only a single person can slip through at a time. Be careful about climbing anything though. Unless your pursuers are a good distance behind you, slowing your forward progress long enough to overcome an obstacle may let them close too much of the gap you have created. After all, in the time it takes you to scale a ten- to twelve-foot fence a pursuer can cover twenty to fifty feet of territory. If he or she can grab your legs before you make it over the top, you are in a world of hurt. Not only have you been captured, but also you will undoubtedly be slammed onto the ground as you are dragged off the fence you were trying to climb.

If you know your neighborhood and are friendly with the local canine population, hopping fences can provide and extra level of safety—assuming the dogs will leave you alone and harass your pursuers, of course. If you have a choice, going over a fence at the corner where four yards meet is an excellent location. That way, if you choose unwisely and the dog or neighbor is not as friendly as you expected, it is just a short hop into a safer yard. In areas that are less familiar to you, you must be especially cautious about what is on the other side of a fence, however. If you cannot see through the fence, you may wish to choose an alternate route. After all, it would not do to hop over a fence only to discover an angry Rottweiler, land in an empty pool, become entangled in thorny rosebushes, or break your ankle from an unexpectedly long drop.

Crossing a busy street is another good way to escape pursuers. To be most successful, be sure to run parallel to traffic, choosing your best moment to act before crossing. If there are multiple lanes, you can implement this run parallel then cross

*A great argument for regular aerobic conditioning as part of your normal workout routine.

methodology for each lane. If you have ever played the video game "Frogger," the real-life strategy works similarly. Cars and trucks hit a whole lot harder than feet and fists so be cautious about your timing and angle of approach. It may even be useful to point where you intend to run to give oncoming drivers a heads-up, sort of like the hand signals that bicyclists and motorcyclists use.*

If someone is chasing you in a car, he or she can travel a whole lot faster than you can. He can also use it as a weapon to squash you. Be sure to cut 90 degrees at your first opportunity, bolting between parked cars, through any convenient business, housing complex, narrow alley, or other area that the pursuing vehicle cannot easily pass through. Travel a couple of blocks then change directions again so that your pursuers cannot simple go around the block and catch sight of you all over again. Be cautious if you see or hear some of your pursuers leaving the vehicle because they may be able to split into more than one search party. Knowing that they have done so will influence which directions will remain available for escape.

Choose your friends wisely; hanging out with people who like to cause trouble will eventually catch up with you. If you are part of a group and find yourselves in a hazardous situation, the best policy is that either you all run at once or everyone stays to fight. Running away together, even if you flee in opposite directions, leaves no one in a tight spot. If the person you were counting on to cover your back flees, on the other hand, you could be in a world of hurt. Similarly, you should not leave your friends to the wolves either.

Once you have made your initial escape it may be time to hide. Hiding, as most of us learn during our childhood is a bit of an art form. Try not to hide anywhere that you cannot escape from quickly if your pursuers stumble across you. People in general are good at spotting human-shaped forms regardless of the surrounding terrain and extremely good at spotting other people's eyes. Ditches, rooftops, woods, vehicles, and a whole host of obstacles can make good temporary hiding places. Be cautious about your silhouette, however. Do your best to keep your arms and legs tucked in behind cover, hunch as necessary to disguise your profile, and be careful not to stare at pursuers if they get close. Odd as it may seem, many folks can feel the weight of your gaze and may notice you because of it.

The best way to hide is often somewhere along the lines of what people expect to see. I once played a game of paintball against a group of folks whose team included a former Army Special Forces soldier. As I was chasing after him, he managed to pull ahead just enough for me to lose sight of him beyond the crest of a small hill. Once out of sight he immediately hid along the edge of the wooded trail simply by lying on top of some very short grass and weeds and remaining immobile. It was such an open spot that my mind refused to believe that anyone could be hiding there, seeing more grass rather than his camouflage covered form. Assuming he was still on the

---

*Don't worry about your pursuers spotting your signals—they'll figure out what you are planning anyway. If you time things right you'll still be safe and the oncoming traffic will slow your pursuers' facilitating your ability to escape.

run, I raced ahead in hot pursuit. Moments after I nearly stepped on him he rose up silently and shot me in the back with his paintball gun.

There are a several reasons why this trick worked so well. First of all, since he remained totally immobile I saw what I expected to see—grass and weeds alongside the trail. Second, his head was facing away from me so I did not notice his eyes peering out behind the camouflage either. And third, it was not an obvious hiding place. I saw an empty trail and raced along it. Had he tried to hide in the same manner in some sort of a dead-end like a box canyon I would have immediately noticed that he could not possibly still be on the run and would have become more attentive. The best hiding places are subtle, easily missed by those that believe their quarry is still on the run.

Be sure to hide somewhere you can rapidly flee from if your pursuers ultimately do find you again. Hiding in a dumpster, under a vehicle, or in a blind alley can be dangerous. While you might get away with it, these are fairly obvious hiding places—ones that might attract attention and additional scrutiny if there is nowhere else to which you could logically have continued to run. Further, they are all places that take time to extricate yourself from. If your pursuers catch up to you and you cannot escape quickly enough, you are back to evading or fighting your way clear once again. Trying to fight your way out of a dumpster or from under a vehicle is problematic at best.

Should You Run If He's Got a Gun?

As stated previously, running is often your best option. You may be asking yourself, however, if fleeing from a bad guy with a gun is also a good idea. Generally, perhaps even counter-intuitively, yes. We can use a simple example to illustrate this point. Let's pretend for a moment that a bad guy is trying to force you into his car at gunpoint. What might happen to you if you immediately turn and run?

For the sake of argument, let's say that 50 percent of the time he will decide to fire at you. After all, the initial encounter is in a public place and the bad guy is trying to get you somewhere more private to do his dirty deeds. He may not want to attract the attention that a gunshot will ultimately bring. He may well hold his fire and continue to look for an easier victim, a common enough real-life scenario.

Even if he does decide to shoot you, it is hard to hit a moving target. Trained law enforcement professionals frequently miss moving targets on the street, even at very close range. Our example bad guy is probably not as gun savvy as a highly trained police officer. So even if he does fire, let's say there is a 50 percent chance that he will actually hit you. Further, if you are hit, most gunshot victims survive. For the sake of argument once again, let's say there is a 50 percent chance of your survival once you have been shot.

So, how does this scenario play out? Do the math for 100 encounters; you would be shot at 50 times. Of those 50, only half actually hit you, so that is 25. Of those hits, you survive half the time. That means you have a 12.5 percent chance of mortal danger if you run immediately. If you cooperate and get into the vehicle, on the other hand, you have nearly a 100 percent chance of something bad, perhaps fatally bad, happening to you when you reach your captor's destination.

So how realistic is this little scenario? According to Detective (ret) J. J. Bittenbinder, only two percent of people who run from a gun-wielding assailant actually die. Others have indicated that the actual number is somewhere around four percent. I have not been able to confirm this statistic but the two to four percent range seems pretty reasonable. Whatever the actual number, I suspect it's much better odds than being taken to a secondary crime scene where our bad guy has privacy and time on his side to do bad things to you…

To sum things up, if you run you have a 96 to 98 percent chance of being safe. If you get into a car with a bad guy, you are unequivocally assured of a ride straight to a secondary crime scene with you starring as the victim. In real life, everyone needs to make his or her own choice depending on the unique characteristics of each encounter. As a general rule, however, I am almost certainly going to run.

Okay, so we have established that running is good. Now, how do you go about doing it successfully? While there is more than one philosophy regarding how to run, I have always been taught to run straight* and fast toward cover rather than zigzagging or otherwise dodging around. The theory is that the farther from your attacker you can get the safer you will be so distance is the most important attribute. In the best possible scenario, the gunman will attempt to chase you rather than standing his/her ground and firing.† Experience shows that it is nearly impossible to hit any-

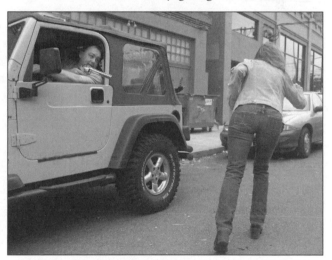

RUN LIKE HELL. EVEN IF THE BAD GUY HAS A GUN, YOU HAVE A ROUGHLY 96 TO 98 PERCENT CHANCE OF BEING SAFE IF YOU FLEE IMMEDIATELY RATHER THAN ALLOWING HIM TO TAKE YOU TO A SECONDARY CRIME SCENE WHERE HE WILL MOST ASSUREDLY HARM YOU. IT IS SOMEWHAT AMUSING TO NOTE THAT WHILE WE WERE SHOOTING THESE OUTDOOR PICTURES A BYSTANDER WALKED UP AND, WITHOUT BATTING AN EYE, PULLED OUT A PAIR OF HANDCUFFS, ASKING IF WE WANTED TO BORROW THEM… ONLY IN SEATTLE'S CAPITAL HILL DISTRICT. MOST ANYWHERE ELSE, THE GUNS WOULD HAVE FREAKED PEOPLE OUT.

---

*At an angle from the shooter, not directly away.
†That assumes that you'll outrun him or her, of course.

thing when both the shooter and the target are moving, even for trained law enforcement officers who are generally better shots than most criminals or ordinary civilians.

The FBI reports that, between 1994 and 2003, 82 percent of law enforcement officers feloniously killed with firearms were shot at a distance of less than 21 feet. Fifty percent were murdered at a distance of less than five feet yet only seven percent were killed at a distance of greater than fifty feet from their assailant. This may not be entirely applicable to civilians who generally do not wear body armor, but it certainly does lead one to conclude that the farther away from a shooter you are, the safer you are likely to be.

When deciding where and how you run will need to take the distance to available cover into consideration as well. Right-handed shooters are almost universally better at tracking and hitting moving targets that move from right to left rather than vice versa. Whether you do choose to zigzag or run straight, your best bet would initially be to move from left to right if the attacker is right-handed and right to left if he or she is left-handed. Either way, gaining distance and cover quickly or closing to counterattack immediately is important. Hesitation can get you killed.*

Concealment and Cover

"Finding nearby cover can save your life. If possible get something substantial between yourself and your attacker… Inside use an upturned table, substantial piece of furniture or thick door. Outside, use a tree, car or other vehicle, metal mailbox, phone booth stand, or even a stone wall." [9]

– *Christopher Caile*

You may remember seeing this famous shooting incident on the news: Attorney Gerry Curry frantically dodging around a tree as his distraught attacker, William Strier, chased after him firing shot after shot from a handgun. Wounded and bleeding, Curry frantically ducked and dodged, trying to keep a medium-sized tree between him and a continuing barrage of bullets. When he finally ran out of ammunition, Stricr was tackled and promptly arrested by an off-duty sheriff's deputy who ran toward the scene.

Before the incident, Curry had never even met his attacker who approached him on the street in front of the courthouse, asked his name, and then once his target was confirmed fired point blank into Curry's neck. Luckily, the elderly attorney was neither killed nor disabled by the initial attack and had the presence of mind to seek the dubious shelter of a nearby tree. This quick thinking and use of cover ultimately saved his life.

---

*It's not hard to hit a man-sized standing target at close range.

Furious that Curry was going to be paid from his trust fund for representing Evelyn Murphy, a trustee whom he claimed was withholding money he needed for medical care, Strier attempted to kill Curry on the California courthouse steps. A cameraman at the scene for another trial caught the whole incident on film and it received a whole lot of attention in the national news.

As the preceding incident aptly demonstrates, concealment or cover can save your life in a gunfight or most any violent confrontation for that matter. Concealment hides you from an enemy's sight, but offers little or no protection from projectile weapons (e.g., bullets, rocks) or other forms of attack. Oddly enough, the vast majority of untrained people will not try to shoot through many forms of concealment such as windows or drywall, though you probably do not want to count on that fact if things get ugly. Concealment is good, cover is better. It simultaneously hides and protects you. A secure hiding place with a solid, lockable door may serve as cover from many forms of physical assault, yet drywall and residential framing is only concealment if an assailant has most any type of gun.

Indoor cover can include certain items of heavy furniture, as well as some walls, doors, stairwells, and alcoves. Hollow core doors found in most residential construction, on the other hand, will not even stop a determined fist let alone a bullet. Outdoor cover can include trees, vehicles, rocks, retaining walls, buildings, garbage bins, and even metal mailboxes. Beware of glass from vehicle or building windows that could either fail to stop a projectile and/or become shrapnel causing additional damage to you.

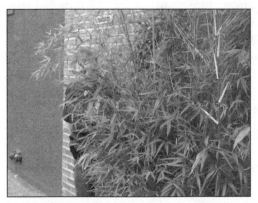

CONCEALMENT, SUCH AS HIDING BEHIND A BUSH, KEEPS THE BAD GUYS FROM SPOTTING YOU BUT AFFORDS NO PHYSICAL DEFENSE.

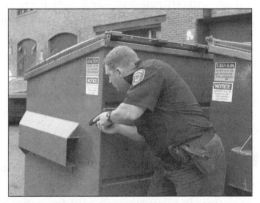

COVER, SUCH AS HIDING BEHIND A STEEL TRASH BIN, WALL, OR OTHER SOLID OBJECT NOT ONLY KEEPS THE BAD GUYS FROM SPOTTING YOU BUT ALSO AFFORDS A PHYSICAL BARRIER BETWEEN YOU AND YOUR OPPONENT'S WEAPON.

Summary

"Insisting on perfect safety is for people who don't have the balls to live in the real world." [10]

– Mary Shafer

The more dangerous you are, the less you should need to prove it. Ego notwith-standing, it is far better to withdraw than it is to face the consequences of causing or allowing an argument to escalate to the point of physical confrontation. Even if a person legitimately uses force in order to escape imminent and unavoidable danger, they still have to live with the physiological, psychological, and litigational results of doing so.

Important principles of personal safety include (1) making yourself a hard target, (2) denying privacy, (3) attracting attention, and (4) taking action as appropriate to your circumstances. The more prepared you are and the more confident you look, the better your odds of avoiding unwarranted attention from bad guys who look for easy prey.

Since violence almost never happens in a vacuum, you can take proactive steps to keep yourself safe from it. Do your best to avoid perilous locations, dangerous times, and hazardous people. Glaring, staring, shoving, arguing, threatening, yelling, or other clear signs of escalation precede the vast majority of violent encounters. Insults and other forms of verbal abuse are common precursors to a fight. As a trained martial artist, you simply cannot afford to play that game.

During the escalation process there are several force options available to help stave off violence: (1) presence, (2) voice, (3) empty-hand restraint, (4) non-lethal force, and, ultimately, (5) lethal force if required. This continuum is similar to that used in many police departments. The first two levels can prevent violence before it begins while the last three take place after you have already been attacked.

Once you are prepared to react to a potentially violent encounter it is important to plan what you will do. Even if you initially need to physically defend yourself, your ultimate goal should be to escape to safety. Simply running, however, is not good enough. It must be done strategically. Evasion deals with the immediate threat, while escape gets you to safety and prevents your assailant from following you to continue his or her attack.

Concealment hides you from an enemy's sight, but offers little or no protection from projectile weapons or other forms of attack. While concealment is good, cover is better. It simultaneously hides and protects you.

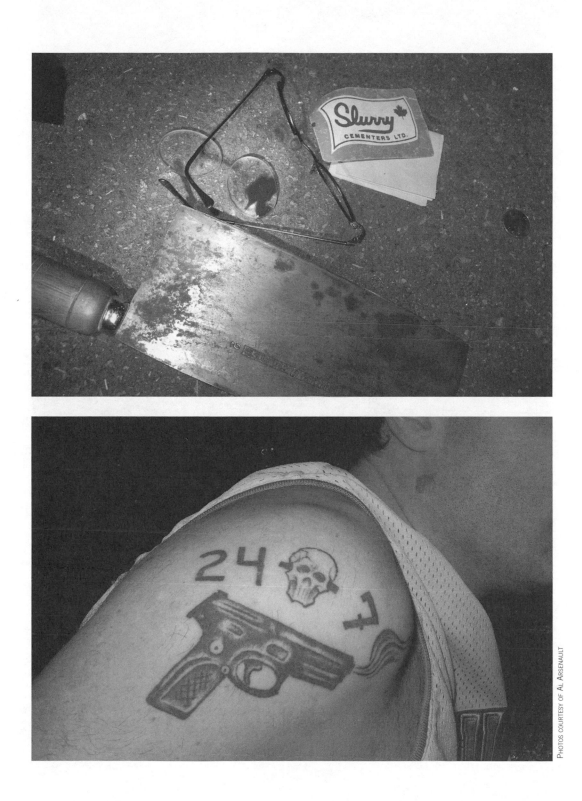

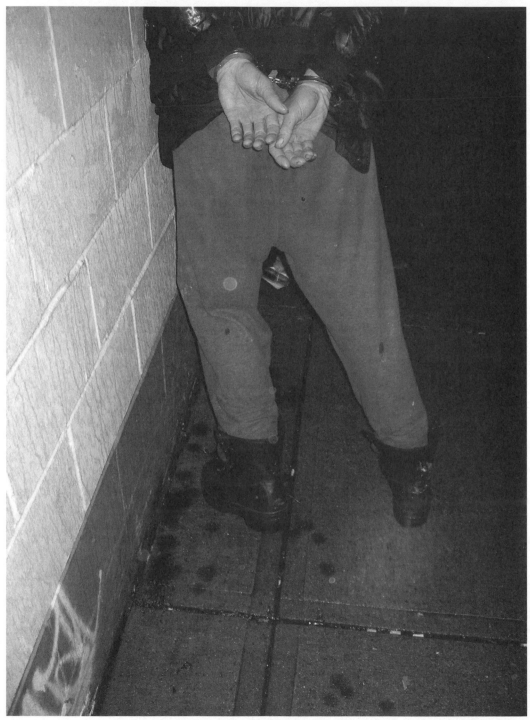

CHAPTER 3

Scenarios

"In preparing for battle I have always found that plans are useless, but planning is indispensable." [1]

– Dwight D. Eisenhower

This chapter is an extension of the awareness and avoidance topics grouped around specific scenarios that practitioners might encounter in their daily lives. Each scenario delves in depth into unique characteristics, concerns, and safety strategies so that you will have a good idea of what you can do to protect yourself should you encounter an armed aggressor in any of these situations. While you can run into the wrong end of a weapon just about anywhere, these situations are commonly associated with armed perpetrators or, in the case of sexual assault, carry a high risk of severe long-term consequences to the victim. Topics, arranged in alphabetical order, include:

- Carjackings.
- Cash machine safety.
- Hostage situations.
- Intimate violence (frequently called "domestic" violence).
- Planes, trains, and public transportation.
- Sexual assault, rape, and molestation.
- Workplace violence.

Carjackings

"On average, 1993-2002, about 38,000 carjacking victimizations occurred annually, according to victim self-reports to the National Crime Victimization Survey… About 15 murders a year involved car theft, though not all were carjackings, for the theft could have been incidental." [2]

– Patsy Klaus

On March 18, 2005 Ronald Whitehead, a 61-year-old Boeing computer engineer, left for work for the last time. He never arrived. Less than three miles from his home, he was found shot to death, his body pushed from his black 2000 Mustang and left in the middle of an intersection by an apparent carjacker in what police characterized as a random crime. According to police reports, Whitehead was shot at least twice, including once in the head, and three shell casings were found on the pavement near his body. While I only met him a couple of times in the cafeteria and he was not really a co-worker, Mr. Whitehead worked in the same building complex for the same part of the company that I do so this one hit pretty close to home.

Discussing the Whitehead murder, King County Sheriff's Sgt. John Urquhart told reporters, "It is pretty unusual for a carjacking to go this far wrong. They are always traumatic. They're always violent, but not to the point where someone dies." This assertion is substantiated by statistical information I have been able to review. Carjacking is rarely associated with murder.

Carjacking is, nevertheless, a serious problem, typically a crime of opportunity. It is frequently related to another crime, perhaps a convenient getaway, a prelude to an armed bank or convenience store robbery, a gang initiation, or a source of quick cash for drug addicts or other criminals. For some teenagers and young adults, carjacking may be a rite of passage, status symbol, or thrill. It can happen just about anywhere—large cities, suburbs, small towns, and rural areas.

Since most jurisdictions do not define carjacking as a specific category of crime it is often reported as either auto theft or armed robbery. Consequently, victim statistics are a bit hard to come by, though the Bureau of Justice Statistics 1993 to 2002 survey reported an average of 38,000 carjackings or other auto-related abductions per year in the United States. They further reported that 74 percent of all carjackings involved the use of a weapon—firearms were used in 45 percent of carjackings, knives in 11 percent, and other weapons in 18 percent. An average of only 15 carjacking-related murders per annum was reported, however.

Since carjacking is a crime of opportunity, you are most vulnerable at highway exit ramps, intersections controlled by stoplights or signs, isolated garages or parking lots, park and ride lots for mass transit systems, self-serve gas stations or car washes, residential driveways, Automated Teller Machine (ATM) kiosks or bank drive-through lanes, or any other location where you must slow down or come to a stop. Carjackers do not always work alone. A little more than half of all carjackings involve multiple perpetrators.*

Another variation of carjacking is commonly called a "bump and rob." In this version a vehicle, usually with at least two occupants, rear-ends or otherwise bumps into you in traffic. As you get out to check the damage to both vehicles and exchange information with the other driver, one of the perpetrators jumps into your car and

---

*56 percent.

drives off, leaving you stranded. His or her partner drives off in the vehicle they struck you with.

What to do

During the 1993 to 2002 survey, only a quarter of all carjacking victims were injured, with about one percent needing hospitalization. If the carjacker threatens you with a gun or other weapon, your best option is frequently to give him/her your vehicle, leaving the area as quickly as possible. Unless you have to protect a small child or other passenger who cannot escape along with you, it is almost always best not to argue. While it may not feel like it at the time, this is not generally a violent crime against a person. It is a crime directed against property, which is usually insured or otherwise replaceable. Despite the trauma of facing a weapon and the inconvenience of losing your vehicle, your life is worth a whole lot more than your car or your insurance deductible.

If you can, your best bet is usually to run away. As soon as you get to a safe place, write down what the carjacker looked like, taking note of his or her sex, race, age, hair color, eye color, distinguishing features, and clothing. If you have Lojack, OnStar, or a similar vehicle tracking system and report the incident quickly, law enforcement officers will often be able to recover you vehicle in a timely manner. While this system can cost around a thousand dollars and/or require a monthly service fee, many insurance companies offer discounts on comprehensive coverage policies should you purchase one.

Reducing your risk

The majority of carjackings (68 percent) take place at night, especially between 10:00 PM and 2:00 AM. Between 1993 and 2002, males committed 93 percent of carjacking victimizations, while groups involving both males and females committed four percent, and women acting on their own committed about three percent of all carjackings. About half of all carjacking incidents occurred in an open area, such as on the street or near public transportation,* while a quarter occurred in parking lots or garages or near commercial places.† About three quarters of carjacking incidents took place within five miles of the victim's home, while only four percent occurred more than 50 miles from the victim's home. This probably has more to do with how far the average person commutes than anything else, however.

Here are some specific strategies that you can follow to reduce your risk when approaching your vehicle on foot, while driving, and upon arriving at your destination:

---

*Public transportation can include bus stations, subways, train stations, or airports.
†Commercial places can include stores, gas stations, office buildings, restaurants, or bars.

Approaching your vehicle on foot

- Stay alert when approaching your vehicle. As always, awareness and avoidance are your best lines of defense. Keep your keys at the ready when approaching your vehicle. Look around and inside the car before getting in. Be wary of people asking for directions, bumming cigarettes, handing out flyers, or otherwise loitering around where you parked.

- Trust your instincts—if something makes you feel uneasy, retreat where you came from or quickly get into your vehicle, lock the doors, and drive away, whichever seems safest. If you have a garage, use it and remember to lock your doors upon exiting even if you are just going into home rather than commuting somewhere.

While driving

- Do not make it easy for criminals to enter your vehicle while driving. Keep your doors locked, windows rolled up, and sunroof closed no matter how short the trip or how safe the neighborhood you must travel through. Do not forget that most carjackings take place near the victim's home. In hot weather invest in air conditioning or keep windows and/or sunroof partially closed so that it is not easy for someone to reach inside. Even though bullets can easily penetrate auto glass, most law enforcement professionals agree that criminals are more likely to shoot through an open window than a closed one.

- When you are coming to a stop in traffic (e.g., rush hour commute), do not tailgate. Leave enough room to maneuver around other vehicles, especially if you sense trouble and might need to get away. A good way to tell if you are far enough back is that you should be able to see the tires of the vehicle in front of you. An additional benefit of this approach is that you are less likely to accidentally rear-end someone or have your car pushed into another vehicle if someone rear-ends you as well. Drive in the center lane where possible to make it harder for would-be carjackers to approach your vehicle. Avoid driving alone whenever practicable, especially at night. Carpooling not only reduces commuting expenses but also makes you a more challenging target for would-be carjackers. Do not stop to assist a stranger whose vehicle has broken down. Use a cell phone or drive to a payphone in a safe area and call for help.

- If you are bumped by another car while driving, look around before you get out. Make sure there are other vehicles near yours or bystanders who can observe what is going on. Use your mirrors to check out the car that hit you and who is in it. If the situation makes you uneasy, memorize or jot down the other vehicle's license number and description and signal the other driver to follow you. Drive to the nearest police station or hospital* or to a similar busy, well-lit area. If you do get out of your vehicle, always take your keys, wallet, or purse with you and stay alert.

*You can often find law enforcement personnel near hospital emergency room entrances.

- Upon arriving at your destination. As always, park in well-lit areas near building entrances, sidewalks, or walkways where other people may travel. Try to park in an attended garage where practicable. If you use valet parking, leave only your ignition key with no identification.* Avoid parking near dumpsters, wooded areas, large vans, or trucks, or anything else that limits your visibility and hides you from bystanders.
- Avoid unwarranted attraction to your vehicle. Never leave valuables in plain view, even if your vehicle is locked and/or has an alarm system. Put them in the trunk or hide them under a seat, preferably before arriving at your destination so that no one will see you doing it. Even if you are rushed, look around before you get out of your vehicle and always remain alert to your surroundings.

Cash Machine Safety

"To ensure customer safety at ATMs, banks are putting ATMs in areas that are visible by passers-by, trimming landscape to prevent potential criminals from hiding, and installing or upgrading lighting that is bright enough for use at night. Some banks also have installed cameras, rear-view mirrors, panic buttons and special signs. And most banks limit the amount of cash that can be withdrawn on a daily basis" [3]

— *American Banker's Association*

Cash machines offer a real convenience for consumers yet at the same time, they offer an element of risk. Using an ATM safely requires awareness and a little planning. Just because an ATM is open and available 24-hours a day does not necessarily mean that it is safe to use the machine 24 hours a day. Most ATM robberies occur at night between 8:00 PM and midnight. Most ATM robbers used a gun or claim to have a concealed weapon when confronting their victim and demanding their cash. They are usually males under the age of 25 and most work alone. Similarly, most ATM robbery victims are also alone when robbed, though the majority of victims are female. Most claim that they never saw the robber coming.

These people usually position themselves nearby, waiting for a victim to approach and withdraw cash. Be wary of obvious hiding places like shrubbery or overgrown trees near an ATM kiosk. All robbers prefer the element of surprise for their attack, choosing to strike when your attention is focused on your transaction and there are no other witnesses present. Robbers also like good escape routes like nearby freeway on-ramps or high-speed thoroughfares. Some wait for the transaction to be complete while others intervene in process, hoping to increase the amount of cash withdrawn that they can steal.

---

*It's a good idea to separate your house keys from your car keys when you use a valet or drop your vehicle at a mechanic so that no one can make a copy of them without your knowing about it.

Use only ATMs in well-lit, high-traffic areas. Do not use ATMs that are remote or hidden behind buildings, pillars, walls, or otherwise away from the public view unless they are inside a store. Choose an ATM that looks and feels safe, even if it is inconvenient, forcing you to drive a couple of miles out of your way. It is far better to be safe than sorry. When you drive up to an ATM location, scan the area for any suspicious persons. If you see anyone suspicious standing near the machine or sitting in a car, simply drive away.

Try to limit your use to daylight hours. If you must use an ATM after hours, take someone with you if you can, ensuring that they look away from the machine, scanning the surrounding area for trouble. If you are confronted by an armed assailant, resist the temptation to fight with a robber unless your life is immediately at stake. Do not attempt to follow a robber after the crime has been committed either. Do your best to remember the thief's distinguishing characteristics during the robbery,* walk or drive to a safe place, and then call the police.

Have your access card ready before you approach an ATM. Memorize your Personal Identification Number (PIN) to prevent loss and speed the transaction. Never tell anyone your PIN, even someone who claims to represent your bank or credit union. Be sure to shield the keypad with your body while you are entering your PIN so that bystanders cannot observe what you type. After inserting your card and your PIN diligently scan the area and keep an eye out behind you.

Once you have completed your ATM transaction and received your cash, put it away immediately. Extract your card and walk away. Do not count your money in public. It is much safer to count your cash in your vehicle or, preferably, at another location. Keep your receipt, reconcile your transaction in a safe location, and contact your bank should there be any discrepancies. Keep all your transaction receipts and verify each one against your monthly bank statement as well.

Never accept an offer to help or a request for help from another person at the machine. Honestly, how many people have you met that truly do not know how to use an ATM these days? Such requests may be attempts to distract then rob you. It could also be an attempt at "shoulder surfing," where the potential thief simply looks over your shoulder to learn your PIN. He or she can then openly steal your cash card, attempt to pick your pocket, or even use an electronic skimmer to get access to your account.

"Skimming" is when criminals install special equipment over the top of a legitimate ATM to scan your data. This parasitic device enables the download and transmission of information that you swipe from your card. It usually works in conjunction with a hidden camera, perhaps in the information or envelope rack, to watch you enter your PIN. A wireless transmitter captures and sends your data to the thief. Pay close attention to the ATM's you use regularly so that you will have a better

---

*And the characteristics of his/her vehicle if a getaway car is used.

chance to spot any illegitimate modifications. As stated earlier, be suspicious of someone who seems too helpful. Thieves have been known to jam one ATM and then direct consumers to another, where a skimmer has been installed.

This may seem far-fetched, but it is real. For example, Ioan Emil Codarcea, 35, was arraigned on May 10, 2005 on a variety of charges including identity fraud, credit card fraud, and larceny. Codarcea, a Romanian national with reputed Russian mob ties, was accused of installing phony magnetic card readers on doors leading to ATMs, or on the actual machines, in several communities in Massachusetts and in Manchester, New Hampshire. The readers recorded card information while tiny cameras focused on ATM keypads, capturing customer passwords and transmitting the images to a laptop computer.

Codarcea allegedly used the bankcard information to make duplicate magnetic strips, which he and several accomplices used to withdraw money from more than 400 customers' accounts starting in March 2003. Most of the victims did not even know that money was being siphoned from their accounts until their banks notified them. Codarcea was arrested May 1 by the U.S. Border Patrol while allegedly trying to smuggle illegal Pakistani immigrants into Vermont from Canada. He was turned over to Boston police shortly thereafter. Police reportedly trailed Codarcea, taking photos of him installing and retrieving the magnetic card readers loaded with account data.

Even if no one else is present, do not become so focused on your transaction that you lose track of others around you. If anyone suspicious or seemingly dangerous approaches, be prepared to terminate your transaction and leave immediately, even if it means running away and leaving your ATM card in the machine. As long as the transaction has been canceled, the card itself will be no good to a robber. If someone suspicious approaches you can utilize the same approach I took at the QFC, asking him or her firmly but politely to back off and leave you alone.

If you use your car at a drive-through, ATM similar rules apply. Keep your vehicle in gear with your foot firmly on the brake while using the ATM. Keep a close eye on your rear and side view mirrors during the transaction. Robbers almost always approach from the rear on the driver's side of the vehicle. If an armed robber confronts you, your best bet is usually to toss some money out the window and speed away.

Another common ATM scam involves thieves putting a thin, clear, rigid plastic sleeve into the ATM card slot. When you insert your card, the machine cannot read the strip, so it keeps asking you to re-enter your PIN. Meanwhile, someone behind you watches as you type. When you give up, thinking the machine has swallowed your card and you walk away, the thief then removes the plastic sleeve, steals your card, and uses your PIN to empty your account. The way to avoid this trap, you can run your finger along the card slot before inserting your card. The sleeve must have at least a couple of tiny prongs that the thief will use to get it back out of the slot and you should be able to feel them.

The good news about skimming and similar crimes is that law limits the liability of ATM fraud victims to $50.00 in most jurisdictions. That means financial institutions and specialized companies that operate cash machines have to reimburse fraud victims for any loss above that amount. Some even cover the entire theft if it is reported promptly. Unfortunately, the fraud is sometimes so clever that you cannot tell that anything is wrong until long after you have been victimized, so monitor your account regularly. At minimum, closely review your monthly statement. Better yet, access your real-time account data on-line if the service is available. ATM manufacturers are always working on technologies that can prevent this type of theft but it pays to be cautious.

Hostage Situations

"Research by the FBI indicates that very few hostages have been killed on deadline. Most hostage takers know their hostages have value, and violence is not in the hostage taker's best interest. Killing on deadline, when it does occur, most often occurs during political terrorist incidents where there are several hostages." [4]

– Thomas N. Davidson

If you have been taken hostage by someone you probably do not care all that much why he or she are doing it, you just want to be safe and unharmed. Law enforcement professionals, however, seek to categorize a hostage taker's motivations to help determine a course of action in dealing with them. This information can be life saving. In essence, there are three types of hostage takers: psychological, criminal, and political. Psychological hostage takers include suicidal personalities, vengeance seekers, and disturbed individuals.* Criminal hostage takers include extortionists, aggrieved inmates, and cornered perpetrators. While the first two intend to take a hostage as part of their crime, cornered perpetrators wind up taking hostages in the process of failing in some other crime such as a bank robbery. Political hostage takers include social protesters, fanatics, and terrorist extremists.

Trapped suspects can end a hostage crisis by surrendering, escaping, or committing suicide. Homicide can be an option considered in addition to any of the three aforementioned actions. Consequently, such situations are volatile and dangerous. Police negotiators study the following information in great detail, using past incidents to predict future encounters and plan their strategies accordingly.

---

*Typically paranoid schizophrenics or manic-depressives.

Psychological Hostage Takers

Psychological hostage takers include suicidal personalities, vengeance seekers, and other disturbed individuals. Suicidal personalities may not care whether or not they are killed by their actions, frequently taking hostages to draw law enforcement attention in attempted "suicide by cop" scenarios. Vengeance seekers are irrationally upset by something, frequently driven to homicidal rage. Their actions are typically well-planned, frequently requiring active police intervention to end the crisis. Disturbed individuals, on the other hand, rarely plan their actions in advance. The most common mental disorders associated with disturbed hostage-taking individuals are paranoid schizophrenia and manic-depressive (bipolar) disease.

Paranoid schizophrenia is a severe psychotic condition frequently associated with persecution fantasies, delusions of grandeur, or extreme jealousy that often occurs with corresponding hallucinations. It is common for such individuals to hear voices, see things, or otherwise react to stimuli that only they can recognize.

When dealing with such individuals it is important to avoid arguing with their delusions. While they may not represent reality to the rest of us, they are real to the disturbed individual. Try to let them vent, avoid staring or getting too close, and attempt to ally yourself with the person's perspective without seeming insincere. Control the rate, tone, pitch, and volume of your voice. Talk low, slow, and quietly.

Manic-depressive illness is frequently characterized by unrealistic hopelessness, overwhelming feelings of inadequacy, suicidal thinking, and self-defeating behavior. If possible, try to establish rapport with such individuals, reassuring them of their self-worth. As with other mentally disturbed individuals try to avoid staring or getting too close unless you have to physically intervene.

Criminal Hostage Takers

Criminal hostage takers include extortionists, aggrieved inmates, and cornered perpetrators. Extortionists are typically motivated by greed, hoping to exchange a victim for their family's money. They frequently demand direct communication with the family threatening dire consequences should law enforcement become involved. These folks are frequently sociopathic in nature, caring only about themselves. When dealing with such individuals, ego stimulation and ego threat are prime motivators. It may be possible to convince such individuals that your release is in their best interest.

Aggrieved inmates may attempt to take over a prison facility or capture prison personnel either through spontaneous protest or via planned stratagem. Cornered perpetrators wind up taking hostages in the process of failing in some other crime such as a liquor store or bank robbery. These folks often have inadequate personalities, very low self-esteem, and a history of bungling personal and professional relationships. When dealing with these types of individuals it is important to find a resolution that helps them "save face."

Political Hostage Takers

Political hostage takers include social protesters, fanatics, and terrorist extremists. Social protesters are frequently young, relatively highly educated individuals trying to eliminate some perceived social injustice. They will to go to extreme means to try to raise consciousness about some issue or make some political point but rarely actually want to seriously harm anyone. A fanatic, on the other hand, is willing to kill and die for his or her cause. A terrorist extremist attempts to demonstrate to the public that their government is incapable of protecting its citizens. The odds of terrorists killing hostages are high, though they are typically looking for adequate media coverage first.

It is extremely difficult for individuals to succeed in negotiating with fanatics or terrorists. This area is especially tricky and ought to be the purview of professionals whenever possible. The key to negotiating with terrorists is the ability to convince them that their point has been well made, their demands thoroughly understood, and that killing the hostages would serve to discredit their cause in the eyes of the world.

Hostage Guidelines (what to do)

So what should you do if you are taken hostage? It is good to have a plan ahead of time since hostage crises incidents are tense, dynamic, and dangerous. For clarity, a hostage situation is a little different from an active shooter situation. In the former, there is typically time for negotiation, police intervention, escape, or some other non-violent response on the part of the hostage. In the latter, you are in imminent danger and must act immediately to save yourself.

It is important to consider that frequently when a hostage taker feels a loss of power or control he or she may be more willing to resort to violence. Additionally, a hostage taker who makes no substantive demands may be contemplating a homicide/suicide scenario, especially if he or she expresses irrational anger at the hostage. Sometimes it is better to wait for events to play themselves out and sometimes it is better proactively to try and to resolve the situation yourself, typically through violence. In choosing whether or not to act, it is important to ask yourself the following questions:

- Is action necessary? The first 15 to 20 minutes of a hostage crisis are typically the most dangerous. Should you act immediately or can you wait and hope for non-violent resolution of the situation? You may have a different answer when faced with a mentally disturbed individual or a cornered perpetrator as opposed to a terrorist extremist.

- Is the action risk effective? If you act now, will the potential consequences outweigh the consequences of not acting? Once the use of force has been attempted by you or by law enforcement personnel, negotiation almost always ceases to be a viable option.

- Is the action acceptable? Is it legally, morally, and ethically acceptable for you to act? If other hostages are also involved, your action or lack thereof may affect them as well. This is a tough moral dilemma. For example, if law enforcement is not aware of the situation it is often better to escape and run for help even if you have to leave family members behind. The longer a perpetrator has privacy in which to conduct his/her crime, the worse off you or your loved ones may ultimately be.

If you are truly convinced that your captor is going to kill you, try to escape at an opportune moment, or possibly even immediately. In many cases, however, it is far better to do nothing offensive, letting professional police negotiators handle the situation. Unless you feel your life is immediately on the line, you may choose to sit tight while attempting to gather intelligence that may aid law enforcement personnel upon your release. Should you choose this strategy, it is important not to glare, stare, make suggestions, argue, moralize, threaten, negotiate, conspire, or otherwise attempt to draw undue attention to yourself or play the hero. Do not speak unless spoken to; then be polite, calm, and friendly to the extent possible.

Try to let your captor do most of the talking. People generally feel better about conversations in which they do the majority of the talking while the other person listens attentively. Try to establish common bonds, helping the perpetrator see you as an individual. If you are disobedient or uncooperative and your captor decides to gag and blindfold you, your peril will be significantly higher as you become easier to eliminate and will have less opportunities to escape if your captor gets sloppy. Similarly, try not to turn your back on a hostage taker as it is psychologically much easier to kill someone who is not looking at you then it is to kill someone who is. Always look for avenues of escape but do not attempt to utilize them unless you are absolutely convinced of success or certain that you will be killed if you do not attempt to escape.

Most hostage situations are resolved through negotiations rather than through armed rescues. In fact, roughly 80 percent of hostages killed during a hostage situation are killed by the hostage takers or by the police during a rescue attempt so officers will do everything they can to end the situation peacefully before resorting to force. If any hostage is killed, however, the dynamic is different. A counterattack at that point is almost certain. In the event of a police assault, immediately hit the floor, cover your head, and stay where you are until commanded by the police to do otherwise. If you are confused for a hostage taker, you will likely be injured or killed by the officers that are there to save you.

If you spot police barricades as you are being led past a window or out onto a sidewalk, you can be reasonably certain that your captor is in the crosshairs of tactical team sniper's rifle. If you are convinced of your imminent demise this might be a good time to wrench free and drop to the floor. Hopefully you will hear a loud noise followed by the impact of your captor's corpse landing on you.

Information That Will Help the Police

If you witness a hostage taking but are not captured yourself there is some important information that the police will want to know. Similarly, if you are one of several hostages you may be freed in exchange for some consideration or otherwise become able to communicate with law enforcement at some point during the crisis. The following list of questions comes from Thomas Davidson's book, *To Preserve Life: Hostage-Crisis Management*. This information can be of immense value for the authorities:

- What occurred and why?
- Is anyone seriously injured or bleeding?
- Why today or at this time?
- Did anyone see, hear, or threaten the use of weapons?
- What is the number and identity of the suspects (accurate descriptions and clothing are important, especially if hostages and suspects have traded clothing)?
- What is the number and identity of the hostages (accurate descriptions and clothing are important, especially if hostages and suspects have traded clothing)?
- What is the location(s) of the suspect(s) and hostage(s)?
- What are the medical, mental, and criminal histories of the suspect(s) and hostage(s)?
- Are drugs, alcohol, or other intoxication suspected?

Impact of Drug Use

Special problems often arise when dealing with a hostage-taker who is under the influence of drugs or alcohol. It is useful, therefore, to understand (at least in general) the affects that various drugs have on a person's nervous system. If you are able to accurately report symptoms of drug use to law enforcement personnel it will be helpful for their planning efforts. There are five main drug groupings to consider: narcotics, depressants, stimulants, hallucinogens, and cannabis.

Narcotics: Narcotics can include drugs such as heroin, methadone, opium, and morphine, which can cause euphoria, drowsiness, respiratory depression, and constricted pupils among other things. Symptoms of withdrawal include sweating, cramps, and nausea.

Depressants: Depressants include substances such as barbiturates, methaqualone, solvents, and alcohol, which cause disorientation, dizziness, slurred speech, delusions, hallucinations, and, of course, euphoria. Symptoms of withdrawal include tremors, delirium, and convulsions. These substances decrease dexterity and increase the users' potential for accidental injury by five to fifty times.

Stimulants: Stimulants include drugs such as cocaine, crack, amphetamines, and methamphetamines, which can cause hyper alertness, excitation, euphoria, and insomnia. Symptoms of withdrawal include irritability, depression, and disorientation. Crack, a popular street drug, frequently causes rapid, intense euphoria followed by a sharp crash, often accompanied by violent impulses. Methamphetamines, also popular on the street, can cause intense euphoria, tremendous energy, heightened sexual potency, paranoid impulses, and violent behavior. People in this condition frequently have decreased pain sensitivity.

Hallucinogens: Hallucinogens can include substances such as LSD and phencyclidine, which can cause users to experience time dilation, delusions, and illusions (which can be linked with suicide, self-mutilation, and accidental trauma.

Cannabis: Cannabis can include such drugs as marijuana and hashish, which can cause increased appetite, relaxed inhibitions, and euphoria. Withdrawal symptoms include insomnia and hyperactivity.

The Stockholm Syndrome (or Stockholm Bond)

On August 23, 1973, the Kreditbank in Stockholm Sweden was robbed. Before the escaped convict who perpetrated this robbery could complete his crime, the bank was surrounded by law enforcement officers. Rather than surrendering, he took four bank employees hostage, holding them for 131 hours in an 11' x 47' bank vault. Sometime during this ordeal, his prison roommate was released and allowed to join him in the bank.

By the time the hostages were released, they had formed a close emotional bond with their captors and developed an irrational fear of the police. Whether this unconscious emotional response was brought about by reliance on the captors for survival, by fear to avoid their wrath, or for some other reason, it is commonly experienced by captives in similar situations. This syndrome has become commonly known as the Stockholm bond.

Perhaps the most famous case of this syndrome was that of publishing heiress Patty Hearst. The Americans held hostage in Iran, on the other hand, never showed signs of developing similar attachments. Perhaps this was because they were frequently left alone, isolated from their kidnappers, and allowed to communicate amongst themselves.

This syndrome can be good or bad, depending upon how you use it. The closer the bond between a hostage and his/her captor the more likely that person will be released alive after the ordeal is over in many cases. On the other hand, many hostages have avoided taking perfect opportunities to escape, such as when a tired captor set down his weapon in easy reach of the captive or simply fell asleep from exhaustion, due to this syndrome.

The Stockholm syndrome is characterized by:

- Positive feelings of a hostage(s) toward his or her captor(s).
- Negative feelings of a hostage(s) toward law enforcement personnel.
- Feelings reciprocated by the hostage taker(s).

Hostage Negotiation

It is almost always best to let trained police negotiators handle all communication with hostage takers. Well-meaning friends, coworkers, or family members who attempt to intervene may inadvertently speak certain trigger words or unleash emotional responses that goad the perpetrator to violence. If the person is manic-depressive, the presence of family or friends may provoke feelings of worthlessness and make matters worse. No matter how much you would like to interfere, it is almost always best to leave hostage negotiation to the professionals. Resist the temptation to try backdoor communication channels or trade yourself for one of the hostages.

Thomas Davidson wrote, "The most dangerous possibility is that the very person who is convinced that he is the one who can talk the suspect out is a big part of the reason the suspect is acting out in the first place. There is no doubt that allowing a friend or relative to talk with the suspect may, on some occasions, speed up or facilitate an end to the incident. Even if it takes the negotiator longer to negotiate a peaceful end to the situation, the tenuous possible benefit of ending the situation sooner by using friends or relatives to negotiate with the suspect does not outweigh the risks associated with this strategy."

Here is a list of problematic words and phrases that Davidson suggests should be avoided in hostage situation:

- Hostage negotiator.
- Hostage.
- Surrender.
- Give up.
- SWAT team.
- Jail, prison, hospital, or institution.
- End it.

- Kill or dead.
- Shoot.
- Crime.
- Sentence.
- Give you my best shot.

Here is a list of useful words and phrases that Davidson suggests should be used in hostage situation:

- First I'd like to get to know you better.
- Could you tell me about it?
- I would like to hear your side.
- Could you share that with me?
- I guess that's pretty important to you.
- Tell me about it.
- That's interesting.
- I see.
- Oh.
- Uh huh.

Intimate Violence (Domestic Violence)

"Domestic violence means: (a) Physical harm, bodily injury, assault, or the infliction of fear of imminent physical harm, bodily injury or assault, between family or household members; (b) sexual assault of one family or household member by another; or (c) stalking of one family or household member by another family or household member." [5]

– Revised Code of Washington

On February 24, 2005, David Hernandez Arroyo, Sr. opened fire outside a Tyler, Texas courthouse killing his ex-wife and an armed bystander who intervened to protect the couple's 23-year-old son. Police estimated that Arroyo, who had a history of spousal abuse and weapons violations, shot 50 rounds in the historic town's square. He was wearing a military-style flak jacket and a bulletproof vest. The 43-year-old gunman was killed in a subsequent gun battle with law enforcement officers after fleeing the scene of the original shooting in which his son and three law enforcement officers were wounded.

Despite earlier warnings, Maribel Estrada, Arroyo Sr.'s 41-year-old ex wife apparently did not believe that he was a threat. The couple had divorced in January 2004 after a 22-year marriage. According to reports, the couple's son, David Jr., was wounded trying to act as a mediator between his parents before his mother was killed. A sheriff's deputy, Sherman Dollison, age 28, was rushed to the hospital in critical condition with wounds in the liver, lungs, and legs after the incident. A sheriff's lieutenant and a Tyler police detective were both treated for minor injuries and released from the hospital shortly thereafter.

Authorities credited the bystander who died, Mark Alan Wilson, age 52, with saving the younger Arroyo's life. Wilson, a concealed weapons permit holder, intervened after Arroyo started shooting, hitting the attacker several times with his own pistol but his bullets did not penetrate Arroyo's body armor. He was quickly wounded by his attacker and fell to the ground. "The gunman walked up to Wilson and shot him while he was on the ground," said Nelson Clyde III, a witness who saw the shooting from a nearby restaurant. He told reporters. "I couldn't believe what I was seeing. It was sickening."

As this outrageous incident illuminates, intimate or domestic violence can be a serious crime. It can affect adults, children, and even pets. Psychologists state that domestic violence is a learned behavior, typically involving controlling actions that encompass different types or levels of abuse such as physical harm, imminent fear of physical harm, sexual assault, or stalking among individuals who have had some type of intimate relationship. Intimate relationships include people, biologically related or unrelated, who are presently residing together, or who have resided together in the past, or have had a dating relationship. It is important to understand that the perpetrator causes domestic violence, not substance abuse, not the victim, and not the relationship.

Since domestic violence is for the most part a learned behavior it is important to understand, and where possible, break the cycle before it spins out of control. Young children who grow up with abuse are much more likely to become abusers themselves. It is important to teach them to respect classmates and family members, avoiding controlling or belittling behaviors. Kids who are taught to deal with anger in a positive manner without resorting to violence or humiliation grow up with the ability to utilize those skills as adults.

Domestic violence is very serious. It can happen to almost anyone. Consequences can include anything from a few bruises to outright murder. While intimate violence commonly involves a male assaulting a female such as Scott Peterson killing his pregnant wife Laci, men can become victims too. Arguably, the most famous instances of this type of abuse involve dismembering rather than outright murder. Examples include acts perpetrated by Lorena Bobbitt who cut off her husband's penis and tossed it from a moving car in 1993, or Kim Tran who tied up her boyfriend, cut off his penis, and flushed it down the toilet in 2005.

Intimate violence situations tend to escalate, with several minor incidents preceding dramatic ones. The victim's behavior in such cases can help either ensure their survival or lead to their destruction. One of the most important things a domestic abuse victim can do is get away from the perpetrator before things get worse. Danger to the victim (and their children, if any), however, is likely to increase at the time of separation so you have to be careful about how you do it.

If you feel threatened in a relationship, it is essential to take action right away. Perceived barriers to separation can include economic or support issues such as lack of housing, loss of income for self and children, loss of health, loss of health insurance, or lack of transportation. Other inhibiters include religious, cultural, or family values that the family unit feels must be preserved at all costs. Another factor can be victim blaming by service providers, law enforcement, or even the courts. Despite these obstacles, there are plenty of resources to help you do the right thing and keep yourself safe. In most communities, there are both government and private agencies such as battered women's shelters that can help you work through these issues, providing relocation, temporary housing, medical assistance, and attending to other needs as appropriate.

Warning Signs

So how do you know that something bad is coming? Here are some warning signs of an abusive relationship that may predict eventual domestic violence:

- Your partner frequently yells at you, reprimands you, or demeans you in public or otherwise causes you to fear his/her temper, or causes you overt concern about what kind of mood he or she is in on a regular basis.
- Your partner isolates you, prevents you from getting or keeping a job, keeps you from seeing friends or family, or otherwise alienates your friends or family so that they feel uncomfortable being around that person.
- Your partner keeps you from leaving your house or locks you out of your house.
- Your partner threatens to hurt or kill you, your children, your family, your friends, or your pets.
- Your partner hits, slaps, pushes, or shoves you, pulls your hair, or inflicts unwanted physical injury on you in any way.

Restraining Orders

If you want to get out of a bad relationship and fear that your partner will try to stop you there are legal avenues that might help. Restraining orders can be issued by a judge to help protect those who fear for their safety due to overt actions by an abusive partner. They are by no means a silver bullet, but can be an important part of taking action to make the situation better in certain instances. Essentially, a restraining order prohibits an individual from an action that is likely to cause harm. It usually prevents any contact or communication between two or more people.

A restraining order differs from an injunction in that it can be granted immediately, without a hearing and without any notice to the opposing party. Restraining orders are temporary; they are intended to last only until a hearing can take place. If you have been granted one due to a domestic violence situation, a copy of your restraining order should always be in your possession. A copy should also be on file with the police departments in whose jurisdictions you live and work, and filed with other counties where you regularly spend time. If a restraining order is violated, call 9-1-1 or your local emergency number and report the situation immediately. The violating party can be arrested and taken into custody.

Let your employer, neighbors, close friends, and family know about the restraining order. Ask that they contact the police if they see the other party near you. Be sure to protect your children as well by notifying school administration, teachers, childcare centers, babysitters, and neighbors of the restraining order and requesting that they contact police if they suspect the order is being violated.

Protecting yourself after a restraining order has been issued

A restraining order, no matter what its weight in court, is really just a piece of paper. If it is violated, there will be a time lag, no matter how small, between when the incident is reported and when law enforcement personnel arrive. It is important, therefore, to take additional steps to remain safe beyond that document. Suggestions include:

- Harden your home, making it more challenging for someone to break in. Change your locks, replace any hollow-core doors, and reinforce sliding glass doors by installing a lock and/or placing a piece of wood in the track. Add interior window locks so that windows cannot be opened or removed from their tracks from the outside of the house. Install motion-sensitive lighting to identify unwarranted movement outside your home. Consider installing a monitored security system.

- Plan an emergency escape route from all areas of your home, including upstairs, and make sure all family members are aware of the plan. Include family pets or other animals in your safety and escape plans. Animals are often targeted by a batterer or stalker as a means of controlling, terrorizing, or punishing human victims. If it is not safe for you to remain at home, it is likely not safe for your animal(s), either.

- If you have small children, teach them how and when to call 9-1-1. Teach your children how to make a collect call to you or family members in case they are abducted. Tell your children not to unlock the door if the respondent tries to get into your home. If possible, purchase a cellular phone or cordless telephone and take it with you as you travel to different rooms in your residence so that it will be immediately available.

- If you work outside the home, consider informing your supervisor of the existence of the restraining order and of any concerns you may have for your safety at your place of employment. Park in well-lit areas or ones where there will be other people around and try to leave work in the company of at least one other co-worker.

- Vary your routine. Make yourself harder to detect and follow by using different grocery stores and shopping malls and regularly changing the hours you shop. Alter your route to and from work as well. Avoid walking in unlighted or isolated areas. If you are being followed while driving or riding in a vehicle, proceed to the nearest police station or look for a police officer. Do not drive straight home.

- Avoid alcohol and/or drugs as they can affect your ability to react quickly and make rational decisions.

Planes, Trains, and Public Transportation

"By staying alert and reporting any problems on buses or at bus stops and shelters, you can help make Metro Transit safer, friendlier and better for everyone." [6]

– Public Safety Partnership

On March 2, 2005, Cumberland City (Tennessee) school bus driver Joyce Gregory was shot to death with a .45 caliber handgun as she drove along her route. The alleged perpetrator was a 14-year old male student. The bus, which was carrying 20 kindergarten through 12th grade students at the time, crashed into a utility pole. Two weeks before the incident Gregory told family members that she was having trouble with students chewing tobacco on the bus. After several warnings, she reported them to school administrators. The suspect was one of those students. Luckily, the bus was moving slowly along a residential street at the time of the shooting and no one else was seriously hurt by the crash.

There have been many other cases over the years, however, where a bus driver was assaulted in transit and there were passenger fatalities from the subsequent crash. A dramatic example occurred when a Metro Transit bus slammed through a guardrail and plunged off the Aurora Bridge in Seattle (Washington) on November 26, 1998. As the 60-foot-long Metro bus crossed the bridge, a mentally disturbed passenger, Silas Cool, stood and pulled out a pistol. Without saying a word, he shot the driver

Mark McLaughlin in the torso and then shot himself in the head. Fatally wounded McLaughlin lost control of his bus. It burst through a guardrail, plunged 40 feet,* tore through several evergreen trees, and then glanced off an apartment building. A 69-year-old passenger, Herman Liebelt, died in the crash. All 32 other passengers were injured, some severely, yet all recovered.

Public transportation such as airplanes, buses, trains, and taxicabs can present unique self-defense challenges. Such environments are captive, mobility impairing, and somewhat dependent upon the actions of the driver, engineer, or pilot to assure your safety. By captive, I mean that you cannot always get off when and where you want to, even to avoid a fight, so escape may not be an option. By mobility impairing, I mean that you cannot move around much during combat should things escalate to that point. Consequently, if you have to fight on a bus, plane, or train your fighting environment will be different than you would find in most other venues.

Because of these unique challenges, it is prudent to delve a little deeper into the peculiarities of each situation. While public transportation in some locations is more precarious than in others, the following information will be generally relevant no matter where you live.

Flying on Airplanes

Despite 9/11, airplanes remain the safest form of public transportation, roughly 50 times safer than driving a personal vehicle such as a truck or car. The challenge is that despite the fact that in the United States there are an average of about 38,000 fatal vehicle crashes every year accounting for approximately 42,500 annual deaths, the handful of airline accidents that also occur get much, much more publicity. It is important to keep things in perspective. Between 1959 and 2003, for example, there were 786 fatal incidents involving commercial airliners that resulted in a total of 25,807 deaths. Looked at this way, we conclude that 44 years of worldwide aviation has killed roughly 60 percent of the number of people that die driving every year in the United States alone. Each death is a significant tragedy, of course, yet headline-grabbing air accidents might lead one to improperly conclude that it is not safe to fly.

So what about terrorism? Aviation accidents are actually a much more common cause of passenger injury or death than overt hostile acts. In fact, the 44-year average sabotage/terrorist rate per million departures has historically run at about 0.3. There were no such incidents at all in 1992, 1995, 1997, 1998, 1999, or 2003.[7] Boeing's (retired) chief safety engineer Earl Weener put it this way: "If you were born on a U.S. domestic airliner and never got off, you'd be 3,000 years old by the time you encountered your first fatal accident and you'd have a fifty percent chance of living through it." Pretty good odds, huh? Nevertheless, contemplating an airline incident is still scary. The good news is that both operational safety and security screening appear to be improving over time.

---

*Fortunately it was near the end of the bridge. If the bus had gone through the rail at the center of the bridge the fall would have been 197 feet.

Let's focus on security. While airline security has gotten a whole lot better since 9/11, few people claim that it is perfect. Screeners do not catch every weapon every time. Unruly passengers still disrupt operations on occasion. Some flights have armed air marshals while most do not. Even if a bad guy does sneak a weapon onto a plane, however, the best defense a pilot has is the hardened security door that separates the cockpit from the passenger cabin. These doors can withstand fists, feet, crowbars, axes, and even bullets, safely securing the pilots against most any physical assault. Unfortunately, the doors must occasionally be opened so that the pilots can exit the cockpit to use the lavatories during a flight. Furthermore, not all pilots secure the doors properly while in the air.

I personally witnessed a shocking lapse of security recently. Returning from a Dallas (Texas) conference, I took American Airlines flight 1587 back to Seattle on March 16, 2005. During that flight, one of the pilots opened the cockpit door, propped it open with his foot, and proceeded to have a 3 minute and 48 second conversation with one of the flight attendants. Despite the fact that she was very good looking, this was an egregious security breach in my opinion.

Over those nearly four minutes, three passengers from the economy class cabin used the lavatory in first class, something they are not supposed to do under the airline's security policy. Furthermore, one of the first class passengers was standing near the forward entry door in arms length from the pilot the entire time. This particular passenger was about six foot six inches tall and weighed around 250 pounds. A former college basketball star, he is big, strong, and could easily have overpowered the smaller pilot and accessed the cockpit. Now I happen to know that this guy, whose name is Phil, would never have done that since I know him well and have worked for him for several years, but the pilot certainly had no way of knowing that he was harmless.

While my boss rode in first class, I watched the entire incident from coach. Fortunately, nothing untoward happened, but there are fire extinguishers, cans, flashlights, and various other improvised weapons readily available in an airplane that anyone could have used in an attempt to overpower the pilots and crash the plane. Even worse, I seemed to be the only passenger who was concerned about what happened. I strongly suspect that had something untoward occurred that my fellow passengers would have attempted to intervene but I am not sure whether or not anybody could have reacted in time. I was certainly too far away to do anything quickly.

Airport security is odd too. For example, after you pass through the security screening area at SeaTac airport you will come across a deli-style Asian restaurant on the main concourse. They have a large table with napkins, condiments, sauces, and various utensils. Since metal forks and knives are banned from flights, they include plastic ware. Yet they also provide chopsticks. These chopsticks are full size, somewhat sharp bamboo utensils, each roughly a ¼" thick—a pretty sweet impromptu weapon that comes in a convenient two pack. In the right hands, those sticks could be used to mess someone up easily.

Despite the fact that airlines are not 100% secure, as passengers we are certainly not helpless. The famous "shoe bombing" case is a good example of where astute crewmembers and passengers worked together to thwart an attempted terrorist attack. Richard C. Reid (a.k.a. Tariq Raja, a.k.a. Abdel Rahim), an Al Qaeda terrorist, tried to blow up American Airlines Flight 63 over the Atlantic on December 22, 2001 by igniting a bomb built into his shoes.

The routine flight from Charles De Gaulle International Airport (near Paris, France) to Miami International Airport (in Miami, Florida) was interrupted when a flight attendant saw Reid attempting to light a match on the tongue of his tennis shoe. She tried grabbing his shoes, but was thrown to the floor where she began screaming for help. When another flight attendant joined in the struggle to stop Reid, he bit her on the thumb and threw her aside as well. The 6' 4" terrorist was eventually subdued by a group of passengers.

Federal law enforcement authorities later found plastic explosives with a triacetone triperoxide detonator, hidden in the lining of his shoes. On January 30, 2003, he was found guilty on terrorism charges at a federal court in Boston, Massachusetts and sentenced to life in prison. During the sentencing hearing, he openly stated that he was an Islamic fundamentalist and declared himself an enemy of the United States.

So what can you do in the unlikely occurrence that something similar happens on your flight? Your best defense, as always, is awareness. Pay attention to your fellow passengers, observing anything unusual or suspicious. Pay attention to impromptu weapons at your disposal such as flashlights, fire extinguishers, belts, books, briefcases, or laptop computers. Your seat cushions not only work as a floatation device in the event of a water landing but also as a shield that can trap an opponent or block an attacker's weapon. Choose an aisle seat if you can and be prepared to act if something untoward actually occurs.

All in all, the odds of another 9/11 style terrorist incident on an airplane are pretty remote since other targets are easier to access and much less well defended. Another piece of good news is that since 9/11, passengers are unlikely to react passively to a future hijacking attempt should one occur. Get to know passengers around you at least a little such that you may be able to act in concert to increase your odds of success and survival.

The down side is that the same security measures that keep us safer can make travel time consuming and more difficult. Heightened airport security measures have increased the time that most people need to get to their flights, creating longer waits at the ticket counter, screening area, and even at the departure gate.

In addition to the familiar metal detectors and x-ray machines, there may be a number of other visible and invisible measures in place at the airport such as bomb detection equipment, bomb sniffing dogs, and even military personnel depending upon the threat level at any given time. Here are a few things you can do to make things go smoother:

- Arrive early: Okay, this one is obvious but most airlines advise arriving about two hours before your scheduled departure. E-tickets can speed up the process while checked baggage, small children, or other special needs may make it longer.

- Have proper identification ready. Government-issued photo identification is generally sufficient though drivers' licenses from certain states may not be acceptable. Be sure to check with your airline about what type of identification is suitable for your flight.

- Skip the ticket line if possible. If you can use an e-ticket and avoid checked baggage, you may be able to skip this line entirely. Most airlines limit passengers to one carry-on item and one personal item such as a briefcase or laptop computer.

- Be easily screenable. Be sure your carry on bags are orderly and presentable. Wear shoes that are easy to remove. Place loose change, wallet, keys, or other metal items into your carry-on bag or jacket pocket. Be cautious not to bring any prohibited items into the airport. If you have a laptop computer be sure that it is easy to remove from your carrying bag. Keep your identification and ticket readily accessible.

- Relax and enjoy the ride. The lines are longer and the security is stronger. While it may be a nuisance, it is all in place to help keep you safe (or at least feel safer about flying). Get there early, follow the rules, and relax. The more polite you are, the better reaction you'll get from security personnel so keep your cool at all times, even if you are taken aside and given extra scrutiny one or more times by airport security and/or airline personnel. In most cases, this extra scrutiny is simply a random event and not an attempt to impugn your integrity. Roll with it.

Things you should not bring on board

Some items are prohibited in checked baggage, carry-on luggage, or both because of the danger they represent for the passengers and crew. While commonly used at work or home, prohibited items may become hazardous in flight due to changes in temperature or pressure that can cause them to leak, generate toxic fumes, or start a fire. Since the list changes from time to time, it is always a good idea to check with your airline or the Transportation Security Administration (TSA) for the most current list of prohibited items.

As of this writing, knives of any length, composition or description and cutting instruments of all kinds cannot be carried onto the airplane. This includes knitting needles, carpet knives, box cutters, razor blades, ice picks, straight razors, metal scissors, corkscrews, and cigar cutters. Similarly, baseball bats, golf clubs, pool cues, ski poles, hockey sticks, tire irons, and many other solid objects are also banned from the cabin area. They can, however, be checked in your baggage. Most martial arts weapons can also be checked but not carried onto an airplane. Any sharp objects in checked baggage should be sheathed or securely wrapped to prevent injury to baggage handlers and security screeners. If you are traveling to a tournament or demonstration, it is a good idea to place a copy of the event brochure on top of the weapons in your checked baggage to help screeners understand that you have a legitimate reason for having these items. Purchase a TSA certified luggage lock so that they can open your luggage as necessary without damaging it.

Poisons, acids, corrosives, infectious materials, radioactive substances, lighters, lighter fluid, and strike-anywhere matches,* sparklers, fireworks, flares, gunpowder, ammunition or other ordnance, blasting caps, dynamite, loaded firearms,† and flammable liquids are prohibited both as carry-on and as checked baggage. Mace, tear gas, and pepper spray are not only prohibited but also prone to leak at high altitudes due to pressure changes. If you want to carry such items at your destination, you can usually purchase them once after you arrive.

Personal care items containing flammable perfume, aerosols, or other hazardous material can usually be carried on board in limited quantities. Similarly, up to four pounds of dry ice may be carried on board for packing perishables providing the package is appropriately vented. You find the latest and greatest rules at the TSA web site, www.tsa.gov.

Transporting firearms and ammunition

Firearms, ammunition, and firearm parts may only be transported in checked baggage. There are certain limited exceptions for law enforcement officers who are authorized to fly armed by meeting the requirements of 49 CFR § 1544.219. Following is a summary of key regulatory requirements from the TSA web site relating to the transportation of firearms, firearm parts, or ammunition in checked baggage. These regulations are strictly enforced. Violations can result in criminal prosecution and the imposition of civil penalties of up to $10,000 per violation.

- All firearms must be declared to the air carrier during the ticket counter check-in process.
- The firearm must be unloaded and carried in a hard-sided locked container.

---

*Up to four books of regular safety matches are allowed as a carry-on.
†Unloaded firearms and sporting ammunition may be carried in checked baggage packed in special containers (see transporting firearms and ammunition below).

- The passenger must provide the key or combination to the screener if it is necessary to open the container, and then remain present during screening to take back possession of the key after the container is cleared.
- Any ammunition transported must be securely packed in fiber (such as cardboard), wood or metal boxes or other packaging specifically designed to carry small amounts of ammunition.
- Firearm magazines/clips do not satisfy the packaging requirement unless they provide a complete and secure enclosure of the ammunition (e.g., by securely covering the exposed portions of the magazine or by securely placing the magazine in a pouch, holder, or holster).
- The ammunition may also be located in the same hard-sided case as the firearm, as long as it is properly packed as described above.
- Black powder and percussion caps used with black-powder type firearms are not permitted in carry-on or checked baggage.

Air carriers may have their own additional requirements regarding firearms and the amount of ammunition an individual may place in checked baggage. It is, therefore, prudent to contact your carrier regarding their policies before your flight. They frequently require a surcharge to transport firearms or ammunition as well.

Riding the Bus

Use a bus stop you know is usually busy and is well lit, preferably in a good neighborhood. Pay attention to not only where you get on and off the bus, but where it will travel in between as well. There may be several options from which to choose; be familiar with the route and comfortable with the neighborhoods through which you must travel. Know the departure and arrival times and try to let someone at the other end know which bus you plan to catch.

Sit as close to the driver as you can. This not only places you in a position to guard him or her against attack, but also allows you respond should the driver have a medical emergency on the road. There is no sense in being paranoid, but you will always be dependant in large part upon the driver for you safety so you might as well position yourself to be able to act as appropriate if something untoward happens. Many transit agencies have their own police force so there may be undercover law enforcement officers riding along with you similar to air marshals who patrol commercial aircraft.

Pay attention to and report any suspicious items left unattended on the bus. Anything that exudes a liquid or vapor, makes you feel nauseated, has unusual wires, or produces an unexplained odor should be reported immediately. The standard procedure is to isolate the object, evacuate the vehicle, and get help. The driver can stop the bus, order an evacuation, and radio for assistance as necessary.

Be conscious of unusual passenger behaviors. Beyond the normal interpersonal confrontations you can find anywhere, a common challenge on public transportation is the unlawful attempt to separate you from your possessions. If you are bumped or squeezed between people, be wary of pickpockets. Commotions or loud arguments may also be attempts to distract you and take your valuables. If someone starts up a conversation, be pleasant but do not give away any personal information like where you live or work. That friendly rider may be perfectly innocent yet he or she could have something nefarious in mind. It never hurts to guard your personal information.

In certain parts of the world, suicide bombers[8] are a significant concern on public transportation. This tactic has been used by Abu Sayyaf, al Qaeda, Hamas, Islamic Jihad, Hezballah, the Kurdistan Worker's Party, and the Tamil Tigers, among other groups. The typical perpetrator is most often male, unmarried, in his late teens or early 20s, and fanatical about his beliefs. He is often well educated, coming from a middle class background. These individuals are very conscious of media attention, timing attacks carefully to achieve the highest possible level of public impact. Behavioral signs that should raise suspicion can include:

- Unseasonable dress, particularly when conspicuously bulky.
- Protruding bulges or exposed wires under clothing, potentially seen through the sleeve.
- Attempts to wear a disguise or blend into a crowd where the person does not seem to belong.
- Repeated and nervous handling of fashion accessories or clothing.
- Slow-paced movements with intense focus.
- Profuse sweating in excess of what might be expected due to environmental conditions.
- Nervous muttering, mumbling, or praying.
- Attempts to maintain distance from or otherwise avoid security personnel where present.
- Exuding a faint chemical odor.

Taking the Train

Wait on a well-lit section of the platform, close to the exit or where there are other people around. Many stations now have closed circuit television cameras and security staff who are trained to deal with emergencies that they observe on them.

When you get on the train, try to sit in a busy compartment and keep any bags and personal possessions you have next to you. If you feel uncomfortable with those around you switch seats or even consider getting off the train and catching the next one. Only do this if the station where you are getting off is manned and busy in case someone begins to follow you though. Know where the emergency button or cord is situated on the train as well as any help points at the station. Identify the location of emergency exits and intercoms in stations and on trains.

As always, pay attention to and report any unusual passenger behaviors. In addition to what was mentioned in the previous section on suicide bombers, some specific things to look for include people who appear to be:

- Conducting surveillance using a camera, cell phone cam, or video recorder.
- Abandoning an item then leaving the area quickly.
- Openly possessing a weapon or any prohibited or dangerous item.
- Looking nervous, irritated, or sweating profusely.

Look for and report any suspicious or unattended packages, devices, baggage, or suitcases. Do not use a cellular phone or radio transmitter within 50 feet of a suspicious package as your transmission could cause a bomb to detonate. Some specific things to look for include:

- Hidden or abandoned packages of any kind, including large items left in garbage containers.
- Items that are connected to wires, timers, tanks, or bottles.
- Items that appear to be releasing a mist, gas, vapor, or have any unusual odor.
- Items that appear to be suspicious or dangerous, such as a canister, tank, metal box, or bottle.

Catching a Taxi

A woman who won $4,000 at the Argosy Casino in Kansas City was robbed at gunpoint on June 9, 2005 by the taxi driver who offered her a ride home. The driver reportedly dropped off another passenger and then drove the woman to southeast Kansas City, where he pointed a gun at her and demanded money. He then told the woman to get out of the car or he would kill her, firing several shots as she ran into nearby woods. The woman was not injured.

San Francisco police reported a rash of taxi thefts that same week. The thief reportedly picked-up and dropped off passengers in at least six different stolen Yellow Cabs, pocketing the fare money and abandoning the vehicle after his crime. While nothing untoward happened to these passengers, the incident points out a danger many people do not consider; the taxi driver you encounter may or may not be a legitimate operator.

Carry the phone number of a taxi or mini cab firm you know with you in case you will need it. It is always better to choose a specific company if you know one you can trust rather than picking any available cab that happens by. Whenever you book a taxi, ask the dispatcher for the driver's name and the type of vehicle they will be driving. Drivers must post their taxi license and photo identification in many jurisdictions so you can compare the person in the driver's seat with his/her photo to help validate his/her legitimacy.

Try to book the taxi you need to bring you home before you go out so that you will not need to accept a ride from whichever random driver happens to be in the area when you need a lift. Give your name to the dispatcher and make sure the driver knows the name the reservation was booked under. If you have to book your taxi in a public place, do it quietly where people are unlikely to overhear your name and address.

If you are dropping a friend off at a taxi, comment on the driver's name if you can see it or the taxi number so that he or she will know that you will remember them. Even if riding alone, it is a good idea to casually communicate that you recognize the driver and his or her vehicle.

If you can, share a taxi with a friend and have your money ready and keys handy at the end of your journey so that you can enter your home quickly. If ever you feel uneasy in a taxi ask the driver to stop in a busy place that you know well and get out.

Sexual Assault, Rape, and Molestation

"Every two minutes, somewhere in America, someone is sexually assaulted." [9]

– *RAINN*

A sexual assault victim in Albany, Georgia was beaten with a board and raped yet managed to provide authorities with DNA evidence against her attacker by biting off a piece of his finger and holding it in her mouth until she could contact police. Faced with the evidence, Demetrius Clyde, 33, pled guilty on May 18, 2003 to charges of false imprisonment, aggravated assault, criminal attempt to commit rape, aggravated sodomy, kidnapping and aggravated sexual battery stemming from the attack. Clyde was sentenced to 40 years, while an accomplice is serving 10 years for an aggravated sodomy conviction stemming from the same incident.

Rape is commonly defined as the penetration of any bodily orifice without the victim's consent, generally with force or the threat of force. Penetration can be with fingers, foreign objects, or penis to the vagina, mouth, or anus of the victim. In most jurisdictions it is also illegal to have sexual contact with someone who is incapable of giving legal consent because they are intoxicated, drugged, unconscious, mentally incompetent, or under age, even if they ask for such contact.

While females are by far the most frequent victims of such crimes, sexual assault (most often in the form of rape or molestation) can happen to anyone. Rape statistics are a little challenging to decipher since many crimes are not reported, especially when the victim is male. Some studies indicate that only 10 to 16 percent of rapes are ever reported to the police though Bureau of Justice Statistics reports suggest that a 30 to 40 percent range may be more accurate. Regardless, males, females, heterosexuals, homosexuals, and people of all ages, races, and income levels have been perpetrators as well as victims.

More than 60 percent of the rape victims have some acquaintance with the perpetrator before the crime is committed. Many are assaulted while on a date with their attacker. Alcohol or other drugs are frequently involved in such cases: 75 percent of men and 55 percent of women involved in acquaintance rapes were drinking at the time of the incident. Approximately six to eight percent of rape victims are male though this number may be even more underreported than similar assaults on females.

Age of consent is tricky and varies by jurisdiction. In most locations, it is 18 years of age. However, a person under the age of 18 can have sexual contact with others who are as young as 14 years old in some jurisdictions or 16 years old in others, depending upon the number of months of age difference between the two individuals and whether or not they are married.

Date rape and rape by someone with whom the victim has previously had sexual relations can be particularly confusing due to the common assumption that such people are somehow entitled to have sex with the victim. That is clearly not the case. Another pervasive belief which can sometimes pressure people is that once you start something you have to finish it. The underlying assumption behind this belief is that consent for some degree of sexual activity includes consent for all degrees of sexual activity. Again, this is incorrect. Legally, either party to an intimate encounter has the right to ask the other to stop at any time.

As you can see, rape is not always a straightforward crime, especially when it comes to consent. Legally it is easy to understand that you cannot have sex with anyone who flat out says, "No." It gets a little trickier from there though. Consent is generally defined as explicitly communicated, reversible, mutual agreement in which both parties are capable of making a decision.

Unfortunately, men and women both give and receive mixed messages about sex. Women are often taught by Western culture that they are obligated to resist a little bit, even if they really want to have sex. Otherwise, they are treated as promiscuous. Men often believe that a women's initial resistance to sex is to be ignored as a token effort. If they give up at that point they are often considered wimps, unable to "close the deal." Consequently, many men are taught to be persistent and women are taught to accept that their refusals may be ignored. This combination of cultural messages creates confusion over what exactly constitutes consent.

Silence is not usually considered consent. Submission is not necessarily consent. There is a fine line between persuasion and coercion. Having sex with someone who reasonably believes that there is a threat of force meets the legal definition of rape in most jurisdictions. It is important that individuals understand and clearly communicate their personal boundaries to avoid confusion and potential repercussions thereof.

Sometimes nuance is not an issue. There are plenty of violent sexual predators out there too. To stay safe it is important to remain cautious, vigilantly aware of your surroundings. Sexual assaults are serious and violent crimes, not the expression of uncontrolled passion. Since pathogens such as HIV/AIDS and hepatitis can be transmitted during forced intercourse, such crimes might ultimately prove fatal for the victim years after the initial molestation, something to consider when deciding how to respond to such attacks. Other sexually transmittable diseases such as herpes while not fatal are either incurable, or can lead to sterility or physiological or psychological challenges for the victim. Furthermore, incidents that begin with rape can progress to battery or even murder. Sexual assault is serious stuff, just as dangerous as the edge of a knife or the point of a bullet in many cases.

Avoiding Rape

We covered awareness and avoidance in great detail earlier. Nevertheless, it cannot hurt to restate that you must be aware of locations and situations where assaults may occur and avoid them as much as practicable. Observe details about suspicious persons. Taking note of a person's size, coloring, hairstyle, facial hair, scars, tattoos, or accent can help you give a good description if they try to follow you, assault you, or otherwise act in an inappropriate manner. If you feel uncomfortable about a person or location, it is almost always wise to leave immediately.

Many rapes happen in or near the victim's home. If you are a woman living alone, it is a good idea to list only your initials and last name in the phonebook or on your mailbox. Try to have a male friend record your answering machine or voice-mail message to create the appearance that you do not live alone. Install a peephole in your front door and never open it to strangers. Keep a cellular phone nearby when you travel to facilitate contacting the appropriate authorities in case of emergency.

Know who is at the door before opening it. Ask for identification from anyone you do not know or feel uncomfortable about. If a stranger requests to use your telephone to call for help, offer to place the call for him or her rather than inviting the stranger into your home. Know which neighbors you could call or run to in the event of an emergency.

Use caution over the phone. Never reveal your phone number or name to a wrong number caller. Do not reveal to a caller that you are alone. Be wary of telephone surveys, especially ones that ask for personal information. If you do not know who the person is and you feel uncomfortable simply hang up. It is better to slightly offend someone than to give away personal information that may be used against you to commit rape, identity theft, or other crimes.

The majority of sexual assaults are perpetrated by people previously known to the victim rather than by total strangers. One step to creating a safer environment is for both men and women to communicate clearly and openly about what they want and do not want sexually. Clear and open communication is crucial in any sexual situation, not only to avoid unwanted attention but to be sure you get the most out of the experiences that you do want. If there are limits that you want to maintain, state what they are, and stick to them. Clearly ask your partner what he/she wants and listen to each other.

Think about your sexual desires and limits and how you respond to social pressures. Consider too how drugs or alcohol affect your decision-making. Knowing these things before going on a date can help prevent any misunderstandings later. Be aware of non-verbal cues, but do not rely on them. Remember that silence does not always mean consent. If you are not sure, ask.

Communicate clearly and assertively. For some people saying "yes" or "no" outright may be difficult, but it is important. Passive or polite approaches can be misunderstood or ignored. Be direct and firm with someone who is pressuring you to do something that you are uncomfortable with. Decide what you want ahead of time; tell you partner, then stick with your decision. If you are uncertain about what you want, stop and talk about it. It is okay to be unsure, though it typically means that you want to wait. Remember that saying "no" now does not mean that you will never want to have sex with a person and saying "yes" does not mean you cannot change your mind later, but mixed messages can damage a relationship at best or lead to violence at worst so it is important to figure out and clearly communicate what you want.

Listen carefully to what the other person is saying and pay attention to what is happening around you. Are you getting mixed messages? If so, stop. Explain why you are confused. It is far better to ask than to assume. Talk together about what would be most enjoyable for each of you. Always watch for, but do not rely on, nonverbal clues. If you know how to read them, nonverbal clues are actually more accurate indicators of intent or emotion than verbal ones, yet they hold a lot less weight in court. In survival situations, you are usually best off going with your gut.

If you feel uncomfortable during a conversation, perhaps because of hearing dirty jokes or derogatory remarks, stop the conversation. If you feel uncomfortable because of unwanted physical contact, such as massaging your neck, stroking your hair, or touching your thigh without your permission, ask the person to stop. Trust your instincts. Even if you cannot explain why you feel a certain way, you have the right to trust your feelings and have them respected. Be aware that effective and assertive communication may not always work. Sometimes people simply do not listen or do not care. Even if you do everything right you still may need to resort to violence to defend yourself.

Use a buddy system when bar hopping or going to parties. Before you go to the event, agree with your friends when you are going to leave, or under what circumstances you will leave without each other. Agree upon signals to give your friends that will indicate needing an escape or a way out if a situation becomes uncomfortable. Do not be afraid to use a little verbal judo to intervene if you think your friend is in a bad situation. It is far better to nip things in the bud while you can talk your way out rather than resorting to violence.

Plan your travel to and from events too. Always make sure you have enough fuel and your car is in good repair, before you leave for a trip, no matter how short it may be. It is a good idea to never have less than a half a tank of gas in case you are stuck in traffic or are otherwise delayed. Park in a well-lit area, have your keys ready in your hand as you approach your vehicle, examine adjacent vehicles for lurkers, and check the back seat before entering. Lock your doors at all times and keep your windows rolled up when possible. If you suspect you are being followed, drive into a busy, well-lit establishment and call a law enforcement agency. If you know the location of the local police department, you can also drive there and ask for help.

If your vehicle breaks down, remain in your car with the doors locked until help arrives. Make sure that any assistance is legitimate. If another motorist offers help, stay in your car and ask the motorist to call the police or auto club. Do not stop if you see a disabled vehicle on the highway. Simply report it and send help for the driver. With cheap prepaid phones widely available, there is really no excuse for not having a cell phone in your vehicle in case of emergency.

If you are walking, take general precautions to assure your safety such as avoiding secluded places, telling a friend or relative where you are going, and assuring that you have a safe way to get home. Walk with others after dark when possible. Avoid shortcuts through alleys or wooded areas, staying in public places where you can take advantage of lighted walkways or main thoroughfares. Vary your route. Pay attention to footsteps and voices. Notice cars that pull up beside you or pass you more than once. If you are being followed, stay in a lighted area and seek safety in a public building where there are other people.

Surviving the Assault

If you are sexually assaulted, your immediate goal is survival. Your best weapon is your ability to think clearly and put your welfare first. Do whatever you need to escape to safety, biting, kicking, punching, and utilizing pressure point techniques or makeshift weapons as necessary.

Do not forget that talking can effectively defuse many assaults. Speak calmly—do not cry, plead, or moralize. If help is within hearing distance, you may wish to try screaming for assistance. Stalling is an intermediate approach to give you time to recover from initial shock and to assess your situation. Do the unexpected convincingly. Stalling can take many forms: pretending to cooperate, going limp and sinking to the ground, or faking sickness. Sticking your finger down your throat and vomiting on an attacker is not entirely out of the question.

Running away is a great option if you can break free and escape to a safe place. You may have to hurt your attacker to be sure that he or she cannot follow and recapture you however. To be most effective, physical resistance must be sudden, unexpected, and vicious. Since your goal is to survive the assault, resistance should be geared toward facilitating escape. You can use your martial skills, makeshift weapons, or other self-defense tools to counterattack but be sure to aim for vital areas since any weapon you use ineffectively could be captured and used against you. If you plan to fight back, you must be resolute, doing whatever is necessary to disable your assailant so that you can successfully escape. Half measures will enrage your attacker and result in retaliatory violence directed against you.

What To Do If You Have Been Raped

If you have been sexually assaulted, you will want to report the incident, get medical attention, preserve the physical evidence, and contact someone who can help you recover from the experience. The first priority, however, is getting to safety. As soon as you have escaped to a safe place or the perpetrator has left you alone, immediately call the authorities. If you do not report the incident, nothing will happen to keep your attacker from preying upon you once again or shifting his/her attention to someone else.

The next step is to get medical attention. Medical care after a rape can detect injuries, and test for and preventively treat sexually transmittable diseases. In addition, a health care provider can collect evidence that could be used in the pursuit of legal or civil action. In addition to saving genetic evidence, samples of your blood or urine may be necessary to test for evidence of date rape drugs such as Rohypnol or gamma hydroxybutyrate (GHB). If you are female and not currently on birth control, emergency contraceptives can usually be dispensed as well.

It is important to preserve the evidence so that you attacker can be brought to justice. Pack a change of clothes to bring to the hospital or doctor's office. Do not change your clothing unless it is severely damaged and un-wearable. If you must change, place your old clothes in a sealed bag or container, handling them as little as possible. Do not wash or clean your clothing. Do not take a shower, bathe, or otherwise clean up. Do not apply medication or cosmetics to cover your injuries until they have been photographed or documented by the authorities or unless a doctor advises you otherwise.

It helps to talk to someone about what happened. You may feel ashamed or embarrassed, thinking that no one will believe you or that the attack is somehow your fault. No one should ever be forced to have sex against his or her will. Telling someone about the incident can give you an outlet to express your emotions. That person could be a relative, close friend, a spiritual advisor (such as a priest, pastor, imam, or rabbi), or a professional counselor. Rape is a traumatic experience and there is no set formula for recovery. Seek counseling to support and guide you through the healing process. It is natural to feel grieved or ashamed but there are many resources available to help survivors get past these types of incidents.

What to Do If a Friend Has Been Sexually Assaulted

If a friend who has just been sexually assaulted asks for your help, be sure they are out of immediate danger right away. Ensure that the person receives appropriate medical attention and preserves any evidence. You cannot force someone to report the incident to law enforcement personnel but it is a good idea to suggest that they strongly consider that approach. If the person is willing, accompany your friend to the police, staying with him or her until all necessary procedures have been completed.

Anyone willing to talk to you about a sexual assault trusts you implicitly. It is paramount to remain a supportive, reassuring presence to help them get through their trauma. Studies show that a survivor of sexual assault is significantly affected throughout his or her recovery by the actions of and attitudes of the people in his/her support system. Your openness, willingness to listen, and non-judgmental support may be a key factor in his or her progress from victim to survivor.

Try to be non-judgmental. Allow your friend to tell you as little or as much as he/she wants to at his or her own pace. Although it does occasionally happen, few people lie about sexual assaults. No matter what your friend was wearing, how they were acting, or how much they had to drink, they are not responsible for being sexually assaulted. No one asks to be raped. Be cautious of asking questions that might imply otherwise. You will, no doubt, be dealing with someone is emotionally fragile, at least temporarily.

Be supportive. Let the person know that you believe in him/her and that he/she is not alone. Encourage your friend to express his or her feelings about what happened. Be interested and empathic without prying or pressing for details. Try not to criticize or judge. An essential part of a survivor's recovery involves regaining control that the rapist took away. Help your friend determine what options they have, and be supportive of whatever decisions they make.

Although your natural reaction may be to give your friend a hug, after a sexual assault many victims do not feel comfortable with physical contact even from close friends or family members, especially those who are members of the opposite sex. If you reach to hug the victim and then stop because you sense he/she is uncomfortable, your action may be interpreted as judgment or disgust. It is best to be available but not to push.

Hearing about a sexual assault is an upsetting experience. Try not to express your own feelings of anger or helplessness to your friend, or to project them onto him or her. You may even want to talk to a trusted friend or counselor about your feelings too. Once a crime has already been committed and the danger is past, countervailing force is no longer self-defense.

Resist the urge to become a vigilante and let law enforcement professionals take care of the situation. Becoming a vigilante will have consequences. Before you do anything hasty, think about whether or not the victim can afford to lose a caring friend to the justice system on top of physical and psychological damage he or she has already suffered from the original assault.

Rape Recovery

After the initial attack, a person who has been sexually assaulted is likely to experience emotional shock, denial, numbness, nightmares, sleeplessness, changes in appetite, difficulty working and concentrating, flashbacks, or a host of other traumatic symptoms. Feelings of guilt, despair, depression, self-blame, and anger are common. This is followed by a period of recovery that is frequently lengthy. During this time, the survivor may seem to recover completely yet intermittently re-experience the traumatizing effects of his or her assault.

Most survivors want to put the rape behind them and get on with their life as quickly as possible. Working through and talking about their feelings is an important step in accomplishing that goal. Beyond friends and family members, there are many organizations and support groups dedicated to helping victims overcome their feelings of helplessness and vulnerability. Bringing criminal charges and/or civil actions against an assailant helps many survivors restore their sense of personal integrity and power.

It is important that survivors make positive choices to spend time with people who believe in them and support them. They should avoid the temptation to isolate themselves or engage in destructive behaviors. Many find that certain friends or family members have complicated feelings about what has happened. If someone reacts in a way that hurts the survivor, he or she needs to get away from that person, at least temporarily. Survivors should spend time with people who can assist them without trying to control them, people who believe in them, and can help them sort out what they need to do to take care of themselves.

Drugs, Alcohol, and Rape

The vast majority of rapes involve drugs or alcohol or a combination of both substances. Both alcoholic and non-alcoholic drinks can be spiked without your knowledge. Watch your drink carefully at parties, bars, and public places. Do not leave your drink unattended or accept one from someone you do not know well or trust. Beyond alcohol, there are two main drugs commonly associated with sexual assaults: Rohypnol and GHB.

Rohypnol is the famous "date-rape" drug. The street names of this substance include roofies, rophies, and roachies. It is a small, white tablet, covered on one side with the manufacturer's name Roche above the number one or two imprinted on the reverse. The number represents the number of milligrams in the dosage. It is a fast-acting sleeping pill that is both potent and undetectable when slipped into an unsuspecting person's drink. Despite the fact that it has been illegal in the United States since 1996 and the fact that recent changes in the drug's formulation now leave telltale blue tracers and floating particles when mixed with liquids, it is still something to be concerned about.

Like all depressants, Rohypnol reduces anxiety and induces sleep. Users experience intense intoxication at low doses, particularly when the drug is used with alcohol. Common side effects include complete or partial amnesia, rapid mood swings, and violent outbursts of temper. When mixed with alcohol, overdoses are potentially life threatening. Effects of this drug begin 20 to 30 minutes after ingestion and typically continue for 8 to 12 hours. Rohypnol does not stay in the body for a long period of time so if you think you have been victimized by it you must get medical treatment as soon as possible to detect the presence of the drug.

Gamma Hydroxybutyrate (GHB) is a clear liquid with a somewhat metallic taste. Street names for this substance include liquid X, liquid E,* easy lay, and grievous bodily harm (GBH). It was first synthesized by a French researcher in the 1960s where it has been prescribed throughout Europe as a general anesthetic and childbirth aid, as well as for the treatment of insomnia, narcolepsy, and alcoholism.

This drug is structurally similar to the neurotransmitter GABA and triggers a variety of effects in the body, temporarily increasing the supply of both GABA and dopamine in the brain. At moderate doses, GHB induces a state of relaxation, euphoria, and diminished inhibition similar to alcohol. At higher does, GHB can

---

*Due to similarities in effect to the psychedelic drug ecstasy.

induce sleep so deep it has been mistaken for coma. It has been illegal in many states since 1997.

Since GHB occurs naturally in the human body as a chemical precursor in the production of GABA, it is relatively nontoxic though it can irritate the stomach and cause nausea or vomiting. Confusion and impaired motor skills may also occur, particularly at high doses, but food can reverse these effects. Effects begin within 5 to 20 minutes of ingestion and last 1 to 3 hours, though they can be prolonged through repeated dosing. GHB does not stay in the body for a long period of time so if you think you have been victimized by it you must get medical treatment as soon as possible to detect the presence of the drug.

Workplace Violence

"Eighteen thousand people are victimized in the workplace every week in the United States. Every week! While more and more companies are moving forward with innovative ways to control this alarming trend, it is imperative that all employees—office workers as well as those working in warehouses, on oil rigs, in manufacturing plants, and in a host of other workplaces—do all they can to stay safe." [10]

– Lt. Col. David Grossman

According to the National Institute for Occupational Safety and Health, workplace homicide is the leading cause of death among female workers in the United States and the second leading cause of death among men. As the quote above indicates, 18,000 people a week[11] are victimized by some sort of violence in the workplace in this country alone. Understanding how to protect yourself and your employees is indispensable knowledge.

This knowledge is critical even in areas where you generally would not consider yourself in danger such as a courthouse where weapons are prohibited and everyone has to pass through a metal detector before entering the building. On March 11, 2005, Fulton County (Georgia) Superior Court judge Rowland Barnes, 64, and his court reporter were killed in the courtroom by Brian Nichols, 33, who was on trial for rape and kidnapping at the time. According to police reports, he allegedly overpowered the female deputy who was escorting him to the proceedings to gain control of her gun. Nichols then used her keys to enter the courtroom, where he killed the judge and court reporter. From there he fled the building, killed another deputy, and then hijacked a car to effect his escape. He was captured 26 hours later after allegedly committing at least one more murder and kidnapping a woman who eventually convinced him to release her and turn himself in.

In the United States there are an average of 17 homicides in the workplace each week, many of which are largely unnoticed by the national media unless a Fortune 500 company, multiple victims, or high visibility victims like the aforementioned judge are involved. While the cost of policies, procedures, and personnel necessary to thwart this trend is costly, the price of inaction is high as well. Employers are frequently liable for the cost of medical treatment, wage replacement, and disability for injured employees. Beyond psychological and physiological damage to employees, families, and co-workers, and the economic costs thereof, a company's stock typically takes a 15 percent reduction for several weeks following these types of incidents, partially due to reduced productivity, adverse publicity, and anticipated legal costs.

The Washington State Department of Labor and Industries estimates that indirect costs of litigation, lost productivity, turnover, and administration related to these cases often run as high as 20 times the direct costs of medical treatment, wage-replacement, and disability pensions caused by workplace violence incidents. According to Michael Viollis, president of Risk Control Strategies, a New York security consulting company, the typical jury award to victims or surviving family members is about $3,100,000 per person per incident. Legal fees for major cases can easily exceed $400,000.

While such incidents can occur at any time in any location, some industries have a higher propensity for workplace violence than others do. In descending order of danger taxicab drivers, liquor store clerks, gasoline station attendants, protective service employees, public safety officers, retail store employees, hotel workers, and restaurant personnel have the highest incidents of workplace fatalities due to violent acts. Industries with the highest risks of non-fatal injuries include psychiatric hospital workers, residential care employees, nurses, job training service workers, protective services employees, law enforcement officers, social workers, and correctional institution employees.

Risk Factors

An analysis of certain risk factors can help identify circumstances in which workplace violence is more or less likely to occur. For example, organizations that handle large sums of money or liquidateable assets, where employees routinely work late at night, or that take charge of mentally disturbed or criminal subjects have a higher risk of violence than other types of agencies. While not an absolute predictor, the more risk factors the higher the danger. By understanding potential risks, you can tailor prevention measures that are appropriate to your business or workplace. General risk factors can include:

- Unstable or volatile clients (e.g., health care, social services, or criminal justice).
- Public contact or work in community-based settings (e.g., social services, real estate agencies, or retail stores).
- Site located in or near high-crime areas.
- Mobile workplace or delivery of passengers, goods or services (e.g., taxicab, bus, law enforcement, delivery services, or construction trades).
- Employees who work in isolation, late at night, or early in the morning (e.g., gas stations, convenience stores, or delivery drivers).
- Guarding valuable possessions or property (e.g., armored car, bank, or jewelry store).

Violence can be facilitated by the institutionalization of poor interpersonal dynamics in the workplace or by a proliferation of ill-trained or dictatorial management. Lack of policies, procedures, and other controls can also be a factor. While some types of workplaces are inherently more caustic than others, a hazard assessment should help identify risks that can be reduced or prevented. A comprehensive workplace violence program should be in place at every organization.

In developing proactive safety measures, it is often useful to categorize the type of violence employees are most likely to face as the strategies for dealing with each type may differ. While anything is possible, there are four major kinds of violence that can occur at the workplace. Some workplaces are more at risk from certain types than others are. The four types of workplace violence are:

- Stranger violence.
- Customer/client violence.
- Co-worker violence.
- Intimate violence.

Stranger Violence Scenario

Stranger violence involves threatening behaviors or physical assaults by people who have no legitimate business relationship to the workplace. People who perpetrate this type of violence are typically carrying out some sort of criminal act such as a rape or robbery on the premises. Workplaces locations at high risk for violence by strangers commonly include taxicabs and late night retail establishments.

Convenience store workers, for example, are frequently at risk from stranger violence since store hours mandate that someone must work late at night or early in the morning. These employees deal with money, work alone or in isolated locations, and are often located in or near high crime areas. Prevention measures might include de-escalation training for employees, minimizing the amount of cash on hand and posting signs advertising that fact, installing closed-circuit video cameras, enhancing lighting, communicating with police or security personnel, and staffing at least two employees per shift. Training plans should be developed and policies established so that front line workers will know what to do should a violent act occur.

Customer/Client Violence Scenario

Customer or client violence involves threatening behaviors or physical assaults by people who either receive services from or are under the custodial supervision of the affected workplace or victim. Assailants can be current or former customers or clients such as passengers, patients, students, inmates, or criminal suspects. Motives for such acts can include seeking revenge for a perceived injustice by the organization or its representatives, attempts to escape control or custody by an employee, or simply a reaction to psychosocial disorders in the perpetrator. Workplaces at high risk for this type of violence include any place that directly serves the public, including transportation drivers, health care providers, law enforcement, and sales personnel.

Social workers, for example, are frequently at risk from customer or client violence. They tend to work at sites with direct public contact or, at times, visit clients' homes in isolation. Furthermore, they tend to deal with clients who may have histories of mental illness or criminal behaviors. Prevention measures might include providing de-escalation training for employees, ensuring that client history is known to the counselors, eliminating client home visits or conducting such visits in teams, controlling access to the work location, and providing security personnel.

Delivery drivers* and trades people† who must enter other people's homes or businesses must be especially alert for potential dangers. Not only may they be threatened or attacked by others, but also they may be falsely accused of a whole host of crimes including robbery, rape, indecent liberties, sexual harassment, or assault. Deployment of distinctive uniforms, company identification badges, and frequent communication with dispatch personnel may help. It is a good idea to document arrival and departure times at each customer location via radio contact with the dispatcher and by filling out a time log. Be sure to minimize the amount of cash or valuables you carry while working these types of jobs.

Co-Worker Violence Scenario

Co-worker violence includes threatening behaviors or physical assaults by people who are employed by the same company as their victim or by a subcontractor or partner organization that routinely works with the victim. This includes current or former employees at all levels throughout a company. Co-workers who perpetrate

---

*Such as pizza deliverers, process servers, and couriers.
†Such as electricians, plumbers, alarm installers, and cable technicians.

this type of violence frequently seek revenge for something they consider unfair or unjust treatment.

Co-worker violence can happen at any time, but it is especially prevalent during stressful job-disruptions such as policy changes, strikes, mergers, acquisitions, divestitures, or layoffs. Be cognizant of employees who exhibit warning signs. These may include people who are chronic complainers, easily frustrated on the job, manipulative, unwilling to compromise, loners, or otherwise exhibit unprofessional or anti-social behavior on a regular basis. Offenders frequently have higher than average intelligence, less than average communication skills, and a history of run-ins with bosses or co-workers. They may be chronic drug or alcohol abusers, romantically obsessed with a co-worker, severely depressed, or obsessed with weapons, police, or military work.

Although anyone can kill at the workplace, perpetrators are typically long-term employees of a company who exhibit many of the warning signs above. They are most often male, aged 35 to 50, though females and younger and older employees have initiated workplace violence in the past. The vast majority of perpetrators make threats or joke about killing or hurting co-workers before they act. Two-thirds of such individuals kill themselves after committing an extreme act of violence.

Prevention measures might include providing de-escalation training for employees, instituting zero-tolerance policies for violent behavior, developing procedures for effectively dealing with disciplinary issues, offering access to employee assistance programs or counseling services, hiring security personnel, and developing emergency evacuation plans. Disruptive job events such as layoffs, mergers, outsourcing, or offshoring should be carefully planned and well communicated throughout the organization.

Many companies also prohibit weapons on their premises though I would argue that such policies are more likely to do harm than good. Lawbreakers will ignore such rules anyway. Potential victims, on the other hand, will be less able to defend themselves when attacked.

Intimate Violence Scenario

Intimate violence on the job includes threatening behavior or physical assault by someone with whom the victim has a personal relationship outside of work. This could include current or former spouses, lovers, relatives, or friends of the victim. People who perpetrate this type of violence are typically motivated by perceived difficulties in the relationship or by psychosocial factors that are unique to that individual or their relationship.

There is a complete section on intimate violence already in this chapter so we will focus on workplace prevention factors here to avoid being redundant. Prevention measures might include providing de-escalation training for employees, offering access to employee assistance programs or counseling services, offering domestic violence prevention training, controlling access to the worksite, ensuring that management and co-workers are aware of any restraining orders that might be in place, developing emergency evacuation plans, and hiring security personnel. If you know that a co-worker has a restraining order against his or her spouse be extra cautious until his or her situation is resolved.

Violence Prevention Plans

Violent acts generally occur in predictable types of sites and settings so when risks are identified proactive plans can be set in place to reduce or eliminate them. To be effective, a senior executive should be appointed to spearhead the program. Management and employees should work together to develop the plan, ensure buy-in, commit resources, provide motivation to address issues, and provide feedback. Policies should be well thought out, comprehensive, fair, and clearly communicated.

Hazard assessments should examine risk factors and determine vulnerabilities for stranger, customer, co-worker, and intimate violence on the job. Incidents that do occur should be tracked and analyzed to determine what caused the failure and prevent it from happening again. Training, reporting, recordkeeping, and periodic evaluations should be integrated into the plan. Employee welfare should be the first priority.

Procedures should be set in place to ensure a coordinated response if an attack occurs, addressing employee safety, site security, emergency services, and medical triage among other issues. If an incident occurs, site safety must be assessed, medical and law enforcement personnel must be contacted, incident areas must be secured to preserve evidence, and all employees must be accounted for. Provisions for medical and psychological follow-up, medical confidentiality, and payment of salary or benefits after the event must be in place where needed to prevent victims from suffering further loss.

Employer Liability

Employers may face civil claims from the victims of workplace violence as well as from perpetrators, witnesses and others who are peripherally involved. Claims can include, but are not limited to, negligent hiring, negligent retention, wrongful termination, and failure to warn. Measures an employer takes to prevent workplace violence may limit potential liability. Some important steps include:

- Develop and implement a comprehensive risk mitigation plan.
- Provide safety education for employees so that they will understand what conduct is acceptable and know what to do during an emergency.

- Conduct comprehensive background and reference checks for all potential new hires and use credit checks to verify job applicant information.

- Research prior criminal convictions of potential hires that might reasonably relate to job duties as permitted by law. For example, registered sex offenders cannot legally work with or around children in most jurisdictions.

- Secure the workplace, limiting access by outsiders to sensitive areas via the use of identification badges, cipher locks, electronic keys, security personnel, and/or other reliable methods.

- Pre-program emergency numbers into employee phones and cellular devices. For personnel who have not been trained how to react under stress, fine motor skills are lost under the effects of adrenaline making it very difficult if not impossible to do something as simple as dialing 9-1-1. In locations where 9-9-1-1 dialing is required this can be even more challenging as more conscious thought is required to do it correctly.

- Conduct routine drug and alcohol testing where appropriate. This generally means that testing must be job related and consistent with business necessity as permitted by law.

- If employees work with large amounts of cash, provide safe drops to limit the amount of available cash on hand, especially during late evening and early morning hours.

- If employees must make home visits establish specific policies and procedures regarding client contact, ensure the presence of others as appropriate, and establish the right of employees to use discretion in avoiding hazardous situations.

- Ensure that any company vehicles are properly maintained and equip field staff with cellular phones or other communication devices.

Employee Safety

Nothing can guarantee that an employee will never become a victim of workplace violence, yet there are prudent precautions that anyone can take to become more secure regardless of whether or not their company has a comprehensive workplace violence prevention program. Start by learning how to recognize, avoid, or de-escalate potentially violent situations by attending employer-provided training where available or finding private courses to go to on your own. Be sure to alert management of any safety or security concerns you may have and be assertive to ensure that your fears are understood. Additional suggestions include:

- Know your company's workplace violence procedures and emergency plans.
- Be professional, treating everyone you interact with on the job with dignity and respect.

- Carry only minimal money and required identification if you have to travel into community settings on the job.
- Avoid entering any location that you feel is unsafe.
- Report unusual co-worker or customer behaviors to management.
- Use a buddy system so that someone else is prepared to act in concert with you should an incident occur at the job site and so that someone knows where you are at all times if you have to travel to other locations to perform your work.
- Identify hazards, escape routes, alternate exits, and hiding places at your workplace and along any routes you must travel to, from, or on the job.
- Identify areas of cover or concealment where you can hide from an attacker but also be aware that those same areas can also be used by perpetrators for ambushing their victims.
- Be aware of improvised weapons such as hot coffee, fire extinguishers, chairs, tools, lumber, company vehicles, cutlery, scissors, telephones, attaché cases, or car keys that you can easily access in an emergency. If you have a concealed weapons license understand your company's policy regarding weapons in the workplace.
- If something bad does happen on the job, never assume that someone else has already reported the incident. Call law enforcement personnel immediately upon reaching a safe location. Answer questions calmly and concisely, stay on the line, and follow the dispatcher's instructions.
- If you have to run from an attacker, try to keep objects such as furniture, boxes, vehicles or machinery between you and your assailant. Everyone will need to make a personal choice about evading or dodging given the unique characteristics of each encounter, but I'm inclined to just run as fast as I can toward safety, grabbing any improvised weapon I come across that can be picked up without slowing me down for possible use later. If you cannot get out a door, do not hesitate to use a window or even break through an interior wall as necessary to escape an attacker. If you cannot run, you will want to hide, regardless of whether the perpetrator is looking for you specifically or simply attacking random victims.

Summary

"Let the fear of danger be a spur to prevent it; he that fears not, gives advantage to the danger." [12]

– Francis Quarles

This chapter has been an extension of the awareness and avoidance topics grouped around specific scenarios that practitioners might encounter in their daily lives. Each scenario delves in-depth into unique characteristics, concerns, and safety strategies so that you will have a good idea of what you can do to protect yourself should you encounter any of these situations.

Carjackings

Carjacking is typically a crime of opportunity, frequently related to another crime such as an armed robbery or gang initiation. While it can happen just about anywhere, you are more vulnerable at highway exit ramps, intersections controlled by stoplights or signs, isolated garages, and other locations where you must slow down or come to a stop. Another common variation is called a "bump and rob" where perpetrators cause a minor traffic accident in order to commandeer your vehicle.

Carjacking rarely leads to murder yet the two are linked on occasion. If a carjacker threatens you with a gun or other weapons, your best option is frequently to give him/her your vehicle and leave the area as quickly as possible. Despite the trauma of facing a weapon and the inconvenience of losing your vehicle, your life is worth a whole lot more than your car.

Cash Machines

Most ATM robbery victims report using a cash machine at night by themselves before they were surprised by the perpetrator. Consequently, limiting use to daylight hours and bringing a friend to watch your back are two good strategies for remaining safe. Cash machines in stores or bank lobbies are generally safer than stand-alone kiosks. Do not become so focused on your transaction that you lose sight of your surroundings. Awareness is always your best defense.

Hostage Situations

A hostage situation is a little different from an active shooter situation. In the former, there is typically time for negotiation, police intervention, escape, or some other non-violent response on the part of the hostage. In the latter, you are in imminent danger and must react immediately to save yourself. The first 15 to 20 minutes of a hostage crisis are typically the most dangerous. Scenarios that play out longer than that frequently end non-violently.

There are three main types of hostage takers: psychological, criminal, and political. Psychological hostage takers include suicidal personalities, vengeance seekers, and disturbed individuals. Criminal hostage takers include extortionists, aggrieved inmates, and cornered perpetrators. Political hostage takers include social protesters, fanatics, and terrorist extremists. Law enforcement professionals categorize hostage takers in this fashion to help shape an appropriate response.

If you have been taken hostage and are convinced that your captor is going to kill you it is a good idea to attempt to escape at an opportune moment. In most cases, however, it is far better to do nothing offensive, letting professional police negotiators handle the situation. Pay attention to your captors and your surroundings, gathering data that can help the police if you are released or can escape.

Intimate or Domestic Violence

Domestic violence is a learned behavior, typically involving controlling actions that encompass different types or levels of abuse such as physical harm, imminent fear of physical harm, sexual assault, or stalking among individuals who have had some type of intimate relationship in the past. These situations tend to escalate with several minor incidents preceding major ones.

There are several warning signs that may predict eventual abuse such as frequent displays of anger, attempts at isolation, threats, or physical attacks. The victim's behavior in such cases can help either ensure their survival or lead to their destruction. One of the most important things a domestic violence abuse victim can do is get away from the perpetrator before things get worse. There are several public and private organizations that offer resources to assist those trying to escape a dangerous domestic situation.

Public Transportation

Public transportation such as airplanes, buses, and trains can present unique self-defense challenges. Such environments are captive, mobility impairing, and somewhat dependant upon the actions of the pilot, driver, or engineer to assure your safety. Sit near the driver where possible. Pay attention to and report any unusual passenger behaviors. Similarly look for and report any suspicious unattended packages, devices, or pieces of luggage.

Sexual Assault, Rape, and Molestation

Rape can happen to anyone regardless of age, sex, sexual orientation, or income level. A majority of sexual assault victims have some acquaintance with the perpetrator before the crime is committed. As always, awareness is your best line of defense.

So is communication. Be clear, assertive, and open about your expectations, interests, and limits to avoid misunderstandings and respect the wishes of others. No really means no, both legally and morally. Be sure to avoid making yourself an easy target for strangers by taking general precautions about where and when you travel, especially when going out alone. Furthermore, keep a close eye on anything you eat or drink in public places as certain drugs such as Rohypnol may be used to facilitate a sexual assault.

Workplace Violence

While workplace violence can happen to anyone, certain locations, industries, and careers have a higher propensity for this danger than others do. There are four types of workplace violence including acts caused by strangers, customers/clients, co-workers, or intimates. Violent acts at work generally occur in predictable settings and sites so hazards can be identified and prevention plans established to reduce the risk. Employers may face civil claims from victims, perpetrators, witnesses, and even those peripherally involved so a comprehensive mitigation plan is prudent.

Regardless of whether or not your employer has developed an emergency plan there are precautions that all employees can take on their own to make themselves more secure. Be sure to alert management of any safety or security concerns you might have and be assertive to ensure that your fears are understood. Be aware of escape paths and makeshift weapons on the job that you could utilize to defend yourself should things get ugly.

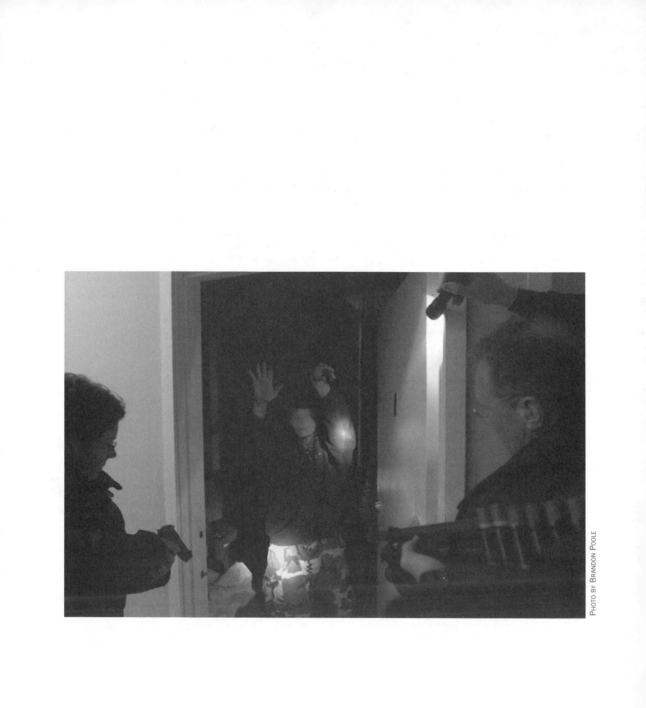

CHAPTER 4

De-Escalation Strategies

"What are you going to do, shoot us?" [1]

– Nicole duFresne

On January 27, 2005, actress Nicole duFresne was shot and killed by an armed robber immediately after uttering her fateful last words, "What are you going to do, shoot us?" This tragedy is an excellent case study in what not to do when confronted by an armed aggressor.

According to news reports, the suspect Rudy Fleming, age 19, and his friends allegedly believed that duFresne and her party would be easy marks for a purse snatching. What was supposed to be a simple property crime turned deadly when the 28-year old actress became confrontational with Fleming after he stole her friend's purse and pistol-whipped her fiancé. She became furious, shoved him, and died shortly thereafter in her fiancé's arms.

Many experts state that robbery is more often about power than anything else. Discussing the duFresne shooting, Alfonso Lenhardt of the National Crime Prevention Council said, "It's a tragedy, but in this case it sounds like the suspect felt he wasn't getting the respect he was due. When a gun is in the hands of a desperate person with low self-esteem, they're going to react that way."

Property is replaceable. Your life is not. If you can satisfy an attacker by giving him/her your wallet, you will be far better for it. After all, anything you live through and learn something from cannot be all bad. Save your righteous indignation for a safer environment after the immediate danger has past. It does you no good to be right yet dead. Having to be right despite the cost or reacting indignantly in the face of a threat frequently guarantees that a conflict will escalate out of control.

Rage is an extreme, energized, and frequently explosive state of anger, typically coinciding with an adrenaline rush, which further clouds the mind. Emotions over-rule your common sense in this state. Like duFresne's righteous indignation, road rage is another instance where an out of control attitude can get you killed. For example, Mark Leidheisl, 39, a regional senior vice president for Wells Fargo, died on April 20, 2005 from a blunt force trauma injury to the head. Sacramento police reported that the incident that led to Leidheisl's death might have been fueled by road rage and that he appeared to have been the aggressor. An unmarked medicine bottle in Leidheisl's car contained Paxil (an antidepressant), morphine (extended tab painkiller), and an unidentified third pill type. Tests later found that he had a blood alcohol level of at least 0.13 (more than the legal driving limit of 0.08) and opiates in his system.

Reports state that Leidheisl allegedly cut off another vehicle while driving out of Arco Arena's parking lot after the Wednesday night game. Leidheisl, a friend and the two men in the other vehicle reportedly exchanged heated words, stopped and got out of their vehicles on a nearby street. During the subsequent fight, Leidheisl fell and hit his head on the pavement, causing the fatal injury. The suspects from the other vehicle, ages 43 and 44, reportedly left but contacted police after seeing news reports about how serious Leidheisl was hurt.

District Attorney Jan Scully told reporters, "After a thorough review of the police investigation, it is clear that Mark Leidheisl died as a result of mutual combat between him and Jeffrey Berndt. One punch thrown in self-defense by Jeffrey Berndt struck Mark Leidheisl in the face, causing him to fall backwards striking his head on the asphalt pavement. This fall fractured Leidheisl's skull, causing his death."

De-escalation is the opposite of escalation, a reduction of the intensity in a conflict. This same phenomenon can be seen in interpersonal, inter-company, and even international relations, as all conflict inevitably stems from disagreements among individuals regardless of what ideology or interest they represent. De-escalation can occur quickly, even spontaneously, especially when a conflict escalates so rapidly that the parties involved fear that any further escalation would be catastrophic and they back off. This only works so long as logic prevails over emotion, however. Enraged people seldom act in their own enlightened self-interest.

A good example of spontaneous de-escalation might be the so-called "Mexican standoff," a common movie cliché where two or more opponents have weapons, typically guns, aimed directly at each other at close range, so that one cannot attack the other without being hurt or killed themselves. Facing certain death, such individuals may be motivated to find a saner alternative. This tension makes movies interesting, but the scenario is not all that common in real life.

The Cuban Missile Crisis[2] was a more realistic example of this sort of thing actually occurring. This same type of phenomenon can also come into play in real-life self-defense situations where we face off against an aggressor who has not yet attacked. There are several strategies we can employ to facilitate de-escalation before things spiral out of control but it does take proactive effort. So long as at least one side believes they can win, de-escalation can be harder to achieve. It is often brought about by changing the context and/or by convincing a predator that it will be too expensive to follow-through on a threat. My laughing at the guy with the knife at the stadium is a good example of a context changing strategy.

Unlike escalation, which often occurs rapidly and unintentionally, de-escalation usually takes effort to bring about. In some circumstances, it may not occur until both parties have reached a prolonged stalemate where neither side can prevail but where both are harmed by continuing the confrontation. Once both sides realize this is the case, they are much more likely to be willing to negotiate at least a temporary (or even a permanent) settlement to the conflict. This sort of thing might be seen during a hostage standoff.

Since it does not usually happen by itself, a variety of approaches is possible to facilitate de-escalation including talking, commanding, co-opting, and submitting.

Talk

"The human race has one really effective weapon, and that is laughter. Against the assault of laughter nothing can stand." [3]

– Mark Twain

It is best to avoid trouble completely via awareness and avoidance. If you cannot simply walk away from a potentially hazardous encounter, however, you may still be able to de-escalate the situation before anything really bad happens. An angry or aggressive person, for example, may just want to vent their outrage. In many instances, you can do a lot of good by calmly listening to them as they rant, all the while preparing yourself to act if attacked, of course. Interject a few choice words as necessary to help them see the situation in a new light.

For example, I stopped at an Arco station to get gas on my way home from work recently. Their price was roughly ten cents per gallon cheaper than anyone else in the area was so they were very crowded. Because the ATM kiosks by the pumps were not working, I had to go into the store, wait in line to pre-pay, and then go back out to fill my tank. After doing so, I had to go back into the store to retrieve a couple of dollars in change.

As I approached the door to retrieve my change I could hear shouting coming from inside. Two women were arguing with the clerk. As I stood in line, I could not help but hear their dispute over the next several minutes. They claimed to have given the clerk $22 to pre-pay and asserted that he put the money on the wrong pump. They said that they had received no gas and wanted him to either restart the pump or give them their money back. He countered initially that they had not paid him, then later that they had told him the wrong pump number and that it was not his fault if someone else pumped gas on their dime. His story changed several times. As the argument escalated, one of the women in line behind me went outside to call the cops. Several others simply left without buying anything. Everyone was very uncomfortable.

The distraught women were African Americans. They were dressed in quality but dirty coveralls, had some sort of ID badges I could not read clipped to their waists, and were very buff. I imagine that they worked as mechanics, maintenance workers, or something similar and had just gotten off work. Neither was a small person. I am 5'10" tall and they were both around my height. The clerk was a dark-skinned Middle Eastern-looking guy, shorter and skinnier than either woman. He had a heavy accent and was a little hard to understand, especially when he raised his voice. Eventually as one of the women called the clerk a liar for the umpteenth time, he retorted that she was a "Fat, uppity bitch." This, as you would probably expect, did not go over too well!

The insulted woman went stiff, then spun on her heel and headed toward the door while her friend continued to argue with the clerk. As she turned past me, I got a good look at her face and jumped several notches up the threat index scale. The last time I saw that "thousand-yard stare" when someone left a building, he returned a short time later with a gun.* Fearing something similar, I decided that I had better do something about it.

As she left, I noticed that she used her right hand to open the door and that she wore a watch on her left wrist so I assumed that she was right-handed. I followed her out as she stalked toward her car. She was not moving very fast so I easily caught up a dozen feet past the door. I figured that she was not armed (yet), so I took a position behind her left shoulder a couple feet back assuming that I would have the most reaction time that way if she did anything untoward.

Having positioned myself where I wanted to be, I calmly said, "You know they have half a dozen video cameras in there. Your transaction must be on tape."

She froze in place but clearly was not really processing what I said so I repeated it again adding, "All you need to do is have the manager review the tape to prove your story. There are cameras out here too so they'll know that you didn't pump any gas." What I did not add was, "... and they'll record anything stupid you're about to do too," but I suspect she figured that out on her own. That was my intent anyway.

She slowly said, "You're right, they do have cameras in there" three or four times. As she did so, I could virtually see the rage draining from her. She turned to face me and said it again, adding, "Thank you."

I replied, "No problem. You probably ought to explain that to your friend." She corrected, "She's my cousin," then said, "Yeah, I'll talk to her."

I followed her back inside. While she pulled her cousin aside and began to calm

---

*I wisely bailed before he returned, reading about the aftermath the next day in the local paper.

her down, I got my change from the clerk. As he handed me the money I pointed out the cameras to him too. He got a goofy look on his face as the realization that everything was being recorded dawned on him too. I honestly do not know who was "right" in this dispute but the look he gave me seemed to validate the ladies' claim. He looked very uncomfortable and real "guilty," something I strongly suspected from his changing story, frustration, and personalization* during the interchange. At the very least, he was unwilling to admit to making a mistake.

The interesting thing is that while the presence of a half a dozen highly visible cameras was obvious to me, no one in the dispute seemed to notice them. Pointing them out changed everyone's context, kicking things down several notches. I will never know for sure if the angry woman was going for a weapon, but I strongly suspect that I prevented something bad, probably something really bad, from happening when I intervened.

I did not stick around to find out how it was all resolved because I had to pick my son up from daycare though I did see a cop car coming toward the place as I was driving away.

Active Listening

I use this tactic a lot because it works frequently and well. There is a trick to it though. Listening, really listening is challenging for most people. In conversations, we often do not truly listen to what others are saying because we are busy formulating our own responses, figuring out rebuttals to the other person's arguments, or thinking up better ways to explain our own perspective. In these instances, we hear but we do not listen. In fact, studies have shown that the typical person devotes less than half of their attention to figuring out exactly what the other person is trying to communicate in a routine conversation.

Active listening is not the opposite of talking. It is a wholehearted attempt to truly understand where another person is coming from. The four principles of active listening include:

- Remaining neutral to the extent possible.
- Giving complete attention.
- Asking clarifying questions.
- Restating the person's main points as necessary to clarify understanding.

Remaining Neutral

Remaining neutral is often harder than it sounds. In stressful situations, it is far better to truly understand the other party first. Examine things from their perspective. Only then should we seek to be understood, presenting our own point of view.

---

*Someone who is unwilling to admit that he or she made a mistake is almost always going to take the argument to a personal level, sooner or later. At that point the conflict is no longer about the mistake.

Jumping to conclusions too quickly may cause you to miss an essential point or may even spark a violent reaction from the other person as they become frustrated with you. Never forget that with few exceptions, no one is evil in his or her own eyes. The other person will often look for justification to make the confrontation your fault, even if they started it from your perspective. He or she may try to get you to say something that can be used as justification to launch an attack.

Giving Complete Attention

Giving complete attention is also easier said than done. This means focusing only on the person to whom you are listening, ignoring all but life-threatening distractions. Since a significant part of communication comes from nonverbal cues, pay attention to your body language. Maintain direct, non-threatening eye contact, lean slightly forward but not so much that you look aggressive, and resist any desire to fidget.

If you are dealing with someone who has spent some length of time in prison direct eye contact may be inadvisable. When dealing with a convict, he or she will usually be more comfortable (and will subconsciously take it as rapport) if your eyes keep scanning the surrounding environment as you talk while standing a little to one side of the person. It is how convicts who trust each other talk while watching each other's backs.

Asking Clarifying Questions

The concept of asking clarifying questions is self-evident, but there is an art to doing it right. Your queries should be used to subtly demonstrate understanding and sympathy for the person's perspective. That does not mean that you have to agree, merely understand. Empathy can go a long way toward eliminating hostility in another person.

Restating the Other Person's Main Points

Restating the person's main points, as necessary, is an excellent way to clarify understanding. It can be a positive way of ensuring that you really understand where a person is coming from. By restating their points in your own words, you can be supportive of them as individuals whether or not you agree with the particular opinion(s) they expressed. Active listening demonstrates respect for a person's perspective. This empathy absorbs tension, de-escalating tense situations most of the time.

Interpersonal Communication

If there is more than one person involved in an escalating conflict, you may attempt to take on a mediation role. In these instances, it is best not to take anyone's side, even the angry person's, unless you know everything about the situation that sparked their anger. Sometimes the angry person is the one in the wrong rather than the victim of someone else's aggression. Sometimes they are right to be upset. You can easily make things worse by taking sides without full knowledge. In the afore-mentioned gas station confrontation, I felt an imperative to intervene and things worked out well. If both people are part of a group and you intervene as an outsider, however they may turn on you. This is not due to bad de-escalation technique but simply because you will be perceived as an interloper.

Be cautious about what you say as you try to de-escalate a tense situation, especially when you are intervening in someone else's conflict. More than half of face-to-face communication comes through non-verbal cues. About 7 to 10 percent of communication comes from what you say, 33 to 40 percent from your tone of voice, and 50 to 60 percent from your facial expressions, body language, and gestures. Most people can detect any disingenuous words you utter, likely making you a target for their anger.

Exercise extreme care whenever someone is inebriated. Indicators of intoxication may include a person whose pupils does not match the ambient light (e.g., pinpoints in a dim room, heavy dilation in sunlight), who is irregularly or heavily breathing, screaming, babbling, using excessively foul language, talking too fast or too slow, moving too fast or too slow, or sweating excessively. Never, ever argue with someone who is drunk or high. The old saying goes, "Reason goes into the bottle faster than the alcohol comes out of it." If you can get away with it, just smile, nod, and say "Yes" or "No" as appropriate.

Do not react to merely provocative words or gestures. Strive to remain calm within the storm of verbal abuse. An old *samurai* proverb states, "When a man throws the spear of insult at your head, move your head! The spear will miss the target, leaving the man empty handed. The spear will be in the wall rather than in you." You will be much better off if you can ignore insulting comments and move on in the discussion. There are a whole lot of people out there who would just love to goad you into striking them so that they can claim self-defense when they trounce you.

Be sure your body language matches your words. Be alert to move if need be, but not aggressively postured. Do not look like a rabbit ready to run or a wolf ready to pounce. Standing in nice, evenly balanced posture with your hands held slightly in front of you is a reasonable compromise to adopting a martial stance. If you do have to use your martial arts skills to defend yourself, there is no point in warning the bad guy that you have been trained how to fight ahead of time. We will discuss this more in Chapter 6 with the "I don't want to fight" stance.

Threats or aggressive and intimidating actions may need to be acknowledged and even confronted. However, be careful about being imperious or arrogant or returning a threat unless you can back it up successfully. It may be better to ask the person to stop using that language or making those gestures as a sign of mutual respect. There can be serious legal consequences if you contribute to escalating a situation that ultimately turns violent, especially if you win. There can other serious consequences if you lose.

Clever Words

Even if you cannot de-escalate a situation simply by talking, clever words can enable you stall until help arrives or the attacker changes his/her mind and leaves. You can also use conversation as a psychological weapon to increase your chances of surviving as well as to create openings for

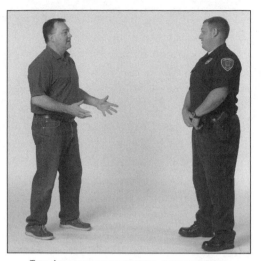

TALK. ACTIVELY LISTEN TO POTENTIAL ADVERSARIES WHILE REMAINING ABLE TO PHYSICALLY REACT IF NECESSARILY.

your physical defenses. Deception, for example, is but one of the tactics you might choose to employ. Any convincing distraction you can create will be to your advantage, such as shouting for nonexistent friends. There is strength in numbers and in making an aggressor believe you are not alone.

If you realize that de-escalation is not working and that you will have no other choice but to fight, it may also be possible to cause your opponent to make a mental twitch, providing a moment of opportunity to counterattack while they mentally shift gears. This twitch is brought about by dissonance between what the person expects and what you actually say or do.

A common example is asking a question. While the bad guy is focusing on your words or thinking about an answer, you have a moment in which to run or strike. This may be particularly useful when confronted with multiple assailants. Ask something completely unexpected like, "What time is it?" or something really odd like, "What was Gandhi's batting average?" or say something disgusting like, "I'm going to rape you!"* Cognitive dissonance is powerful. During the opponent's momentary confusion, you will have an opportunity to act. Similarly, if you can hit an aggressor while he or she is talking it takes about half a second for them to mentally switch gears from communicating to fighting.

---

*Though this won't play too well in court if anyone overhears it.

Command

"More powerful than a standing army is a well spoken word." [4]

— *Napoleon*

Law enforcement professionals and military personnel have an advantage in many encounters where they have the authority to command compliance from an unruly party. Priests and members of the clergy have authority over their parishioners too. When dealing with children or underlings we all have a certain amount of hierarchical authority that we may be able to draw upon to order compliance with our wishes. In certain cultures, senior citizens may be able to exercise authority over younger individuals whether or not they are members of the same family. Just because we have the authority to demand something, however, does not necessarily mean that everyone will comply. The fugitive may resist, the soldier may desert, the employee may disregard, and the child may remain obstinate.

COMMAND. HIERARCHICAL AUTHORITY MAY ALLOW YOU TO COMMAND COMPLIANCE FROM AN UNRULY INDIVIDUAL.

In his book *Verbal Judo*, George Thompson recommends a five-step process for communicating with difficult people. It is an escalation continuum that helps you place context and respond accordingly rather than simply reacting to whatever the other party does. These steps keep you from having to merely restate a request over and over again, a process that is not only prone to failure but also a sign of weakness, which can degrade whatever authority you have. Flexibility and variation, on the other hand, frequently imply strength. The process works like this:

- Stage 1 – Asking.
- Stage 2 – Setting the context.
- Stage 3 – Presenting options.
- Stage 4 – Confirming.
- Stage 5 – Acting.

Asking

In stage one you ask to aggressor to do whatever it is you would like. For example, the person may be threatening you with a knife. Assuming that you see the weapon and he has not already attacked, you are most likely dealing with an intimidation attempt rather than a botched assassination. This is something you may be able de-escalate before it gets really ugly. Your stage one request will undoubtedly be for the aggressor to drop or put away the weapon: "Sir, I want you to lower your weapon."

Be very clear about what you want the person to do. Individuals attacking you may be drunk, intoxicated, or suffer from certain mental conditions that affect their ability to reason. Saying something like, "don't make me shoot you," is not necessarily clear enough for someone who is reasoning impaired to understand and comply with. "Drop the knife now," on the other hand, is pretty hard to misunderstand. Avoid negatives: tell the person what to do rather than what not to do. It would be a shame to have to kill somebody simply because they could not figure out what you were ordering them to do.

Setting the Context

In stage two, you explain why you are making the request. "That's a large knife you are carrying. It places me in immediate fear for my life." This not only ensures absolute clarity about what you want but also shows potential witnesses the severity of the situation, identifying the aggressor and placing you in good legal standing if your de-escalation attempt ultimately fails.

Setting the context can also help the aggressor understand your point of view. On occasion, the person truly does not realize that the consequences of what they are doing or the fact that it is unacceptable or wrong. Furthermore, he or she may not recognize your authority to get them to comply. A concise, logical explanation may be enough where merely asking, in and of itself, is not sufficient.

Presenting the Options

In stage three, you present options in the other person's best interest that help him understand why he should comply. "I am also carrying a weapon. If you put down you knife we can talk about this. If you fail to comply, I'm going to have to shoot you."

This helps the aggressor understand the potential consequences of his or her actions. Never forget that as long as your opponent feels that he can win, he will have little motivation to comply. These situations are very complex; winning is a fluid idea. Once that person recognizes the severity of the situation, on the other hand, he may be more inclined to cooperate.

Confirming

In stage four, you ascertain with certainty whether or not the other person will cooperate. "Now I'd really rather not spend the rest of the evening cleaning up blood and filling out paperwork and I suspect you'd rather be sipping a beer and watching the game than sitting in the hospital so why don't you put down the knife and we'll talk. What is it going to be? Will you drop the knife now?" If you are going to say something like this, however, you really need the body language to back it up or it will likely backfire.

You have already asked the person to comply, explained why you are asking, and presented alternatives that demonstrate that it would be in their enlightened self-interest to acquiesce to your demands. There can be no confusion about what you want the person to do. His or her response to your confirming question will help you understand whether or not force will be required to gain compliance.

Acting

In stage five, you have to act to achieve compliance. If this particular scenario reaches stage five, either you or your attacker will undoubtedly end up getting seriously hurt. I hope that it will never escalate that far but if it does, you will at least know that you tried your best to keep it from reaching that point. This approach may also play out favorably in a court of law as well.

Furthermore, by understanding and practicing this five-step approach you will be able to use it to make calm, rational decisions under severe stress. Even if you do not have hierarchical authority, your physical presence, martial training, or the weapon in your possession may allow you to command compliance with your wishes. Consequently, it is good to understand this five-step process.

Co-Opt

"Because at many times and for many purposes it [the tongue] is the fittest weapon... For the tongue is such a weapon without it be governed, it will cut worse than any sword, sting worse than any nettle, prick deeper than a thorn." [5]

– Joseph Swetnam

If you are a regular civilian like me, especially one who works security or otherwise interacts with the public on the job, the odds are good that you will find yourself in a situation where you can use the threat of an authority figure to gain compliance from a potential adversary. A co-opting strategy attempts to make you look like the good guy, someone who insulates the other party from negative consequences of their actions. In other words, if the aggressor complies or cooperates with you, the "big bad cop" will not be called upon to haul him away. Because you want to be on his side, you will do what you can to let him off the hook if he will just cooperate.

I use this approach all the time at the stadium. Because we are on a college campus, no alcohol is allowed in the facility yet folks smuggle it in anyway. If someone is drinking and disruptive, we generally make an arrest, yet if he/she is merely drinking and causing no trouble, we are a bit more lenient. If the illicit drinker is willing to hand over his/her contraband without any fuss, he or she gets to stay and watch the game. If that person refuses or causes any trouble, he/she is escorted out.

I usually say something along the lines of, "I'm sorry sir, but alcohol is not permitted in the stadium. You are going to have to hand that over to me." If he appears reluctant, I will add, "You know if you give it to me, I'll just toss out the beer and not tell anyone. You get to stay and watch the game. If I have to get the cops, on the other hand, they'll toss you out. In addition, they'll give you a big, expensive citation. Wouldn't you rather just give me the beer?" Stated that way, ninety-five percent of football fans hand over the alcohol and I have no further problems with them. Some even thank me for keeping them out of trouble.

Another co-option strategy I like to employ at the stadium involves an incident report form. I carry around a clipboard or binder with several pre-printed forms that are used to document altercations and incidents for our official record. These notes may be used in court or may simply be recorded as lessons learned so that we can continuously improve our operations. From time to time, however, I use them for another purpose: to calm down an irate fan.

Every so often someone gets upset about something we just cannot fix at the time such as when the roof leaks, the referees blow a call, the concession stand closes halfway through the fourth quarter, or a television camera operator blocks someone's view by refusing to kneel down during a play. When these types of situations arise, I like to give the irate person a form to fill out rather than telling him or her that there is nothing that I can do about their concern. It not only demonstrates that I care about what the person thinks, but it also helps them focus their anger in a constructive manner. They have to articulate their issue, writing it down in a coherent and legible manner.

By the time the person is done writing down their concern nine out of ten are no longer upset. Even if we never follow up on the complaint, the simple fact that the person was able to communicate what was bothering them helps de-escalate the situation. Furthermore, by having a record of the problem, we are frequently able to alleviate it at a future event. There are tons of other ways to demonstrate empathy for another person, most of which can reduce tension and de-escalate conflict.

Another way to co-opt a person is by setting reasonable limits. In the east end zone we frequently have fans from two rival schools sitting in close proximity to each other, one set primarily in the north end and the other primarily in the south end of the bleachers. There is always someone who wants to taunt the other guys, throw things, or simply get in someone else's face in an immature display of school spirit. Typically, these individuals are inebriated and are attending the game with several buddies who want egg them on.

Co-opting is an effective approach here too. I frequently tell the rowdies that so long as they stay on their side of the seats and keep the profanities to a minimum that they can cheer lead, jump up and down, scream, yell, and otherwise blow off as much steam as they would like. I draw the line at the goal post, a convenient demarcation to separate the two sets of fans. I set these rules early, talking to the bare-chested, the paint emblazoned, the overly enthusiastic, and others likely to cause trouble. Because I am seen as reasonable, they generally comply. The first time someone steps over the line, I warn that person that I cannot keep the cops from acting when he or she is caught, nor will I protect him/her if the other fans fight back. That usually helps too.

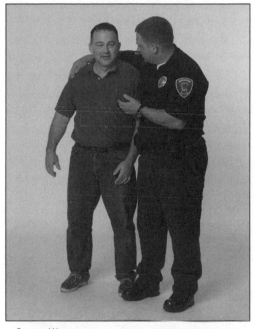

CO-OPT. WHILE THIS GESTURE LOOKS FRIENDLY IT ALSO POSI-TIONS YOU TO PHYSICALLY CONTROL A PERSON WITH LESS EFFORT SINCE YOUR HANDS ARE PRE-POSITIONED.

By setting a reasonable and rational boundary and explaining it ahead of time, most fans are more than happy to comply. Furthermore, if more level-headed members of the group believe that everyone will suffer (e.g., be asked to leave) due to immature actions of a few they tend to help me keep their buddies in line. In this fashion, I am seen more as a mentor or a friend than I am as an authority figure. I ultimately gain more compliance, have happier customers, and a whole lot less arrests that way. Everyone wins.

Submit

> *"It's okay if someone insults, resists or (verbally) attacks you. Laugh it off. Show that it has no meaning, no sting. If you fight back and resist the affront, you give it life and credibility. If you defend yourself you invite counterattack."* [7]

> — *George J. Thompson, Ph.D.*

I received an e-mail recently from my friend Dominic who related an interesting story told by one of his friends who is a Japanese policeman. A restaurant owner had called the police because they were having problems with four Russian sailors. Dominic's friend arrived just past midnight and asked what the problem was. The Russians wanted to pay their bill in U.S. dollars and the owner only wanted Japanese yen. As the owner could not speak Russian and the Russians could not speak Japanese, the restaurant owner had called the police to settle the dispute.

Fortunately, the leader of the Russian seaman spoke a little English so Dominic's friend could communicate with him. While the incident could easily have ended with violence, property damage, and someone being carted off to jail, cooler heads prevailed. The policeman simply asked for 50 dollars from the sailors and gave them 5,000 yen in return which covered the tab. The end result was a resounding win-win where everyone was happy and the officer was able to return to his station without any prisoners.

Give people what they want is a great way to resolve a conflict. Unfortunately if often requires thinking outside the box. The policeman was able to give both parties a winning deal simply by understanding what was going on and exchanging currency. Do not be so caught up in what you want that you also get locked into the way you want to get it. There is more than one way to accomplish just about anything.

Imagine this scenario: you walk out of a store bumping into a huge man carrying a large soft drink causing him to drop it. He is clearly upset, calls you a derogatory name, and takes a swing at you. If your goal is to not get hurt, you can walk away, he can walk away, he can be dragged away on a stretcher, or he can be carried away in a box. All these options accomplish your goal of not being hurt, but some are clearly better than others are.

What might happen if you can scoot away from his punch and say something

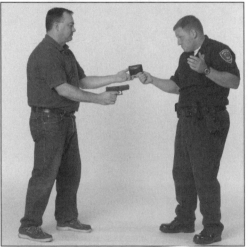

SUBMIT. IN SOME SITUATIONS, IT IS PRUDENT TO GIVE IN.

along the lines of, "Whoa! I am sorry, I did not see you there. Let me help you clean up and buy you a new one." Conversely, what will certainly happen if you immediately begin to fight back?

If you are in error about something, admit it. Honesty is a much better way to de-escalate a bad situation than lying or stubbornly refusing to acknowledge a wrong. It is tough on the ego, but it sure beats an unnecessary hospital stay, jail time, or a premature trip to the morgue.

Try not to insult or embarrass the other person in any way, particularly in public. I do not like being treated that way, I am pretty sure you do not either, and strongly suspect that neither will an aggressive person. Giving someone a face-saving way out affords him or her the opportunity to back down gracefully. Put their back up against the metaphorical wall, on the other hand, and they will ultimately feel forced to lash out at you, striking back (from their perspective) to save their dignity and honor.

Even if you are in the right, it is sometimes prudent to pretend otherwise. Do not let your ego overrule your common sense. Giving your vehicle to a carjacker, your wallet to a robber, or your apology to someone who tries to start a fight hurts a lot less than eating a blade or a bullet because you refused to back down.

Summary

"To win one hundred victories in one hundred battles is not the highest skill. To subdue an enemy without fighting is the highest skill." [7]

– Sun Tzu

De-escalation is defined as the reduction of the intensity in a conflict. It can occur quickly, even spontaneously, especially when a conflict escalates so rapidly that the parties involved mutually fear that any further escalation would be catastrophic, and they back off. This only works so long as logic prevails over emotion, however. There are several strategies we can employ to facilitate de-escalation before things spiral out of control but it does take proactive effort. So long as at least one side believes they can win, de-escalation is harder to achieve. There are four major strategies for verbally de-escalating a conflict: talking, commanding, co-opting, and submitting.

The key aspect of talking is active listening. It is a wholehearted attempt to truly understand where another person is coming from. The principles of active listening include remaining neutral to the extent possible, giving complete attention, asking clarifying questions, and restating the person's main points as necessary to clarify understanding. Speech can be used as a psychological weapon too; facilitating your ability to physically act in self-defense should it be necessary to do so.

Commanding can be done in five stages along an escalation continuum that helps you place context and respond accordingly rather than simply reacting to whatever the other party does. This five-stage process keeps you from having to merely restate a request over and over again, which is not only generally ineffective but also a sign of weakness that can undermine your authority. The five stages are asking, setting the context, presenting options, confirming, and acting.

Co-opting is an attempt to place yourself in a positive light relative to the other person, frequently by insulating them from negative consequences of their actions in the eyes of authority figures or law enforcement. In this fashion, you can be seen more as a mentor or a friend than as an authority figure yet still gain compliance.

Submitting is giving another person what they want as a way to end the conflict. Even if you are in the right, it is sometimes prudent to swallow your pride and apologize or give in to another person's request. Do not be so caught up in what you want that you also get locked into the way you want to get it. There is more than one way to accomplish just about anything.

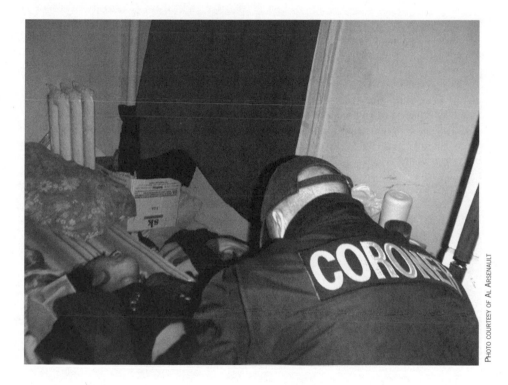

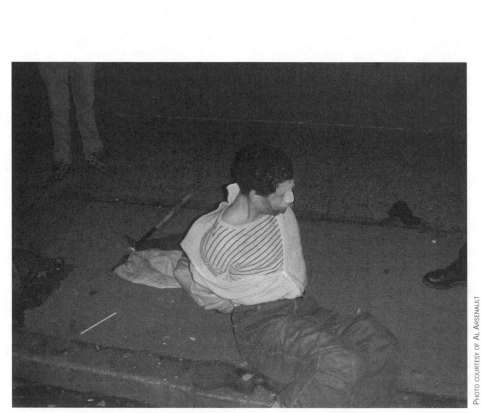

CHAPTER 5

Countervailing Force

"We sleep safe in our beds because rough men stand ready in the night to visit violence on those who would do us harm." [1]

– George Orwell

Physical violence should be last-ditch effort to keep yourself safe after awareness, avoidance, and de-escalation have all failed to do so. Countervailing force, or physical self-defense, is violence applied against an aggressor to keep him or her from hurting you. In the process, you may intentionally or unintentionally injure, maim, or kill an opponent. Because of this possibility, the legal, moral, spiritual, and psychological aspects of self-defense must be explored.

During combat, it takes both physical skills and mental determination to survive. We will also discuss the combat mindset necessary to carry you through a battle as well as the mental triggers that can help you know when there is no choice but to engage an enemy.

Legal Considerations of Countervailing Force

"You may find yourself tangling with criminals or terrorists. Sometimes you'll need to neutralize them until the police arrive, and sometimes you'll be forced to kill. Either way you must act on moral, ethical, and legal principles that are based on the circumstances… use discretion. Remember that you are the good guy and act like one." [2]

– W. Hock Hochheim

Let us face it practitioners of the martial arts, even those whose primary goal is not self-defense, learn dangerous, even deadly techniques. We have an obligation to understand not only how to hurt someone, but also when it is appropriate to do so. Every martial practitioner should have a good understanding of the law as it applies to countervailing force. While the specifics often vary by jurisdiction, the following principles generally apply:

- Adopt a defense-oriented mindset.
- Strive to avoid confrontation.
- Understand self-defense laws.
- Ensure a legitimate claim of self-defense.
- Understand the legalities of deadly force.
- Understand how the courts might rule.
- Never overreact.
- If you must fight, respond judiciously.

1) Adopt a Defense-Oriented Mindset

Most martial practitioners have been taught to avoid conflict. Karate, for example, is first and foremost a defensive art. This essential tradition is best described by Gichin Funakoshi's famous saying, "*karate ni sente nashi*" which translates as "there is no first strike in karate." This convention helps practitioners of potentially lethal arts behave in a manner appropriate to interaction within polite society, something I think we would all agree is a positive thing indeed. This mindset is so important that it goes beyond mere words and is reflected in the training methods and physical movements of the art. For example, every *kata* in *Goju Ryu* karate begins with a defensive technique.

To ensure clarity, however, cutting off an attack before it is fully in play looks like a preemptive strike but is still a defensive movement. In this fashion, practitioners sense that an attack will be forthcoming and then cut it short before the opponent has the chance to transform the mental desire to attack to the physical movement necessary to execute that desire. This preemptive defensive strike is called *sen sen no-sen* for those of you who recognize the Japanese expression.

Martial practitioners study their art for physical conditioning, mental discipline, personal growth, and self-defense purposes. The ultimate goal of the serious *budoka* should never be the ability to go around beating people up. In fact, I would assert that the more dangerous you really are the less you should feel a need to prove it. The best martial artists I know are quiet, unassuming individuals who avoid conflict whenever possible.

2) Strive to Avoid Confrontation

As I have stated previously, the only way to guarantee victory in a physical confrontation is to walk away before the first blow is thrown. Although martial artists train to survive or even triumph in a fight, I believe that practitioners should do everything they can to avoid violence in the first place. Even if you legitimately use force in order to escape imminent and unavoidable danger you still have to live with the physiological, psychological, and litigational results of doing so.

That is not to say that you will never have to use deadly force, of course. If you do engage in a battle for your life, a solid understanding of your local self-defense laws can help you avoid winning the fight only to lose your freedom (and/or everything you own) in the courts afterward.

3) Understand Self-Defense Laws

I am a martial artist not an attorney, neither so nothing in this book should be construed as a legal opinion nor should any of its contents be treated as such. Having said that, however, the classic rule is that self-defense begins when deadly danger begins, ends when the danger ends, and revives again if the danger returns. Neither a killing that takes place after a crime has already been committed, nor a proactive violent defense before an attack has taken place is legitimately self-defense in the eyes of the court.

A person can only resort to deadly force in order to escape imminent and unavoidable danger of death or grave bodily harm. An attacker must not merely have made a threat to attack you (by words and/or actions), but must also be in a position where he or she is obviously and immediately capable of carrying out that threat and/or has begun to do so. A common test is that the attacker must demonstrate intent to attack and have both the means and opportunity to do so.

4) Ensure a Legitimate Claim of Self-Defense

The cornerstone of a legitimate claim of self-defense is the innocence of the claimant. A person must be entirely without fault. If a martial artist initiates a conflict, he or she cannot claim self-defense. If the practitioner allows a conflict to escalate into a lethal situation when it could have been avoided, he or she shares some degree of culpability and, once again, cannot claim self-defense.

This cannot be overemphasized. There are countless stories of martial artists picking fights they regret for the rest of their lives because people were maimed or killed and the practitioners are subsequently sued or jailed or both. You cannot afford to let your ego overrule your commonsense.

5) Understand the Legalities of Deadly Force

Depending on the circumstances, almost any form of physical assault can be considered deadly force. In Washington State (RCW 9A.16.010), deadly force is defined as, "the intentional application of force through the use of firearms or any other means reasonably likely to cause death or serious physical injury."

Other jurisdictions will have similar definitions. In general, any blow delivered powerfully and deliberately to a vital part of the body may be construed as deadly force so long as it can be shown that it was struck with the intention, or predictable likelihood, of killing. Since that is exactly what most of us train to do, we must be prudent in the application of force outside the *dojo*.

6) Understand How the Courts Might Rule

The courts are more likely to interpret a blow as deadly force if the person delivering it is physically much stronger than the victim, a professional fighter, a trained martial artist, or an assailant who attacks with extreme savagery. An example of extreme savagery in the eyes of the law would be gratuitously raining blows upon a fallen opponent who has obviously given up the conflict, even if he or she started the fight in the first place.

While a great majority of deadly force cases involve the use of weapons, martial artists stand a good chance of being charged with a crime resulting from an unarmed confrontation, especially if their training background is uncovered. Knowing that, your best strategy to avoid such unpleasantness is simply never to overreact.

7) Never Overreact

Equal force doctrines require law-abiding citizens to respond to an attack with little or no more force than that which he or she perceives is being used against him/her. In some places, the law clearly specifies that equal force must be exactly equal. The attacked can respond with no more force than that by which he or she is threatened – slap for slap, punch for punch, kick for kick, or deadly weapon for deadly weapon.

Disparity of force between unarmed combatants is measured in one of two ways. It exists if (1) the victim is being attacked by someone who is physically much stronger or younger or (2) the victim is being attacked by two or more assailants of similar or equal size. In such cases, you may legitimately be able to exert potentially lethal force to defend yourself. Regardless, nowhere can a person legally respond to an assault of slight degree with deadly force.

8) If You Must Fight, Respond Judiciously

Practically you will usually want to respond to an assault with a degree of force sufficiently, but not greatly, superior to that with which you are threatened. There are two advantages to this "slightly greater" degree of force doctrine: (1) it places the defender in a more secure tactical position, and (2) it discourages the assailant from continuing his or her attack and escalating into a position where lethal force is warranted.

Some self-defense experts throw out the phrase, "it's better to be judged by twelve than carried by six." I am not personally an advocate of that sentiment because I feel that it trivializes the seriousness of violent confrontations. Never forget that if you are found guilty in a jury trial you will be spending a whole lot of quality time in a confined environment with unpredictable, dangerous neighbors who may be less than friendly as you interact with them. You may also suffer consequences with others in the community, facing challenges from family, friends, employers, and those you wish to interact positively with on a daily basis. Under no circumstances, however, must you let fear of legal consequences keep you from surviving a violent encounter.

A great majority of states require that law-abiding citizens avoid conflict whenever possible. It is best to withdraw, leaving the scene entirely. Retreat from a belligerent party who threatens you unless the attack is so savage that there is not sufficient time to escape or unless withdrawing (or leaving cover in the case of a gunfight) would increase your vulnerability.

The only exception to this rule is within the confines of your own home (or in some places your place of business). In most cases if someone breaks into a person's home and assaults him or her, the homeowner does not legally need to attempt to retreat though in some cases it may be prudent to do so anyway. This is not true in all jurisdictions, however, so check your local laws.

The bottom line is that in the eyes of the court you must also be in reasonable fear for your life or someone else's prior to applying countervailing force. If you are cornered and have to fight, you clearly must use your skills to assure your safety and well-being. It is essential, however, to make a commitment to yourself to use them wisely. Furthermore, ensure that any students whose education is your responsibility will understand how to do the same.

AOJP Principle

"In films murders are always very clean. I show how difficult it is and what a messy thing it is to kill a man." [3]

– Alfred Hitchcock

AOJP stands for ability, opportunity, jeopardy, and preclusion. Another way to ascertain whether or not it is judicious to use countervailing force in self-defense situation is the AOJP principle. If ability, opportunity, jeopardy, and preclusion are all present, you have a good legal case for taking action. If one or more of these criteria are not met, you are on shaky ground.

Ability

Ability means that an attacker has both the physical as well as practical ability to kill or maim you. This may include use of a conventional or improvised weapon such as a knife, gun, or baseball bat. It also includes the physical ability to wield said weapon (or fists or feet for that matter) in a manner that can actually injure you. A small child with a baseball bat probably does not have the same ability to cause harm as a professional ball player.

Opportunity

While your attacker may have the ability to harm you, his ability does not necessarily mean that he also has the immediate opportunity to do so. Your life and well-being must be in clear and present danger before you can react with physical force. For example, a bad guy with a knife has the ability to kill you only so long as he is also within striking range of the weapon or can quickly move into striking range to initiate his attack. A physical barrier such as a chain link fence may protect you from a knife-wielder but not an assailant armed with a gun so opportunity relates not only to the attacker and the weapon, but also to the environment within which they are deployed as well.

Jeopardy

Jeopardy or "imminent jeopardy" as the law sometimes requires, relates to the specifics of the situation. Any reasonable person in a similar situation should feel in fear for his or her life. This distinguishes between a truly dangerous situation and one that is only potentially dangerous. While you are not expected to be able to read an aggressor's mind, you certainly should be able to ascertain his intent from his outward appearance, demeanor, and actions. Someone shouting, "I'm going to kill you," while walking away is probably not an immediate threat while someone shouting, "I love you," while lunging with a knife probably is.

Preclusion

Even when the ability, opportunity, and jeopardy criteria are satisfied, you must still have no other safe alternatives than countervailing force before engaging an opponent in combat. If you can run or retreat from harm's way without further endangering yourself this criteria has not been met.

Ethical/Moral Considerations

"The necessary consequence of a man's right to life is his right to self-defense. In a civilized society, force may be used only in retaliation and only against those who initiate its use. All the reasons which make the initiation of physical force an evil make the retaliatory use of physical force a moral imperative." [4]

– Ayn Rand

The second paragraph of the Declaration of Independence proclaims, "We hold these truths to be self-evident, that all men are created equal, that they are endowed by their Creator with certain unalienable Rights, that among these are Life, Liberty and the pursuit of Happiness." Every person has a fundamental right to life, one that cannot be overridden by anyone save by the consequences of one's own actions or by one's own choosing. To state it in a manner that gets more directly to the heart of the issue, in my opinion, each and every person on earth has the fundamental right not to be killed. This right not to be killed is a human entitlement, a mark of any civilized society.

Of course, there is also a paramount reciprocity factor. It is possible to waive the right not to be killed by murdering or attempting to murder someone else. In other words, you have the duty not to kill or harm others so long as others adhere to the same duty toward you. It is the breakdown of this reciprocal relationship that explains why aggressors fail to have the right not to be killed by their victims, and why you possess the moral right to kill someone in self-defense if there is no other way to resolve a confrontation.

If someone makes an unprovoked attack against you, your friends, or your family, the aggressor is morally at fault for the attack, and all consequences thereof. The defender is both morally and legally innocent so long as he or she acts within the true definition of self-defense, guarding him or herself against a real, imminent, and unavoidable threat of serious physical injury or death.

British statesman and political theorist Edmund Burke[5] wrote, "All that is necessary for the triumph of evil is that good men do nothing." There are times when we are morally impelled to act in defense of others or ourselves. For some—law enforcement officers, soldiers, and security personnel to name a few—it is their job to run toward danger. For everyone else, you must defend yourself if attacked directly, and search your character in determining how to act if you come across an incident of violence toward someone else.

Before you rush into a dangerous situation unnecessarily, think of your kids, your family, your spouse, or other important people in your life. You are not just endangering yourself by your actions; you are potentially affecting them as well. Is there a non-violent way to intervene? Is it possible to de-escalate a situation without becoming physically involved? Are you certain about who the good guy is and who the bad guy is? Before anything actually occurs, it is a good idea to consider various scenarios and search your values. Carefully consider the consequences of taking action versus not taking action, and what type of action you might take.

It is a good idea to ponder these issues before you have to make such decisions on the street, as there is very little if any time for preponderance in the heat of battle. A thorough understanding of your moral values along with a well-thought-out ethical perspective can hold you in good stead. If you are a religious person, you might also wish to examine spiritual teachings to help you decide what to do should you ever be confronted by evil.

You have a fundamental human right not to be killed, even if you must exercise countervailing force to safeguard that right. Further, you have a moral imperative to act in your own defense and possibly in the defense of others as well.

Religious Objections to Self Defense

"He that hath no sword, let him sell his garment, and buy one" [6]

– Luke, 22:36

Anyone who has seen a rendition of the Ten Commandments has undoubtedly read the decree, "Thou Shall Not Kill." Although these words are a common translation, they are, nevertheless, not terribly accurate, distorting the intent of this pronouncement. A more appropriate translation of Exodus 20:13 reads, "Thou Shall Not Commit Murder."

Murder is generally defined as the crime of causing the death of another human being with malice aforethought and without lawful excuse. Killing on the other hand, is that act of causing someone or something to die. It may or may not be justified, depending on specific circumstances. Killing an attacker who poses an immediate and unavoidable threat to your life, executing a convicted felon in accordance with a lawful sentence of death, or defending one's country upon the field of battle are all examples of killings that do not meet the legal or theological definition of murder. In fact, the Bible is replete with stories portraying these three types of events, none of which are admonished. Murder, on the other hand, is clearly and repeatedly denounced.

This difference between "killing" and "murdering" is paramount. Similarly for those who study the New Testament, *Matthew* 5:39 is often mistranslated as well. A common translation reads, "But I say unto you, that ye resist not evil: but whosoever shall smite thee on thy right cheek, turn to him the other also."

A more accurate translation according to many biblical scholars should state, "But I say to you, do not resist evil with evil (or in a like manner)..." There is a huge difference between a command to not resist evil and to not resist with evil. Turning the other cheek is a metaphorical way of telling people not to seek vengeance for or respond violently to insults, very sound advice. It is not a literal requirement to stand there and let someone beat you to a pulp. Evil must be resisted, even evil impulses in yourself as well as evil actions from others.

Whoever is attacking you has almost certainly assaulted someone before. The more times he or she gets away with it the more dangerous that person is likely to become. If you successfully defend yourself against an armed assailant you not only save your own life but likely that of the criminal's next victim as well. Good and moral people ignore insults and avoid seeking revenge yet that does not mean that they passively stand by and allow themselves or others to be slaughtered by evil doers.

Killing in self-defense is neither a violation of God's laws nor man's. As stated earlier you have the fundamental right not to be killed. Hopefully you will never be called on to proactively defend that right but it is important to understand that you do not necessarily have to jeopardize your soul in order to do so.

Psychological Considerations

"Bravery is being the only one who knows you're afraid." [7]

– *Col. David Hackworth*

Unfortunately, survivors of violent confrontations frequently pay a psychological price for the actions that they must take to stay alive. The same thing can happen to those who fail to intervene when their inaction leads to another person's death.

According to Lt. Col. David Grossman, most participants in close combat are literally frightened out of their wits. Once conflict escalates to violence, we stop thinking with our forebrain (prosencephalar areas, especially the neopallium) and our midbrain takes over. Development of the forebrain is what makes us uniquely human, creating the physiological basis for many of our unique skills related to memory, planning, conjecture, fabrication, and complex cognition. The midbrain or mesencephalon is archipallian in origin, sharing its general architecture with the most ancient of vertebrates and even insects. Dopamine produced in the subtantia nigra plays an important role in the motor system, motivation and non-associative learning processes of every species.

In extreme stress situation, the midbrain typically overrules the forebrain, mobilizing the body for survival. This fight or flight reaction is a valuable, hard-wired survival mechanism. After all, if you see a snake it is simply not prudent to figure out what kind of snake it is until you are safely beyond its striking range.

In conflict situations, this primal midbrain processing creates a powerful resistance to killing one's own kind, at least in emotionally healthy individuals. This is an essential survival mechanism that prevents a species from destroying itself during conflicts such as territorial disputes and mating rituals. Nature provides excellent illustrations of how this works. Piranhas, for example, fight their own species with flicks of their tails yet use their vicious teeth unrestrained against other creatures.

This resistance to killing one's own species is an important factor in understanding the psychological cost of combat. Soldiers, for example, train to overcome this natural reluctance to kill other human beings by using realistic, man-shaped targets that pop up to present a "threat" and fall when hit with a bullet. This kind of powerful operant conditioning reliably influences the primitive, midbrain processing of a frightened soldier, facilitating his or her ability to take another person's life in battle. Soldiers, law enforcement professionals, and many martial artists train in simulated conditions that desensitize us to attacking and potentially killing our fellow human beings should we be called upon to do so.

According to Grossman, any conditioning that overrides our innate resistance to killing has enormous potential for psychological backlash. Throughout history, every warrior society has developed some sort of purification ritual to help returning warriors deal with their guilt, reassuring them that whatever they did in combat was good and proper, necessary for the safety and security of their tribe. In primitive societies, this generally involved ritual bathing, separation, and ceremony designed to reintegrate warriors back into their tribe. Similarly, soldiers returning from modern wars frequently find parades, medals, monuments, psychological counseling, and the unconditional acceptance of family and/or society waiting for them upon arrival back home.

There are other historical ways of assuaging one's guilt after a battle. *Wergild*, in Norse, Anglo-Saxon, and Viking culture was a reparation payment made to the family or clan of someone a warrior killed from his own tribe or nation. The word can be translated as "man price," an important custom that warded off disruptive feuds and long-standing cycles of retribution. The size of the payment was based upon the social rank of the victim. Thralls and slaves, for example, technically commanded no *wergild* though it was commonplace to make a nominal payment nevertheless. To the ancient Celts, this payment was called *ericfine*, to the Slavs it was *glowczyzna*; in Islamic and Arab traditions, it was simply called blood money, a concept that exists in some countries to this day.

Without some type of purification ritual or societal mechanism for diminishing guilt, many combat survivors have a challenging time reintegrating back into society. Further, the midbrain's hijacking the forebrain in combat can also result in erratic, uncontrollable physiological reactivity such as flashbacks that occur later on. Such unwarranted physiological reactivity can cause a person to dread further incidents, an unhealthy cycle of anxiety that creates fear, which creates more anxiety.

For example, most returning Vietnam veterans were attacked and condemned in an unprecedented manner due to the unpopularity of that war in American culture. The very conditioning the soldiers received in training that helped them survive the horrors of battle were magnified by societal condemnation and physiological reactivity which created a circumstance in which approximately one million veterans became victims of post-traumatic stress disorder (PTSD), a condition that has always occurred in warfare, but never previously recorded at such magnitude.

PTSD is a psychological condition caused by exposure to or confrontation with highly stressful experiences, typically involving participation in or witnessing of death or serious physical injury. This stressful experience, when combined with feelings of intense fear, helplessness, or horror may lead to PTSD, particularly when the experience is caused by another person. For example, the last time I climbed Mount Rainier, a member of our party was struck by a falling boulder that broke his leg. A few of months later he was back on the mountain again, climbing as if nothing untoward had happened. Had the exact same injury been caused by a tire-iron wielding thug on the street his emotional recovery may very well have been affected.

Symptoms can include re-experiencing phenomena via nightmares and flashbacks, emotional detachment (or hyper control), sleep abnormalities, irritability, excessive startle (hyper vigilance), and uncontrolled rage among other indicators. Experiences likely to induce this condition include most any form of combat or violent physical attack, rape, emotional abuse, or even catastrophic natural disasters. PTSD often becomes a chronic condition but can usually improve with treatment (or, rarely, even spontaneously). There is also the possibility of other psychiatric disorders that may be experienced simultaneously.

PTSD is primarily an anxiety disorder and should not be confused with normal grief and adjustment after traumatic events. For most people, the emotional effects of such incidents tend to subside after a few months. If you have been involved in a violent altercation, it is a good idea to consider professional counseling which can facilitate a healthy recovery. If symptoms last longer than a few months, you may need professional diagnosis to see if you have developed a psychiatric disorder. Regardless, most people who experience traumatic events will not develop PTSD, though it may have a delayed onset of years or even decades if you do develop this disorder. Delayed triggers usually come in the form of life changing events such as the death of a relative or close friend or diagnosis of a serious medical condition.

The good news is that PTSD has been thoroughly studied and there are a variety of clinical techniques that mental health professionals and clergy members can use to help victims make a full recovery. With counseling survivors of traumatic events are able to confront their memories and emotions, while working to de-link them from any kind of physiological response. Autogenic breathing techniques[9] and structured debriefing sessions are helpful in this process.

Another challenge of traumatic situations is that they are frequently associated with memory impairment, a condition commonly described as "critical incident amnesia." The greater the stress, the greater the potential of memory problems as victims have difficulty in transferring information from short-term memory to long-term memory. There are several root causes for this phenomenon, including sensory overload, tunnel vision,* and adrenal stress.†

Combatants frequently encounter post-incident amnesia immediately after a traumatic experience, failing to remember the majority of the information they observed during the encounter. After a healthy night's sleep, there is usually a significant memory recovery, resulting in an ability to remember a majority of what occurred. This is the period at which you will have the most reliable memories of what occurred. The most complete recovery, however, will happen within about 72 hours, but it will inevitably include at least partially reconstructed (and therefore somewhat contaminated) information. Inevitably, an individual who has experienced some level of memory loss will discuss the event with others and seek retrieval clues from external sources such as media reports.

Human memory is a fallible process. It includes active construction in which prior experiences, knowledge, beliefs, prejudices, and expectations are constantly shaping, filling in the gaps, and potentially distorting our perception of what actually occurred; a reason that eyewitness testimony is not always reliable. Since memory is a product of perception, it can become distorted whenever our perception becomes distorted or disrupted.

Vision is a huge contributor to memory since it is the primary mechanism by which we observe the world around us. Hearing, touch, taste, and smell play a role too, of course, but not to as great a degree in most people. Under extreme stress, visual exclusion or tunnel vision narrows our field of view by as much as 70 percent. Similarly, stress-induced pupil dilation can disrupt our ability to focus (especially on close objects), degrading our depth perception.‡ Since the visual field is disrupted or narrowed, the amount of information we collect from it will be incomplete.

We are constantly bombarded by stimuli from the world around us, much of which is disregarded as unimportant and not transferred from short term to long term memory. Even in individuals with so-called "photographic memories," focused

---

*Fixation on some particular aspect of a situation to the exclusion of most everything else.
†Especially at levels that drive your heart rate above 175 beats per minute. We will talk more about accounting for adrenaline in Chapter 6.
‡This is a significant challenge for shooters since we lose the ability to focus on the front gun sight.

attention is required to ensure that transfer. Focused attention to certain stimuli can preclude attention to others, resulting in a flashbulb-like effect where only certain aspects of an event are actually remembered (e.g., something new or unusual).

Immediately after a traumatic incident, much of what occurred is still in the brain, but it has not been processed in such a manner that it can be retrieved. One of the key factors in being able to access such information is sleep. The brain focuses on problem solving and the resolution of emotional concerns during sleep, particularly during REM sleep (which is when most dreaming occurs). This sleep cycle helps the brain consolidate unusual information that requires a good deal of adaptation in order for it to be absorbed. In fact, REM sleep cycles happen more frequently and last longer for individuals who are placed in circumstances in which they must process great quantities of new information. Although you may not remember much about a traumatic incident right after it occurs, you should experience significant memory recovery after a good night's sleep.

If your initial night's sleep is disturbed, however, memory recovery may be disrupted. Further, if you were rendered unconscious or injured to the extent that you require an operation involving general anesthesia, there is a good possibility that normal memory recovery will be greatly disrupted. Your ability to remember crucial details about a violent incident and subsequently to defend yourself in court is greatly influenced by the memory recovery process. Do everything you can to safeguard your first night's sleep after any violent encounter.

Combat Mindset

"Stand your ground; don't fire unless fired upon, but if they mean to have a war, let it begin here." [10]

– *Captain John Parker*

Perusing the headlines, you can easily find evidence just about every day that evil exists, or at least truly evil people. Some crimes simply boggle the mind. For example, in December of 2004, a Missouri woman was strangled and her baby cut from her womb by a Kansas woman who had been faking pregnancy. The baby was later found alive, and the attacker charged with kidnapping resulting in death.

In February of 2005, Sarah Brady a resident of Fort Mitchell Kentucky was attacked in what may have been a copycat crime attempt. This 26 year-old, nine-month pregnant woman fought off and killed a knife-wielding attacker, Katherine Smith, who was allegedly trying to steal her unborn baby. Brady was then taken to the hospital to receive treatment for her wounds, from which she later recovered.

Investigators reported that Smith, age 22, had been falsely telling neighbors for weeks that she was pregnant. A search of her apartment after her death revealed a baby nursery.

Smith methodically set Brady up for slaughter. On the Tuesday preceding the incident she called Brady, whom she apparently did not know beforehand, and asked her to come over and pick up a mistakenly delivered package. The next day, Smith called once again, asking Brady to pick up another package. When she arrived on Thursday at Smith's apartment, she was attacked. The unarmed, heavily pregnant woman still managed to overcome and kill her armed assailant. Police reports indicated that the killing was justifiable self-defense and that no charges would be filed.

As mentioned previously, the most common type of knife fight is an ambush attack. With a set-up like the aforementioned package pick-up, it would be difficult to predict and avoid violence ahead of time. Further, it is quite challenging for a nine-month pregnant person to run from a determined attacker and expect to get away unharmed.

In an unavoidable self-defense situation, one from which you cannot escape, you must commit yourself emotionally and physically to winning at all costs. Any other outcome may very well mean your death. Nothing should enter your mind but the actions of yourself and your opponent. Failing to devote all your concentration to the conflict may prove disastrous.

There is a concept called the fearlessness of no fear. It is about the quintessential martial mindset, total concentration on the moment. The famous story of the tea master and the *ronin* sheds some interesting insight into this concept:

At the insistence of Lord Yamanouchi the *daimyo* of Tosa Province, a reluctant tea master was taken to Yedo* on an official trip attired in *samurai* garb, including the two traditional swords of the warrior class. While running an errand for his master in the city, the tea master was accosted by a *ronin*.† Since he was by himself and dressed beyond his station, this was exactly the thing the tea master feared might happen.

At first, he was so scared that he was unable to speak, yet was finally able to admit that he was not really a *samurai*. Upon discovering that his opponent was merely a tea master and not a fearsome warrior, the ronin was more determined than ever to take his money. The *ronin* declared that it would be an insult to the tea master's province if he did not defend his honor. The tea master replied, "If you so insist, we will try out our skills, but first I must finish my master's errand. Then I will return tomorrow morning for a duel."

The *ronin* agreed and the tea master rushed to complete his errand so that he could talk with the master of a local *dojo* (martial arts school) before his fateful meeting with the *ronin*. He intended to ask the sword master how he might die in the man-

---

*Yedo is the feudal name for the modern city of Tokyo.
†A ronin is a masterless samurai, literally a wave man (one who is tossed about like the waves on the sea). Lacking a benefactor, many *ronin* took up criminal endeavors to support themselves.

ner befitting a *samurai*. The sword master was taken aback by the question, saying, "You are unique. Most students come ask me how to use a sword. You come to me asking how to die. Before I teach you the art of dying, please serve me a cup of tea."

Forgetting about his impending catastrophe, the tea master prepared tea in the manner he always did—as if there were nothing else in the world that mattered except for serving the tea. Deeply moved by the tea master's intense, but natural concentration, the sword master exclaimed, "That's it! That very state of mind is what you will need tomorrow when you go to meet the *ronin*. First think of serving tea to an honored guest and act accordingly. Draw your sword and close your eyes. When you hear his *kiai* (spirit shout), strike him with your sword. The contest will probably end with a mutual slaying."

The tea master thanked the sword master and went on about his business. The next morning when he went to meet the *ronin*, he followed the sword master's advice to the letter. The tea master boldly stood before his opponent, the embodiment of concentration. The *ronin*, who had previously seen a coward, now faced the personification of bravery. Instead of advancing to attack, the *ronin* retreated. Cowed with fear inspired by the superior concentration of his adversary, he turned and fled. After standing awhile and hearing no shout, the tea master opened his eyes to gaze upon an empty street.

This is an example of what the Japanese call *fudoshin* or indomitable spirit. Miyamoto Musashi, arguably the greatest swordsman who ever lived, demonstrated the ultimate evolution of such spirit. In his writings, he related that many opponents fell before his sword simply because they believed that they would, not necessarily, because he was the better warrior.

When your life is on the line, fight not only for yourself but also about those who care about and depend upon you—your children, your spouse, your family, and your friends. In the heat of battle you will not have time to think of anything beyond the immediate but it is wise to consider beforehand what will happen to your loved ones if you do not make it. Sometimes the impact to others can be even more motivating than the impact to yourself. You must make a wholehearted commitment to survive. Here is another amazing real-life example:

On March 7, 2003, Sgt. Marcus Young, an 18-year veteran of the Ukiah, California Police Department received a seemingly routine shoplifting call at a Wal-Mart store. He had a 17-year-old police cadet named Julian Covella riding along with him at the time. They met briefly with store security to understand the situation, collected the suspect, and then proceeded to bring her out to the patrol car.

As Sgt. Young and Wal-Mart security guard Brett Schott put the shoplifting suspect Monica Winnie, 18, into the back seat of the patrol car, her 35-year-old companion Neal Beckman tried to intervene. A dangerous looking individual with small devil horns tattooed on his forehead, he approached the group with his hands hidden from view in his pockets. As Beckman approached, Young commanded, "Take your hands out of your pockets," but received no response. He repeated his command to which Beckman responded, "I have a knife," drew his blade, and began to attack. What Young did not see was the Beckman's gun, a .38 caliber revolver, held in his other hand.

Utilizing both his police training and the skills he developed as a 2nd *dan* black belt in karate, Young quickly wrenched the attacker's arm into a lock but was unable to force him to let go of the knife. As both of them slammed into the side of the car, Beckman began firing, hitting Young in the face, body, and arm. Schott, the unarmed security guard, leapt into the fight wrenching the revolver away from Beckman. Before he realized that the gun was no longer loaded, the suspect stabbed him in the chest with his knife, collapsing his lung. Weakened by the massive chest wound, Schott disengaged, trying to find cover.

As this occurred, officer Young regained his feet and tried to reach for his own gun only to find that his humerus (upper arm bone) had been shattered paralyzing his gun arm from nerve damage. He tried to draw with his left hand only to find that it had been ripped apart during the struggle, its separated tendons visible through the opened skin.

Deprived of his weapons, the suspect then dove into the front seat of the police car, closed the door, and frantically began searching for the hidden switch that would release the loaded Remington shotgun and HK sub-machinegun locked therein. As Beckman tried to free the heavy weapons, Young turned to his cadet Covella, saying, "Take my gun out and put it in my hand." The boy quickly released the safety strap and placed the firearm into Young's mangled hand.

Kneeling to steady himself, he tried to shoot the suspect through the closed door to no avail. Re-aiming through the closed window, he managed to place two rounds into the suspect, dropping him. He then asked the cadet to call for assistance and began deliberate controlled breathing exercises to keep himself calm, conscious, and alive until medical personnel could respond.

The heroic security guard Schott recovered from his horrific injuries. Both he and police cadet Covella received numerous awards for valor from their roles in the incident. These included heroism citations from the Veterans of Foreign Wars and the American Legion, and dual Citizen of the Year awards from the California Narcotics Officers' Association. Covella has since been accepted as a cadet at the United States Naval Academy at Annapolis.

As of late 2004, Sergeant Young was on light duty, still recovering from his severe physical injuries and facing more surgery. He was awarded the National Rifle Association's honor as Police Officer of the Year for 2003, as well as the Mayor's Medal of Valor. He was also nominated for the Presidential Medal of Valor and the California Attorney General's Office Medal of Valor. His incident has been included in a fear and anger management classes at the California Police Standards and Training council.

Young reported that he felt he owes his survival not only to Schott and Covella, but also to the many instructors who trained him over the years. "They taught me to shoot from awkward positions if I was wounded," he related, "and they taught me to be resourceful and keep thinking and keep fighting no matter how I might be injured. They taught me to never give up."

Never give up. Focus on neutralizing the immediate threat and worry about how badly you are hurt after the incident is over and you are safe. As Sarah Brady and Sergeant Young have demonstrated, resourcefulness, clear thinking, and a burning desire to remain safe at all costs can carry you through amazing challenges. Never forget that if it hurts, you are still alive. If you are still alive, you can continue to fight.

Triggers

"Dangerous is wrath concealed. Hatred proclaimed doth lose its chance of wreaking vengeance." [11]

— Seneca

Use of countervailing force is an individual decision based on each unique situation, taking into account legal, moral, ethical, religious, and psychological considerations. While there are several factors to take into account, let us assume that you will only respond with violence when it is prudent to do so. Having said that, before you find yourself tangling with an aggressor on the street, a certain amount of introspection is still required to help you determine how and when you should respond.

Ask yourself the following questions:

- Given a clear, present, and unavoidable danger to yourself or your loved ones, could you kill in self-defense? Really think about that. Could you crush the life out of another human being with your hands, feet, or a makeshift weapon? This kind of violence is very close and very personal. Could you crush someone's throat, bash in his head, impale his heart, or ventilate his lung, and watch him or her die from your actions?
- Given a clear, present, and unavoidable danger to yourself or your loved ones, could you maim someone in self defense? Could you gouge out an eye, shatter an eardrum, dislocate a joint, knock out teeth, or otherwise cause permanent injury to another human being, even if he/she started the fight?

Even with the legal right and moral obligation to act, some people are simply incapable of applying countervailing force. Even some parents are incapable of violence to protect their own children, something that many people can do even if they would not actively defend themselves. If you fall into this category, it is far better to know that now than it is to figure it out in the heat of battle.

If you do have to kill someone, no matter how justified, you will likely pay a psychological price for doing so. The same thing can happen however if you fail to take action, which leads to another person's death. It is important to think about this before anything untoward happens.

If you cannot visualize yourself harming another human being, even at risk of your own life or well-being, you should not even consider carrying a weapon for self-defense. It will undoubtedly be used against you. Furthermore, never deploy a weapon you do not intend to use. If you draw, you must be prepared to fire.* You have to not only be right to act, but also willing to act in self-defense. Clearly, you would rather not have to act, but if you are merely bluffing, an opponent may figure that out and punish you for it, perhaps fatally.

There are a wide variety of possible triggers that can help you know it is time to act. Everyone will respond based upon his or her individual circumstances, character, and psychological make-up. If you find yourself in a situation of extreme violence, you will have an easier time reacting if you have considered what to do ahead of time. Here are some scenarios to consider. Any or all of these may be appropriate triggers:

- You face an armed attacker and know that you are about to die if you do not act, and possibly even if you do. You have nothing to lose by fighting back.
- You are faced with clear, present, and unavoidable danger of death, dismemberment, or significant harm to yourself.
- Your spouse is faced with clear and present danger and cannot escape without your intervention.
- Your child is faced with clear and present danger and cannot escape without your intervention.
- You discover a pregnant woman or small child who is faced with clear and present danger and cannot escape without your intervention.
- You are confronted with an aggressor who attempts to force you into his/her vehicle or otherwise take you to a secondary crime scene.
- You are about to be raped.
- You are about to be tied up or handcuffed by an aggressor.†
- You are ordered to turn your back or are about to be blindfolded by a captor.

---

*Or stab or whatever your weapon does.
†Since your options will become severely limited once you are encumbered this may be a good time to act.

• You are taken captive by someone you believe is a vengeance seeker, terrorist extremist, fanatic, or other hostage taker who sincerely intends to kill you.

Bystanders

"Oh my God, he stabbed me! Please help me! Please help me!" [12]

— Kitty Genovese

The infamous murder of Catherine "Kitty" Genovese shocked the nation in 1964. Genovese, a 28-year-old, 105-pound woman was brutally stabbed, robbed of $49, and left to bleed to death in front of her New York apartment. While more than 40 people overheard her desperate pleas for help, or actually watched her being stabbed and/or bleeding to death, no one bothered to call for an ambulance or inform the police until more than 30 minutes later. By then it was too late.

While Kitty Genovese's neighbors were New Yorkers, they were not necessarily any more heartless, apathetic, or different from witnesses to thousands of other crimes across the country. The problem was and is that while each witness was waiting for someone else to do something, no one did anything. There is an interesting phenomenon commonly called the Bystander Effect. Research has consistently found that as the number of bystanders increases the likelihood that any one of them would help a victim in trouble decreases. People help others more often and more quickly when they think they are alone. There are a couple of reasons for this.

To begin, the more bystanders present, the more likely it is that any individual person will assume that someone else has called for help or that someone else will intervene. A person by himself or herself cannot assume that someone else is responsible for taking action. The larger number of bystanders, the less obligated each is likely to feel that they have an imperative to intervene.

Secondly, anyone who did not see an incident from the beginning may be unsure about what is going on. Who is the bad guy and who is the victim? To the extent that we are unsure about what is going on or the situation is ambiguous, we are more likely to look to others for help in defining whether or not intervention is appropriate or necessary. If others do not get involved, we may decide that whatever is happening does not require our assistance. That is one reason why first aid/CPR students are taught to look a specific person in the eye, describe the emergency, and tell that person to dial 9-1-1 for assistance.

Many people try to avoid showing outward signs of worry or concern until they see that others are alarmed as well. After all it would be quite embarrassing to be worked up about something everyone considers a non-event. This sort of caution encourages bystanders to appear nonchalant about a potential emergency inhibiting everyone's urge to help. The larger the number of people who appear unconcerned about a situation, the stronger that inhibiting influence will be on everyone else, a cycle that feeds upon itself. The converse is also true. The more people who appear alarmed the more likely that someone would decide to intervene.

In a more recent case, at least ten people allegedly saw 18-year-old Rachel Burkheimer bound and gagged, lying on the floor of an Everett (Washington) garage in September 2002 shortly before she was murdered. None of them stopped to help. None of them even called the police. Legally, none of them had to. An attempt was made in March of 2005 to pass a law requiring bystanders to notify the police of crimes they witness yet house Bill 1236 did not make it through the legislature.

Be wary of bystanders. Good Samaritans who may be drawn to your aid could just as easily be frightened away over concern for their own personal safety. You simply cannot count on receiving any help unless they are folks whose job it is to act, such as emergency services personnel and law enforcement officers. In fact, the presence of bystanders can be good, bad, or neutral. They may be inclined to help you, they could ignore your plight, or they may even be inclined to hurt you, especially if they are friends of your assailant. Even if bystanders do not get directly involved, they may be called upon to testify to your actions in court. Refer to Chapter 8 for important information about creating witnesses.

Summary

"I say, you died a good death if your life had inspired someone to come forward and shoot your murderer in the chest—without asking to be paid." [13]

— *Chinua Achebe*

As trained martial artists we have an obligation to understand not only how to hurt someone, but also when it is appropriate to do so. Every martial practitioner should have a good understanding of the law as it applies to countervailing force. While the specifics often vary by jurisdiction, the following principles generally apply: adopt a defense-oriented mindset, strive to avoid confrontation, understand self-defense laws, ensure a legitimate claim of self-defense if you have to act, understand the legalities of deadly force, figure out how the courts might rule, never overreact, and if you must fight, respond judiciously.

Another way to ascertain whether or not it is judicious to use countervailing force in self-defense situation is the AOJP principle. If ability, opportunity, jeopardy, and preclusion are all present, you have a good legal case for taking action. If one or more of these criteria are not met, you are on shaky ground.

Every person has the fundamental right not to be killed. There is also a paramount reciprocity factor. It is possible to waive the right not to be killed by murdering or attempting to murder someone else. In other words, you have the duty not to kill or harm others so long as others adhere to that same duty toward you. It is the breakdown of this reciprocal relationship that explains why aggressors fail to have the right not to be killed by their victims, and why you possess the moral right to kill someone in self-defense if there is no other way to resolve a confrontation.

While many people know the biblical commandment, "Thou Shall Not Kill," a more accurate translation of Exodus 20:13 reads, "Thou Shall Not Commit Murder." The difference between killing and murdering is paramount. You can legally, morally, and ethically take another person's life in self-defense if there is no other alternative but to do so.

If you do have to kill someone, no matter how justified, you will likely pay a psychological price for doing so. The same thing can happen if you fail to take action that leads to another person's death. Post Traumatic Stress Disorder (PTSD) is a psychological condition caused by exposure to or confrontation with highly stressful experiences. Symptoms can include such things as nightmares, flashbacks, hyper control, sleep abnormalities, irritability, hyper vigilance, and uncontrolled rage. Experiences likely to induce this condition include most any form of combat or violent physical attack, rape, emotional abuse, or even catastrophic natural disasters. Witnessing or responding to these events can trigger the same reaction. PTSD often becomes a chronic condition but can usually improve with treatment.

PTSD is primarily an anxiety disorder and should not be confused with normal grief and adjustment after traumatic events. For most people, the emotional effects of such incidents tend to subside after a few months. If you have been involved in a violent altercation, it is a good idea to consider professional counseling which can facilitate a healthy recovery.

In addition to the possibility of PTSD, combatants frequently encounter post-incident amnesia immediately after a traumatic experience, failing to remember the majority of the information they observed during the encounter. After a healthy night's sleep, there is usually a significant memory recovery, resulting in an ability to remember a majority of what occurred. This is the period at which you will have the most reliable memories of what occurred. The most complete recovery, however, will happen within about 72 hours, but it will inevitably include at least partially reconstructed information.

Use of countervailing force is an individual decision based on each unique situation, taking into account legal, moral, ethical, religious, and psychological considerations.

While there are several factors to take into account, let us assume that you will only respond with violence when it is prudent to do so. Having said that, before you find yourself tangling with an aggressor on the street, a certain amount of introspection is still required to help you determine how and when you should respond. You should have a pretty good idea ahead of time what triggers will indicate that it is prudent to engage in a physical altercation.

If a situation does escalate to violence, be wary of bystanders. They can be good, bad, or neutral. They may be inclined to help you, they could ignore your plight, or they may even be inclined to hurt you, especially if they are friends of your assailant. Even if bystanders do not get directly involved, they may be called upon to testify to your actions in court.

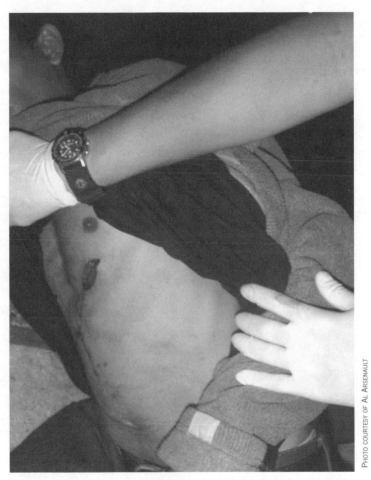

A STABBING VICTIM.

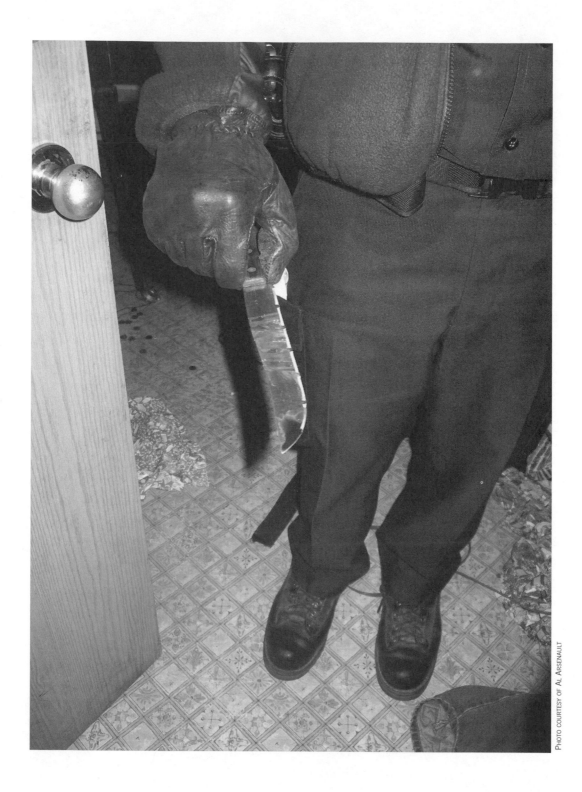

CHAPTER 6

Armed Conflict

*"Many that live deserve death. And some die that deserve life. Can you give it to them?
Then be not too eager to deal out death in the name of justice, fearing for your own safety. Even the wise cannot see all ends."* [1]

– J.R.R. Tolkien

By the time a confrontation has escalated into armed conflict, you know that you
are in serious trouble. After all, awareness, avoidance, and de-escalation have already
failed. Non-violent techniques for controlling the confrontation have likewise been
unsuccessful. Your demeanor, voice, presence, and/or body position has not been
enough to dissuade your attacker.

You are now in survival mode. This kind of thing is totally different from an
unarmed fistfight. Any time you are touched by an opponent's weapon you may be seriously injured, crippled, maimed, or even killed. Under these extreme conditions, you
will have to rely on your courage, training, creativity, and determination to survive.

Levels of Force

*"The first right of every human being is the right of self-defense. Without that right, all
other rights are meaningless. The right of self-defense is not something the government
bestows upon its citizens. It is an inalienable right, older than the Constitution itself. It
existed prior to government and prior to the social contract of our Constitution."* [2]

– Senator Larry Craig

A continuum of force should be applied judiciously to preserve your safety as the
situation warrants. There are no absolutes in self-defense but your ultimate goal is to
apply sufficient force to effectively control the situation and keep yourself from
harm. In general, you may legally use reasonable force in defending yourself.
"Reasonable force" is considered only that force reasonably necessary to repel the
attacker's force.

Unfortunately "reasonably necessary" is a vague term usually associated with what the "reasonable person" would think necessary. The so-called "reasonable person" is a fictitious composite of all the reasonably prudent people in a given cross section of life.

Whether the ordinary person acted reasonably will likely be judged against the reasonably prudent, similarly situated ordinary person in the appropriate geographic area. Everyone starts out at this level, but other personal attributes may heighten their required standard of care.

Whether a martial artist acted reasonably in a fight will likely be judged against the reasonably prudent fighter of similar skill and training in that general geographic area.*

The reasonable person standard is not necessarily used in all criminal proceedings nor is it universally applied in all civil proceedings. On the other hand, some standard of reasonable and right are embedded in the mind of every person, including those sitting in the jury box. The reasonable person standard will likely also be used in any civil suit (e.g. wrongful death) filed after a criminal decision.

A trained fighter is usually held to a higher standard of "reasonableness" than the average person in a court of law is. The martial artist's training gives him or her better understanding of the application and consequences of using a certain amount of force. Thus, where a less skilled individual might be able to shoot a club-wielding attacker, it may only be reasonable in the eyes of an undereducated jury for the martial artist to use his or her hands for defense. For non-practitioners, most folk's understanding of martial arts is limited to unrealistic movie and television stunts.

Crimes generally revolve around the "intent" to do something bad, or the "reckless disregard" of the consequences of doing something that turned out bad in retrospect. Reasonableness also enters criminal proceedings to help resolve issues surrounding intent or reckless disregard. You can never know what someone intended yet the courts can infer what was intended from evidence and circumstances. This inference involves knowledge, skill, training, and state of mind of the participants as applied to the evidence and circumstances at hand.

Exceeding a reasonable level of force may well turn a victim into a perpetrator in the eyes of the court. Justifiable self-defense is a victim's defense to a criminal/civil charge. If one's intent were to defend his or her self then a reasonable person would only do so using reasonable force. Using a higher level of force infers intent to needlessly harm the other. This allows the perpetrator turned "victim" to use your defensive actions against you, the victim turned perpetrator. Even if a criminal prosecutor dismisses your actions, a civil court may not do so. Consequently, a dynamic scale from defensive to offensive to survival applications can help you put things into perspective to avoid over- or under-reacting.

---

*This works the same way for other experts as well. For example, whether a doctor acted reasonably in medical care will be judged against the reasonably prudent doctor of similar skill, training and specialty.

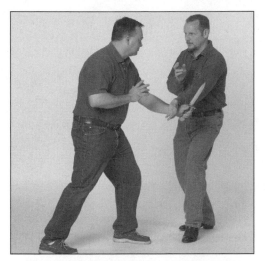

DEFENSIVE TECHNIQUES. BLOCKING A KNIFE TEMPORARILY PROTECTS AGAINST BEING CUT BUT DOES NOTHING TO PREVENT FURTHER ATTACKS. THIS IS AN INSUFFICIENT RESPONSE IN AND OF ITSELF FOR THIS SCENARIO.

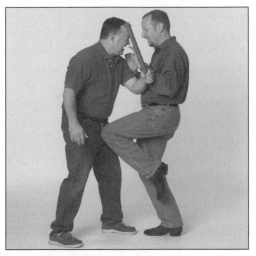

OFFENSIVE TECHNIQUES DISCOURAGE AND/OR DISABLE AN OPPONENT'S WILLINGNESS AND ABILITY TO CONTINUE THEIR ATTACK. THEY ARE TYPICALLY NON-LETHAL.

Defensive Techniques

Techniques for defense such as blocking, dodging, or evading may protect you from harm as you try to escape an assailant. A purely defensive strategy cannot last long, however. If you cannot immediately get away from an attacker, remaining solely defensive allows the assailant to control the fight and ultimately cause your grievous bodily injury or death.

Offensive Techniques

The only way to stop a determined opponent you cannot get away from is with offensive techniques that discourage and/or disable their willingness and ability to continue attacking you. Offensive techniques include punching, kicking, shoving, tripping, and all the usual martial arts applications such as strikes, chokes, locks, and even certain pressure point techniques. When weapons are used to protect yourself, offensive applications may also include the use of stun guns or chemical sprays, or if you are in law enforcement, water cannon, bean bag guns, Tasers, and other typically non-lethal control devices.

Regardless of what the advertising states, people occasionally die from "non-lethal" devices or techniques so they should not be deployed unless you are truly in jeopardy. For example, on May 3, 2005, an unidentified Phoenix (Arizona) man suspected of assaulting a law enforcement officer died after being shocked multiple times with Taser stun guns during a struggle with police.

According to news reports, the 24-year-old man had run out a back door of his apartment when officers tried to arrest him. A female officer caught up with the man and shocked him. When the suspect continued to resist arrest, another officer shocked him with his stun gun as well. The suspect became unconscious and was later pronounced dead at the hospital. While there is little evidence of Tasers alone causing accidental death,* some states are beginning to pass laws controlling the use and ownership of stun guns and similar devices.

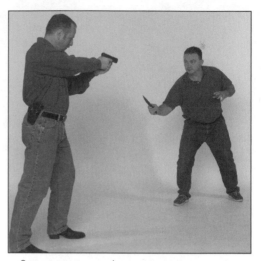

SURVIVAL APPLICATIONS. IN CERTAIN CIRCUMSTANCES, NON-LETHAL DEFENSIVE AND OFFENSIVE APPLICATIONS ARE SIMPLY NOT ENOUGH TO ASSURE YOUR SURVIVAL. NOT ALL SURVIVAL APPLICATIONS ARE LETHAL YET THEY TYPICALLY CAN BE.

In another example, on October 22, 2004 Victoria Snelgrove, a 21-year-old journalism major at Emerson College, was hit in the eye by an FN303 pepper ball projectile fired by police who were trying to break-up a mob unruly baseball fans near Fenway Park who were celebrating the Red Sox winning the American League pennant at Yankee Stadium. The pepper balls, a usually non-lethal projectile, are designed to break apart on impact, acting in a manner similar to OC spray. Snelgrove subsequently died at Brigham and Women's Hospital later in the day from the head injury.

Fights are dynamic and unpredictable. Combatants have died from falls, improperly applied chokes, and other typically non-lethal restraints. Consequently, your best defense is not being there in the first place.

Survival Applications

While non-lethal defensive and offensive techniques are appropriate in certain situations, defending against an armed assailant almost always requires you to kick things up another notch. Survival applications, while not always lethal, typically can be. For the martial artist there are vital area strikes, pressure point manipulations,† and other fight-stopping techniques. You can also utilize makeshift weapons, knives, firearms, and even vehicles as the situation warrants. Keep in mind the moral, ethical, and legal considerations previously discussed as you determine how to act.

---

*Forensic studies typically find other contributing factors such as heavy drug use.
†Pressure point manipulations in and of themselves do not always work so they should be considered "extra credit" rather than relied upon as a primary technique.

Principles of Defense

"There is a large variety of dangerous people carrying knives, some of whom are highly skilled in a variety of fighting styles and some of whom are not. But whether a blade is wielded by a master or a stupid drunk, it can still cut you, and cut you badly. Even if it's flailed haphazardly, it can sever an artery or, as your mother used to warn, take out an eye." [3]

– Loren Christensen

When fighting an armed assailant it is essential to control the weapon, disable the weapon delivery system (your attacker), simultaneously attack and defend, and never stop for any reason until he is incapacitated enough that you can safely get away. After the first defensive move, your next technique needs to be, if not immediately lethal, at least severely disabling. Aim for vital points such as eyes, ears, throat, solar plexus, groin, knees, and ankles. Use all your strength and skill. You never know which blow will land so make each one count. The shorter the fight the safer you will be.

Train realistically, hard, and often. *Dojo* training can help you develop skills necessary to survive on the street. As the great sage Aristotle once wrote, "Excellence is an art won by training and habituation. We do not act rightly because we have virtue or excellence, but rather we have those because we have acted rightly. We are what we repeatedly do. Excellence, then, is not an act but a habit." Make rigorous, realistic training one of your daily habits for survival.

Real fights rarely happen in the *dojo* however. Training in the *dojo* is essential, of course, but practicing outside the *dojo* on occasion can help realistically prepare practitioners for real combat. It is important to understand how you might apply your martial techniques should you be fighting on a hill, around furniture or other obstacles, in a stairwell, under water, in a crowd, or in any other unusual situation, you won't find in the *dojo*.

Be sure to practice in street clothes so that you will understand the benefits and limitations that come with your wardrobe. For example, the clothes that most people wear are simply not conducive to the extreme leg movements necessary to kick above their waist. While that may be obvious with dresses or long skirts, it often holds true for jeans and slacks as well. Certain types of footwear such as steel-toed boots, on the other hand, can increase the potency of kicking techniques (though you may have to hold your toes differently).

There are several principles that can help you defeat an armed attacker, regardless of what type of weapon that he or she employs against you. Those include:

- Keep it simple.
- Get off line.
- Control the person holding the weapon.
- Aim for the target.
- Never underestimate the opponent.
- Fight as if your life depends on it.
- Cheat to win.
- Account for adrenaline.

Keep it Simple

Do not get fancy, especially against an armed assailant. On the street, there are no points for executing a technique with perfect form. Do whatever it takes to win no matter how messy or sloppy it becomes. Once the fight begins, adrenaline will affect your fine motor skills so you have to keep things simple if you wish them to be effective. Use well-directed, efficient techniques—things you know you are good at and can rely on under extreme stress. There are techniques you know, techniques you can do, techniques you practice, and techniques you would be willing to bet your life on. Apply only the latter in a real fight. Any mistake you make could be your last.

Hick's law states that response times increase in proportion to the logarithm of the number of potential stimulus-response alternatives. That is a fancy way of saying that the more choices you have to make the longer it takes to make a decision. While you may know and even practice hundreds of techniques in your martial training, a limited subset is required in self-defense situations. During the OODA loop, the orientation and decision flow time will be adversely affected if you think too much, ultimately leading to disaster.

Try to simultaneously attack and defend, using body movement for evasion coordinated with strikes that work like blocks. For example, if you can blow out someone's knee with a joint kick you simultaneously upset their balance, reduce their ability to fight, and spoil their aim. To have the greatest opportunity for success, you should strike or defend with your body part (e.g., hand, elbow, knee, foot) closest to your adversary. Defensive movements must cut off the attacker's technique before it gains too much speed and power, catching it as close to their body as possible and causing as much disruption to their plans as achievable. Offensive techniques must afford the opponent as little reaction time to counter as possible.

Get Off Line

Most martial artists are simply not skilled enough to go toe to toe with an armed aggressor and not get hurt. Move away from the strength of their attack, preferably away from the weapon. It is imperative to not only get off line, but also to keep your attacker from being able to reorient immediately at the same time. In a typical martial arts example, we might call this "closing." Closing is done by moving to the outside while blocking across the opponent's body to tie-up his or her limbs, forcing him/her to reposition before successfully counterattacking.

It is even better if you can get behind your adversary. Use movement and distraction to imbalance and overcome. Stay balanced, upright, and mobile, keeping your weight centered over your feet. Body positioning and mobility not only keep you out of harm's way but also afford opportunities to counterstrike. Good balance is also needed if you are to generate powerful, effective techniques.

Control the Weapon

Controlling the weapon is more complicated than it sounds. This does not necessarily mean disarming the opponent. Traditional locks, control techniques, and disarms do not always work, even when you are highly skilled. To be prepared you must accept that depending on what he or she is pointing or swinging at you, it may not be possible to remove a weapon safely from an attacker's control. You may be able to keep it from hitting you however, which is all that really matters. Use body

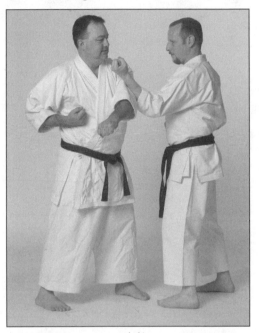

CLOSING BLOCK (*CHUDAN UKE*). NOT ONLY IS THE ATTACKER CLOSED BUT THE DEFENDER HAS ALSO MOVED OFF HIS LINE OF FORCE. THE ATTACKER MUST REPOSITION HIS BODY IN ORDER TO CONTINUE FIGHTING. DURING THIS SPLIT SECOND OF DEFENSELESSNESS, A WELL-EXECUTED COUNTERATTACK IS NEARLY UNSTOPPABLE.

positioning, movement, and judicious martial applications to keep the weapon away from you while defeating the person holding it.

Someone brandishing a weapon is likely trying to scare or threaten you. Someone attacking you with a weapon, on the other hand, is almost certainly trying to kill you. Disabling the weapon's delivery system is essential. You must stop them as quickly as possible before they can critically injure, permanently maim, or kill you.

Do not forget to use both hands. You may have your own weapon in one hand

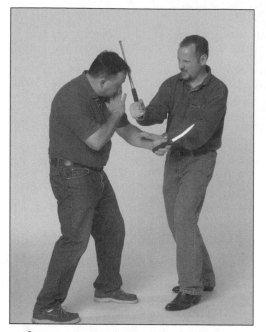

CONTROL THE ATTACKER'S WEAPON, USING ONE OR BOTH HANDS AS APPROPRIATE. IN THIS EXAMPLE, ONE HAND PARRIES TO DEFLECT THE OPPONENT'S BLADE WHILE THE OTHER IS FREE FOR A COUNTERSTRIKE USING AN ASP BATON. NOTE THAT THE DEFENDER HAS MOVED OFF LINE AS WELL FOR ADDED SAFETY.

yet the other remains free to deflect, parry, check, grab, or otherwise control your opponent and/or their weapon. Some knife fighting systems, for example, use the concept of a "live hand" to control an opponent's weapon while others use a "dead hand" to receive their attack saving your more vital areas from damage. I rather prefer the mentality associated with the "live" concept, but either way both hands come into play. Do not get so caught up in using your weapon that you forget about your other hand.

Aim for the Target

Certified fight director Michael Jerome Johnson[4] once said, "If you're going for the weapon, its stage combat. If you're going for the target, it ain't." I like that quote. There is a huge difference between movie fights and real ones, of course, yet all too often newcomers and even some experienced martial artists aim for their opponent's weapon rather than trying to hit the person they are fighting. This phenomena stems in part from procedures we put in place to train safely, fear of hurting our training partner, and our inherent trepidation of weapons we know can hurt us.

This may be okay to a certain extent in the *dojo*, but it is a bad habit we must break to survive on the street. I remember holding my sword to one side leaving a gigantic gap in my defense only to have student after student continue to aim at the weapon during one seminar I taught to some new fighters in a medieval recreation group. In disgust, I finally tossed my blade onto the ground and said, "Hit me now." Since I was wearing real armor and we were using wooden swords made from rattan I was in no danger of seriously injury from that little stunt, but it did effectively drive the point home. They finally got the message: aim for the person who is attacking you.

It is the person not his or her weapon that will kill you. While you may certainly have to parry at times during a fight, never forget that your opponent is your most important target. If you are fighting for your life, you must make every blow count. Aim well.

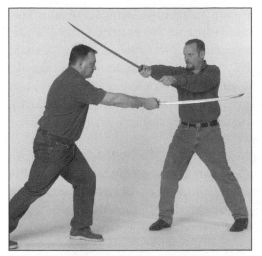

AIM FOR THE OPPONENT NOT HIS/HER WEAPON. THE WEAPON IS HARMLESS BY ITSELF; IT IS THE ADVERSARY WHO WILL KILL YOU. IN THIS EXAMPLE I AM DODGING THE SWORD THRUST WHILE COUNTERATTACKING WITH MY OWN BLADE. IF I HAD TARGETED THE SWORD, I WOULD HAVE NEEDLESSLY BLOCKED AND FORGONE AN OPPORTUNITY TO SUCCESSFULLY COUNTER-ATTACK. OPPORTUNITIES SUCH AS THIS OPENING ARE RARE IN A REAL FIGHT; THEY MUST BE TAKEN ADVANTAGE OF.

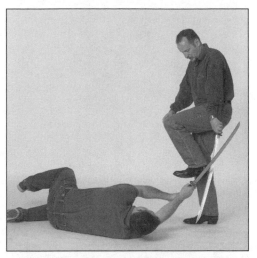

REMAIN VIGILANT UNTIL YOU ARE ABSOLUTELY CERTAIN THAT YOUR ADVERSARY IS NO LONGER A THREAT. AS THE OLD CHINESE PROVERB STATES, "DEAD TIGERS KILL THE MOST HUNTERS." HERE, THE OPPONENT HAS BEEN KNOCKED TO THE GROUND YET CONTINUES TO PRESS HIS ATTACK.

Never Underestimate an Opponent

By definition, an attacker is dangerous. He or she has almost certainly successfully ambushed and possibly even killed someone else before attacking you. Do not assume that you are more skilled or better trained than your opponent is. Consistent, high-quality training is the best way to ensure that you will have the skills and confidence necessary to prevail if an attack occurs, but it does not necessarily prepare you for all the unpredictable things your adversary might do. Be prepared for anything, never letting your guard down until the confrontation is completely over and you have escaped to safety.

The Japanese have a martial arts concept called *zanshin*, or continuing mind. It is a state of enhanced awareness that should exist just before, during, and right after combat. A martial artist in this state should be hyper-aware of his or her surroundings and prepared for anything. In Western terms, he or she is working in an alpha brain wave state. In slang terms, dude is in the zone.

Be mentally and physically prepared to fight or continue a fight at a moment's notice, always keeping your opponent in sight. Even if your blow knocks an adversary to the ground, remain alert for possible continuation of his or her attack. Do not get caught by surprise, that is a good way to die. Street attacks often involve multiple assailants many of whom are seasoned fighters who know how to take a blow and

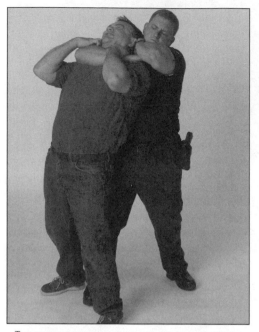

THIS CHOKEHOLD IS GENERALLY A NON-LETHAL RESTRAINT YET IT CAN EASILY KILL IF IMPROPERLY APPLIED OR HELD FOR TOO LONG. ANYONE WHO ATTACKS YOU IS DOING SO FOR A REASON. YOU CANNOT COUNT ON HIS OR HER GOOD GRACES TO LET YOU SURVIVE WITH ONLY A BEATING. WHEN FACING AN ARMED ATTACKER THE DANGER IS EVEN MORE SEVERE. YOU MUST FIGHT AS IF YOUR LIFE DEPENDS ON IT.

shrug off the pain. Be mindful of additional assailants and be prepared to continue your defense as long as necessary. Remain vigilant until you are absolutely certain that your adversary is no longer a threat and that no one else is prepared to take up the battle on his or her behalf.

Fight as if Your Life Depends On It

You can never tell for certain what an attacker's intentions are, but an armed aggressor certainly means to do you some harm. Even when someone only intends to scare you, injure you, or otherwise "teach you a lesson," they might still inadvertently cripple, maim, or even kill you. Some criminals intentionally kill for no apparent reason, perhaps just for the thrill of it. You cannot assume that they will limit their actions voluntarily, beating rather than killing you. You must make them stop. Your survival is at stake. Use every tool at your disposal. Be prepared to use real or makeshift weapons to even the odds.

Cheat to Win

There are no rules in a street fight. Anything goes, including biting, spitting, hair pulling, eye gouging, and punching or kicking targets that would get you disqualified from a tournament match. You must be firmly resolved to do whatever it takes to survive. Try to distract or disorient an assailant or otherwise trick your attacker into letting his or her guard down.

Grapplers such as judo, jujitsu, and wrestling practitioners, for example, are conditioned to stop all movement when an opponent taps out, signifying defeat. If someone has you in a choke, joint lock, or pin from which you cannot quickly escape, you can try to tap him three or four times with your fingertips,* wait until he hesitates or release the hold, then hit him with everything you've got. This technique frequently works even when someone realizes you are doing it because they are so conditioned to let go when an opponent taps, signifying submission.

You might also try to do something that is out of place, unexpected, loud, or dis-

*Or your foot if your hands are entangled.

gusting. Anything that surprises an opponent will aid your defense. One of the best examples of this I have seen was when two male fighters were tangled up, one leaned forward, planting a wet, sloppy kiss on the other's nose, then kneed his opponent in the groin as he instinctively flinched away from the kiss.

I have also seen *judoka* pick their noses and pretend to wipe the snot on an opponent's uniform to get him to flinch away. While this is certainly a violation of tournament etiquette, it can be effective on the street. Even a properly delivered spirit shout or *kiai* can momentarily freeze an opponent leaving him or her vulnerable to your attack.

Account for Adrenaline

When I took a defensive handgun course several years ago, I was taught to train for handling the survival stress reaction commonly associated with actual combat. To simulate the reaction we had to do as many pushups as we could as fast as we could for one minute. Immediately after completing the pushups, we sprinted to the parking lot and raced around the building four times as fast as we could go, covering close to a mile in the process. We then sprinted back into the building and attempted to accurately fire down range under the watchful eye of our instructors.

While I could normally hit the bulls-eye of a static paper target much of the time at 25 feet during shooting competitions, and always put every shot in the black, the first time I attempted to do so after this stress test I missed the paper completely. It was an eye-opening experience.

Once they taught us breath control techniques to help us recover from the affects of adrenaline I found my targeting much less diminished. This breathing was similar to *ibuki* breathing in martial arts, breathing in through the nose and out through the mouth following a 4-count process for each step—inhalation, hold, exhalation. In other words, each cycle of combat breathing includes:

- Inhale for a 4-count.
- Hold for a 4-count.
- Exhale for a 4-count.

The more comprehensive and realistic your *dojo* training is, the better you will perform in actual combat since conditioned responses can help you counteract, or at least work through, the affects of adrenaline. Conversely, the more stressed you are through exertion, fear, or desperation, the harder it is perform. In a violent encounter, your heart rate can jump from 60 or 70 beats per minute (BPM) to well over 200 BMP in less than half a second. Here is how accelerated heart rates can affect you:

- For people whose resting heart rate is around 60 to 70 BPM, at around 115 BPM many begin to lose fine motor skills such as finger dexterity making it difficult to successfully dial a phone, open a lock, or aim a weapon.
- Around 145 BPM most people begin to lose their complex motor skills such as hand-eye coordination, precise tracking movements, or exact timing, making complicated techniques very challenging if not impossible.
- Around 175 BPM most people begin to lose depth perception, experience tunnel vision, and sometimes even suffer temporary memory loss.
- Around 185 – 220 BPM many people experience hyper-vigilance, loss of rational thought, and inability to consciously move or react. Without prior training, the vast majority of people cannot function at this stress level.

Angles of Attack

"There is only one tactical principle which is not subject to change; it is to use the means at hand to inflict the maximum amount of wounds, death, and destruction on the enemy in the minimum amount of time." [5]

– General George S. Patton

More than two decades ago in Society for Creative Anachronism (SCA) and Realm of Chivalry (RoC) sword training, I learned nine distinct angles or planes of attack from which a weapon might approach. My instructor described them as a plus, an 'x', and a poke. Later on with live steel choreography, I discovered the same basic angles were used to explain the forms. Later still while practicing *arnis* in the Philippines, I was taught those same nine angles once again.

It may be beneficial to think of these nine angles as planes through which the weapon must travel to reach you. Each angle can be aimed at any section of your body—head, torso, groin, and so on. Though some systems use as many as 13 or even 20 planes of attack, I think that anything more than nine is really semantics. For all intents and purposes, I think that this approach realistically defines the angles from which you may be attacked and helps identify what you might do to engage or evade a weapon coming at you from those angles. The key concept is that you can expect a weapon to travel along one of these planes of attack as your opponent delivers the blow. Even with trickery and fancy movements designed to disguise the direction of the strike, all blows eventually end up coming toward you from one of these nine planes.

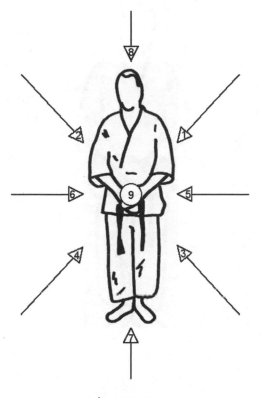

ANGLES OF ATTACK.
(ILLUSTRATION COURTESY OF KRIS WILDER.)

The Japanese have names for these planes of attack, combining the level of the attack with the angle of the attack to describe its trajectory. Upper level strikes are called *jodan*, middle strikes called *chudan*, and lower level strikes called *gedan*. Vertical strikes are called *uchi*, sideways strikes are called *yoko*, diagonal strikes *naname*, and thrusts *tsuki*.

Combining *jodan* (upper), *chudan* (middle) and *gedan* (lower) with *yoko* (side), *naname* (diagonal), *uchi* (strike), and *tsuki* (thrust) is a useful way to describe the nine planes of attack, one that is a little more distinct than simply naming the angle. In this fashion, a diagonal head strike (planes 1 or 2) is called *jodan naname uchi* in Japanese, while a straight shot down into the head (plane 8) is called *jodan uchi*. A horizontal baseball bat style strike would be *chudan yoko uchi* if aimed at the midsection, or *jodan yoko uchi* if swung at the head. Similarly it would be *gedan yoko uchi* if aimed below the waist. This concept can help practitioners figure out what kind of attack they face and how best to respond.

Using Japanese terminology, we can also differentiate a shorter jabbing thrust

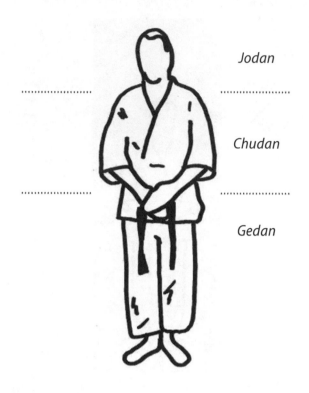

Jodan

Chudan

Gedan

LEVELS OF ATTACK (ELEVATION).
(ILLUSTRATION COURTESY OF KRIS WILDER.)

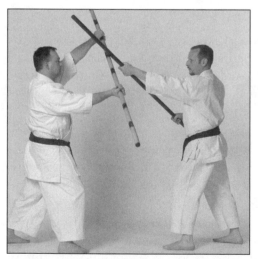

THE ANGLE AND ELEVATION DESCRIBE AN OPPONENT'S ATTACK. THIS IS A DIAGONAL HEAD STRIKE OR *JODAN NANAME UCHI* WITH A *BO* STAFF.

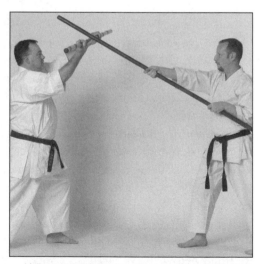

HERE IS A HEAD STRIKE OR *JODAN UCHI* WITH A *BO* STAFF.

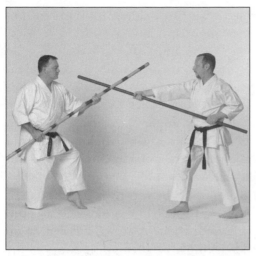

TSUKI WITH BO STAFF, HANDS HELD FIXED AT EVEN THIRDS.

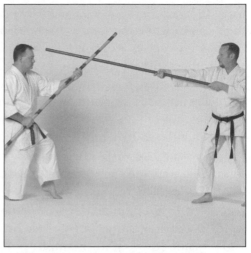

NUKIBO WITH BO STAFF, POOL CUE STYLE WITH HANDS
AT ONE END.

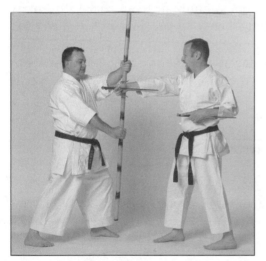

TSUKI WITH A SAI TSUKAGASHIRA (BUTT END). NOTE THAT IN
THIS INSTANCE THE HAND HOLDING THE SAI IS STRUCK BY THE
BO DURING THE BLOCK.

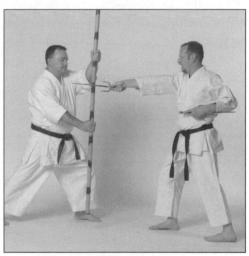

NUKI WITH A SAI SAKI (TIP OR POINT OF THE SAI). IN THIS
INSTANCE THE HAND HOLDING THE SAI REMAINS SAFER.
FURTHERMORE, THE TIP OF THE SAI CAN BE DEADLIER THAN
THE BUTT (DEPENDING UPON HOW IT IS USED).

(*tsuki*) from a longer range strike (*nuki* or *nukibo*).* With a *bo* staff, for example, the *tsuki* is performed with both hands firmly on the weapon, spaced evenly (typically one third of the way from each end) for maximum speed and control. The *nukibo* strike, on the other hand, is more of a pool cue-style shot where the *bo* is held firmly at one end and slid between the fingers of the lead hand for maximum distance with a slight loss of precise control. There is a significant range difference between

---

*Nuki means thrust. *Nukite* is a finger thrust; *nukibo* is a thrust from a *bo* staff, and so on.

these to blows. With a *sai*, the *tsuki* is performed with the *tsukagashira* (butt end) of the weapon while the *nuki* is performed with the *saki* (tip).

Some weapons work more effectively along certain lines of attack than they do along others. Baseball bats, for example, can be used to thrust with but that maneuver does not play to any special strength of the weapon as it would with a spear. Bats are generally used to swing at an enemy.* They are also easier for most people to swing at an opponent at a downward or sideways angle rather than upward. Consequently, you are probably not going to be as concerned with angles 3, 4, 7, and 9 as you would be with others should your opponent have a baseball bat. That is not to say that you will never see an upward strike from a bat, only that it is less likely.

Knowing which angle a blow is coming from can help you react appropriately, especially if your opponent is armed and you are not. In such circumstances, the ability to evade and immediately close or escape is important. A straight down or up strike (planes 8 or 7), for example, can be evaded simply by turning sideways to the blow such that it lands in front of you. Similarly, you can shift or lean away from a diagonal blow (planes 1, 2, 3, or 4). You can duck, jump, or scoot backward from a horizontal blow (planes 5 or 6) depending on where they are aimed (*jodan*, *chudan*, or *gedan*).

In general, it is best to evade while moving toward your opponent so that you can counterattack, control the weapon, or otherwise stop any follow-on strike. It may be possible to evade and immediately escape but that is somewhat chancier if your adversary has not been disabled first.

Stances and Footwork

"Never fight the suspect toe-to-toe. Continually sidestep the attacker or step in a 45-degree angle away from the trajectory of his blade, so that he has to turn toward you. This gives you a little more time to deliver blows to his throat and eyes." [6]

— *Loren Christensen*

Body positioning and footwork is crucial to surviving a street assault. An ill-timed slip may put you out of position to defend yourself thereby ensuring your swift demise. Strength of technique and ability to move to attack or defend rely on proper footwork and good balance regardless of the fighting environment or terrain. Despite the common misconception that stances are just for *kata*, the postures that you practice in the *dojo* can hold you in good stead on the street if you use them properly.

Proper body alignment is critical in a fight. Lose your balance and you likely lose the battle. Further, you can attack your opponent's feet, ankles, and knees simply by

---

*Or a ball for that matter.

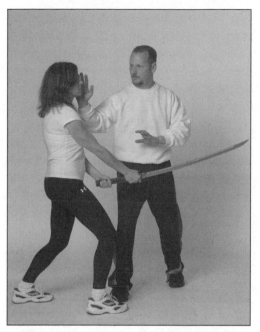

Turn sideways to avoid a head strike from a sword (plane 8). Note that I have moved toward my opponent to position myself for a counterattack before she can strike at me again.

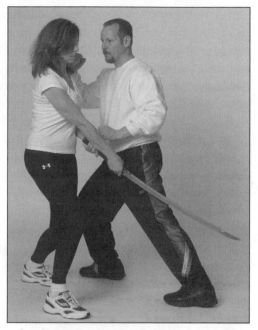

Shift/twist to avoid a diagonal strike coming in from my left (plane 1). Again, I am attempting to move toward my opponent to counterstrike.

engaging with proper stance, balance, and body alignment, unbalancing him or her with your lower body while simultaneously striking with your fists or elbows. Combining leg and hand techniques into one swift attack can be devastating and very hard to defend. Further, proper stance facilitates maximum power for your strike. Without it, you are at a serious disadvantage.

The most commonly used stances in martial arts that can be utilized in actual combat include *sanchin dachi* (hourglass stance), *zenkutsu dachi* (front forward stance), *shiko dachi* (*sumo* or straddle stance), and *neko ashi dachi* (cat leg stance). Each stance has a different purpose with different dynamics.

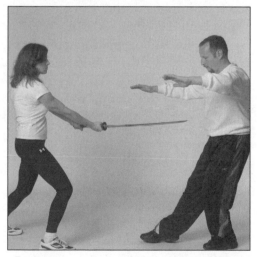

Evade, pulling stomach out of the way, to avoid a horizontal blow coming from my left to my right (plane 5). My intent would be to immediately shift back in and jam her arms to stop a follow-on blow while counterattacking.

Sanchin dachi is a well-balanced stance used for close-quarters fighting. It is performed with feet shoulder-width apart; weight distributed about 55/45 front to back. The forward foot is about one step ahead of the rear foot. Toes are pointed slightly inward, especially on the front foot, where it is more pronounced. The knees track straight ahead, aligned with the hips. Back is straight, spine aligned, with the pelvis pulled forwards and upwards to straighten the lower back as well. Shoulders sit straight above the back with head centered above that such that a straight line goes from the top of the head straight down through the center of the body.

Zenkutsu dachi is a strong forward stance designed for deep distance-covering lunges or to receive driving attacks such as tackles by an opponent. It looks a lot like a hurdler stretch and is performed with the feet shoulder-width apart, forward leg bent about 120 degrees at the knee, rear leg straight and extended approximately two shoulder-widths behind lead foot; the torso is erect. If you drop to a kneeling position from this stance, you will discover that your back knee aligns with your front heel (assuming that you are doing it correctly, of course). Weight is distributed approximately 75 percent on the front leg and 25 percent on the back leg.

Shiko dachi is used to uproot an attacker from beneath his center and is commonly used in Japanese *sumo* wrestling (hence the nickname). To execute it correctly you must be touching an opponent's body with yours. This stance is too immobile to be used successfully at

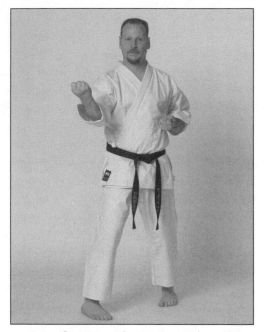

SANCHIN DACHI (HOURGLASS STANCE).

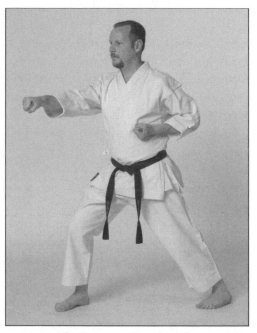

ZENKUTSU DACHI (FRONT STANCE).

any distance. It is performed with feet spread approximately two shoulder-widths apart, toes pointed outward at 45 degrees. Weight is distributed evenly over both legs so it is a fairly stable stance. Knees are bent deeply and pulled back as far as possible with the torso erect. Lower legs/shins are approximately vertical. Pull your shoulder blades together, keeping your upper body vertical. You generally fight at a 45 degree angle over one knee.

Neko Ashi Dachi works off the natural flinch reaction. Rear knee is bent, with foot flat on ground, and toes facing to the outside. The front foot rests lightly (~10 percent) on the ground approximately one shoulder-width forward of the rear leg. Toes face forward, flat on ground, with the heel of foot raised. Crouch slightly, with front leg in center of body, bent a little at the knee. If you slide the front foot behind you, it should clear the back foot rather than entangling it. Keep your torso erect while thrusting backwards with your buttocks.

This does not mean that you must always use the exact same stances in combat as you would in performing your *kata* (forms), however. *Zenkutsu dachi*, for example, is often performed as *shozenkutsu* (half-front stance) in street combat, a shortened, more mobile version of the longer stance seen in many *kata*. You must, however, exercise great caution in making these types of changes, ensuring that your alteration is strategically supportable and consistent with proper stance dynamics.

For example, *zenkutsu dachi* is commonly used to close distance much like a

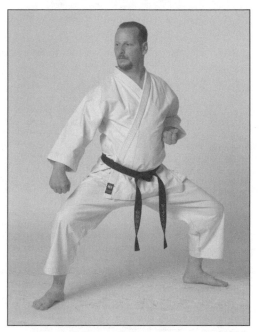

Shiko dachi (sumo stance).

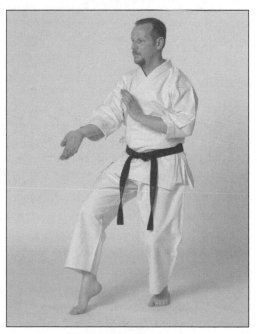

Neko ashi dachi (cat stance).

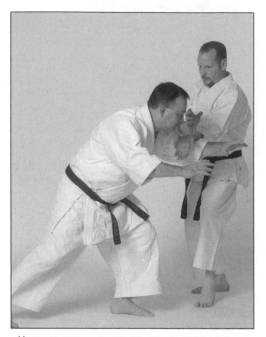

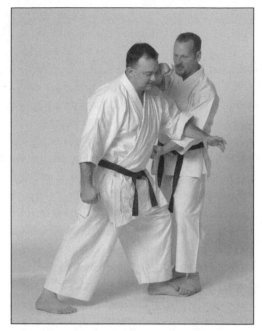

HERE IS AN EXAMPLE OF SHIFTING OFF-LINE, USING *NEKO ASHI DACHI* TO REDIRECT A BULL RUSH CHARGE. THIS STANCE IS USED FOR RAPID DIRECTION SHIFTS. IT IS FLEXIBLE AND QUICK BUT NOT STRONG. THIS TECHNIQUE WILL ONLY WORK IF YOU GET OFF YOU OPPONENT'S LINE OF FORCE WHILE STAYING WITHIN STRIKING RANGE.

AFTER REDIRECTING YOUR OPPONENT IN *NEKO ASHI DACHI*, IT IS ESSENTIAL TO IMMEDIATELY SHIFT FORWARD AND COUNTER-STRIKE. *SANCHIN DACHI* IS A GOOD STANCE TO USE FOR THIS FOLLOW-UP MANEUVER. IT IS WELL-BALANCED, EASY TO SHIFT INTO, AND PROPERLY ALIGNS YOUR BODY TO DELIVER A POW-ERFUL BLOW (IN THIS CASE A *MOROTE TSUKI* DOUBLE PUNCH).

lunge-thrust in fencing. Shortening the stance to *shozenkutsu* in this application may require two steps when only one should have been necessary, ceding valuable momentum to an opponent. This stance is also used to receive strong forward attacks such as a tackle while counterattacking with movements like a clavicle strike and hammer fist to the head. If your stance is not deep and strong enough in such situations, you will be bowled over whether your counterstrike is successful or not. *Zenkutsu* can also be used to add power and momentum to an attack, which is more readily accomplished with a deeper stance than *shozenkutsu* for many applications.

Similarly, some stances such as *shiko dachi* are difficult to perform in certain types of street clothes. To off-balance an opponent with the greatest mechanical advantage, however, you must get below his or her center of gravity. Inability to perform this stance correctly limits the scope of your tactical response. If your clothing selection limits the stances you are able to perform, you must choose applications that can be properly executed with what you are wearing. Such issues notwithstanding, practitioners must have proper body alignment and good stance in order to optimize their techniques in battle.

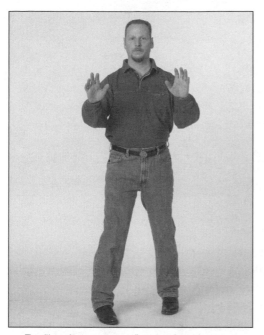

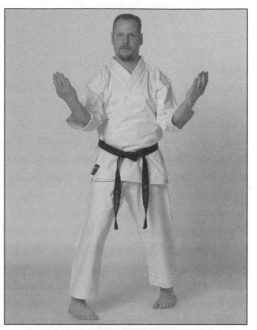

THE "I DON'T WANT TO FIGHT" STANCE. IN THIS POSITION YOU ARE READY TO FIGHT BUT DO NOT LOOK PARTICULARLY AGGRESSIVE OR PREPARED. YOUR WEIGHT IS BALANCED SO THAT YOU CAN MOVE IN ANY DIRECTION QUICKLY WHILE YOUR HANDS ARE IN POSITION TO ATTACK OR DEFEND, ALL WITHOUT APPEARING THREATENING. YOU CAN ADD TO THE EFFECT BY MOVING YOUR HANDS BACK AND FORTH A LITTLE IN A WARD-ING GESTURE WHILE YOU SPEAK, WORKING TO DE-ESCALATE THE SITUATION. SINCE YOUR HANDS ARE ALREADY MOVING IT'S EVEN EASIER AND FASTER TO BRING THEM INTO PLAY IF YOU ARE ATTACKED.

SANCHIN MOROTE KAMAE. THE "I DON'T WANT TO FIGHT" STANCE IS VERY SIMILAR IN STRUCTURE TO THE *SANCHIN MOROTE KAMAE* POSITION SHOWN HERE. THIS POSTURE BEGINS MANY TRADITIONAL *KATA* (OBVIOUSLY, THE PALMS ARE REVERSED BUT THE STANCE AND BODY ALIGNMENT IS ALMOST THE SAME). A SLIGHT ADJUSTMENT IS ALL THAT IS NEEDED TO TRANSFORM THE "I DON'T WANT TO FIGHT" STANCE INTO A FIGHTING POSTURE.

Your ability to move rapidly in any direction, utilizing good timing is important. Your best tactic is to move away from the strength of your opponent's attack without completely disengaging, particularly when weapons come into play. The bull rush is a good example. If a larger opponent is charging you, it is challenging, if not impossible, to stand your ground and receive the attack without being bowled over. Shifting off line, on the other hand, can provide a tactical advantage, which allows you to redirect the opponent's force and simultaneously counterattack.

To be clear, the aforementioned stances are typically used after the fighting actually starts. Rather than adopting a martial-looking stance that warns potential opponents of your training and might even provoke a conflict during the preceding escalation process, however, I suggest using the "I don't want to fight" stance while there is still a chance to talk your way out of a confrontation. It is a non-aggressive posture that can almost instantly turn into a fighting stance.

The "I don't want to fight" stance is performed by standing with one leg slightly in front of the other, weight evenly balanced. The hands are out and moving slowly back and forth in a warding gesture, elbows down. To the untrained bystander it looks very much like someone who really and truly does not want to fight. Even a trained opponent may mistake this for an innocuous posture.

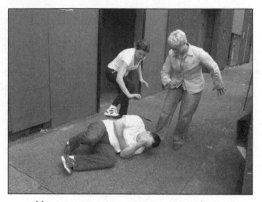

MOBILITY IS ESSENTIAL TO STREET SURVIVAL. IF YOU GO TO THE GROUND, YOUR OPPONENTS CAN STOMP YOU WITH IMPUNITY.

The trained observer will note that this stance is quite similar to the *sanchin morote kamae* (*sanchin dachi* stance with a double block) ready position used in many traditional *kata*. From here, you can readily attack or defend with hands or feet.

Good stances and body alignment facilitate fighting power, graceful movement, and agile footwork. Footwork is important in any fight but it is even more critical in a tandem ambush than it is in a solo encounter. Criminals often work together where one person distracts or holds down the victim while the other robs or kills him (or her). Dealing with multiple attackers is very challenging. If you are forced to fight, you can realistically only engage one adversary at a time. Once the first opponent has been defeated, you can move on to defeat the next attacker.

Defense against a large group is generally handled by strategically engaging one person at a time in a manner that confounds the other's ability to reach you. You can only do that, however, if you remain balanced, upright, and mobile. Without stance integrity, you lose vital mobility. Should one opponent drive you to the ground, for example, the others can simultaneously engage and defeat you.

Range Considerations

"Never kick the blade. A martial artist I know was jumped by an assailant armed with a knife. My friend launched a kung fu kick at the blade only to have the attacker do a fillet on his ankle, calf, and thigh before he could retract his foot. A hand holding a knife is too fast to kick." [7]

– Loren Christensen

The decision to run or fight and what tactics you can use will be based in part by the weapon you face, how it is deployed, and how far away you are at the beginning of the encounter. Similarly, if you are armed, range considerations will determine whether or not you can deploy your own weapon in self-defense or if you will have to attempt to control your enemy's weapon first. In Chapter 9 we will discuss various weapon types in detail but for the moment it is important to note that some are more effective in certain ranges (e.g., grappling, close, or short) than they are in others (e.g., mid, long, or extreme).

In grappling range, for example, you may be able to stop an opponent from drawing a gun or even wrest it away from him even if you do not have time to deploy your own weapon in return. In short or mid range, on the other hand, you may be better off fleeing or deploying your own weapon as your assailant will have an easier time shooting you than you will have striking him with your body. Such decisions will need to be made in a split second so *dojo* practice with realistic scenario training is a good idea.

Preventing weapon deployment is an excellent example, something you can practice with a training weapon and real holster. Conversely, if you have the weapon, you can practice handgun retention techniques to facilitate your ability to deploy the weapon and/or prevent being disarmed and killed with your own device. Trying such scenarios at full-speed with a partner can help you get the hang of it. I suggest starting out slowly and working toward that ultimate goal of realistic intensity so that no one gets hurt, however.

Here are some things to consider. If the bad guy is wearing a shoulder holster, he will have to reach across his body to draw the weapon. Similarly, if he has a hip holster, he will have to reach back, down, and then up again to withdraw it. In either case, you may be able to press-block (*osae uke*) his arm, temporarily pinning it in place for long enough to strike. In order to block successfully a person from drawing their weapon you will need to have good stance integrity and strong forward pressure, another reason why posture is important on the street. Your opponent only needs to clear a small amount of space to free his or her weapon, something you cannot afford to let him/her do.

A fanny pack or pouch-style holster takes two hands to operate. One hand opens the pouch while the other withdraws the weapon. Unlike a traditional holster that requires only one hand, it is usually easier to prevent a person from drawing their weapon from a pouch-style holster because of this structure.

Range considerations also affect the tactics you can employ in combat, regardless of whether or not you have a weapon. In grappling range, you may employ your elbows, knees, or arms while in close range you may have an easier time using your fists and feet. Similarly, if you are armed you will want to operate in your weapon's most effective range or conversely in your opponent's least effective one. If you have

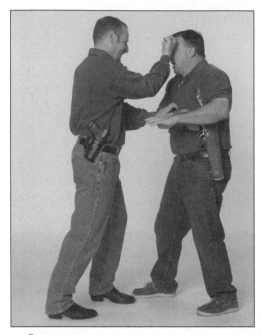

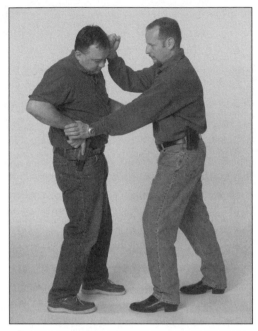

BLOCKING SHOULDER HOLSTER DRAW WITH AN *OSAE UKE* (CROSS-BODY PRESS BLOCK) AND SIMULTANEOUS *URAKEN UCHI* (BACKFIST) COUNTERATTACK. NOTE THAT FORWARD PRESSURE CONTROLS THE OPPONENT'S MOVEMENT.

BLOCKING HIP HOLSTER DRAW WITH PRESS BLOCK AND *TETSUI UCHI* (HAMMER FIST) COUNTERATTACK. NOTE THAT FORWARD PRESSURE CONTROLS THE OPPONENT'S MOVEMENT.

a walking stick or staff and are squaring off against a knife-wielding assailant, for example, you will want to maintain distance from your attacker. If the roles were reversed, you would want to close distance to deploy the blade.

Certain tactics such as high kicks are not very effective in a real fight. They look great in tournaments and movie choreography but are simply too dangerous and impractical to try in real life. To begin with, no matter how flexible you are, it is fairly difficult to execute a high kick at full speed and power with cold muscles. Further, you are probably not going to be wearing a loose-fitting *gi* the next time you find yourself in a real-world life or death encounter.

Further, street combat is typically close, fast, and furious. High kicks require range, speed, and distance for success. A better kicking tactic in such encounters is to chop away at your opponent's knees, shins, ankles, and/or feet. Such attacks are quick and vicious and require very little range to employ. They are difficult to see, even harder to avoid, and cause significant physiological damage with minimal effort. Once you have entangled your opponent's feet with your kicks, you will have a much better chance of landing upper body blows with your hand strikes. If you are tied up really close, knee strikes become easy to execute and hard for your opponent counter.

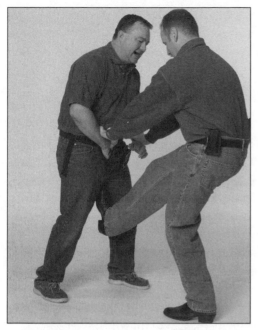

BLOCKING FANNY PACK HOLSTER DRAW WITH PRESS BLOCK AND COUNTERSTRIKE *MAE GERI* (FRONT KICK) TO THE GROIN. IT IS IMPORTANT TO STRIKE UPWARD TO CRUMPLE YOUR OPPONENT RATHER THAN OUTWARD WHICH MIGHT PUSH HIM AWAY FROM YOU, GIVING HIM ROOM TO DEPLOY HIS WEAPON (EVEN IF ONLY FROM THE GROUND).

Hanging back and firing at the head with your foot, on the other hand, can be disastrous. Not only does it take longer for your attack to get there, but also you leave yourself unbalanced during the time that all your weight is on one foot. Moreover, your leg is vulnerable to whatever weapon your opponent has deployed.

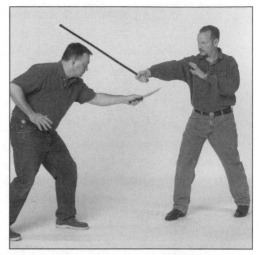

KNIFE VS. WALKING STICK. WHILE THE BLADE MAY BE A DEADLIER WEAPON, THE SHORT STAFF HAS A DISTINCT RANGE ADVANTAGE. YOU CAN INCREASE YOUR ODDS OF SURVIVAL BY PLAYING THE STRENGTHS OF YOUR WEAPON AGAINST THE WEAKNESSES OF YOUR ADVERSARY'S.

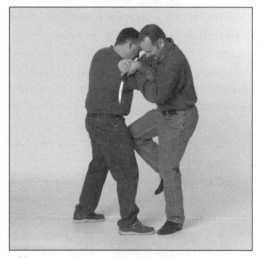

HIGH KICKS RARELY WORK SUCCESSFULLY IN STREET COMBAT. A KNEE STRIKE, ON THE OTHER HAND, CAN BE VERY EFFECTIVE WHEN TIED UP WITH AN OPPONENT IN GRAPPLING RANGE. SLIGHTLY FARTHER OUT A TRADITIONAL LOW KICK CAN BE EXECUTED TO SIMILAR EFFECT.

Empty Hand-to-Weapon vs. Weapon-to-Weapon Combat

"I don't care what anybody else says, if you find yourself facing a weapon bare-handed, get out of there as fast as you can." [8]

— Marc MacYoung

Fighting an armed opponent is very dangerous. It is vastly preferable to avoid such encounters entirely, but if you have to fight against a weapon, you should ideally have one yourself as well. The major exception to this rule is when you do not have sufficient time to deploy your own weapon before being attacked. Even if you have a knife or a gun, you may have to defend yourself with your fists or feet before you can deploy it.

Empty-hand combat versus an armed opponent is extraordinarily challenging. If you cannot prevent your opponent from deploying his or her weapon or bring your own into play before it is too late, you will have to disable him/her immediately. Beyond not being hit yourself, your first response must be either lethal or severely disabling. Any delay in dispatching your opponent may get you injured or killed.

Improvised weapons such as rocks or sticks are generally not as effective as designed weapons such as knives or guns but are usually preferable to having no weapon at all. Regardless of the type of weapon you use, stopping power is an important consideration. Remember that you goal is to avoid being injured and remain safe, not to kill your assailant. Sometimes, however, lethal force is the only viable way to keep yourself safe. Both the ability of your weapon to generate damage and the time it takes to do so are important in such encounters.

Bullets do not always stop a determined opponent, at least not on the first shot. Neither do knives, swords, nor most blunt instruments short of a Mack truck for that matter. It is important to both move and strike, getting off your opponent's line of attack in case your response is not effective on the first try. Even mortally wounded opponents do not always drop immediately. This fact was well known in the old West where they coined the term, "Dead man's ten." It referred to the ten seconds or so a fatally wounded gunfighter still had to kill his opponent before falling over dead. The same concept was observed in Bowie knife duals as well.

Some weapons take longer to deploy than others. Reaction time, both yours and your opponent's is another factor to consider. Since action is always faster than reaction, your opponent will frequently have the initial advantage, another good reason to remain mobile during a fight. In some cases, you may choose to deploy a less effective improvised device that you already have in your hands such as a briefcase, cane, or radio over a designed weapon such as a gun that takes time to draw and deploy.

Summary

"Whoever fights monsters should see to it that in the process he doesn't become a monster." [9]

– *Friedrich Nietzsche*

A continuum of force should be applied judiciously to preserve your safety as the situation warrants. There are no absolutes in self-defense but your ultimate goal is to apply sufficient force to effectively control the situation and keep yourself from harm. A dynamic scale from defensive to offensive to survival applications can help you put things into perspective and avoid over- or under-reacting.

When fighting an armed assailant it is essential to control the weapon, disable the weapon delivery system (your attacker), simultaneously attack and defend, and never stop for any reason until he or she is incapacitated enough that you can safely get away. After the first defensive move, your next technique needs to be, if not immediately lethal, at least severely disabling.

There are several principles that can help you defeat an armed attacker, regardless of what type of weapon that he or she employs against you. Those include keeping it simple, getting off line, controlling the person holding the weapon, never underestimating the opponent, fighting as if your life depends on it, cheating to win, and accounting for adrenaline.

There are nine angles or planes of attack from which a weapon may be deployed. Some weapons work more effectively along certain lines of attack than they do along others. Knowing which angle a blow is coming from can help you react appropriately, especially if your opponent is armed and you are not. In such circumstances, the ability to evade and close or escape is crucial.

Body positioning and footwork is crucial to surviving a street assault. Strength of technique and ability to move to attack or defend rely on proper footwork and good balance regardless of the fighting environment or terrain. Despite the common misconception that stances are just for *kata*, the postures that you practice in the *dojo* can hold you in good stead on the street if you use them properly. The most commonly used stances in martial arts that can readily be deployed on the street include *sanchin dachi* (hourglass stance), *zenkutsu dachi* (front forward stance), *shiko dachi* (*sumo* or straddle stance), and *neko ashi dachi* (cat stance).

The decision to run or fight and what tactics you can use will be based in part by the weapon you face, how it is deployed, and how far away you are from it at the beginning of the encounter. Similarly, if you are armed, range considerations will determine whether or not you can deploy your own weapon in self-defense or if you will have to attempt to control your enemy's weapon first. It may even be possible to disrupt an opponent from accessing his/her weapon if you are close enough when the fight begins.

Fighting an armed opponent is very dangerous. It is vastly preferable to avoid such encounters entirely, of course, but if you have to fight against a weapon, you should ideally have one yourself as well. The major exception to this rule is when you do not have sufficient time to deploy your own weapon before being attacked. Even if you have a knife or a gun, you may have to defend yourself with your fists or feet before you can deploy it. Empty-hand combat versus an armed opponent is extraordinarily challenging. If you cannot prevent your opponent from deploying his or her weapon or bring your own into play before it is too late, you will have to disable him/her immediately.

Reaction time, both yours and your opponent's, is another factor to consider. Since action is always faster than reaction, your opponent will frequently have the initial advantage, another good reason to remain mobile during a fight. In some cases, you may choose to deploy a less effective improvised device that you already have in your hands such as a briefcase, cane, or radio over a designed weapon such as a gun that takes time to draw and deploy.

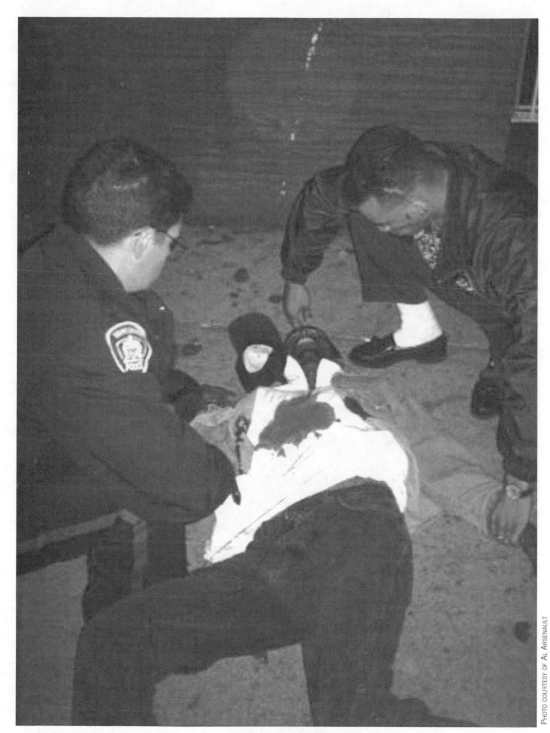

VIOLENT CRIME VICTIM'S LAST BREATHS.

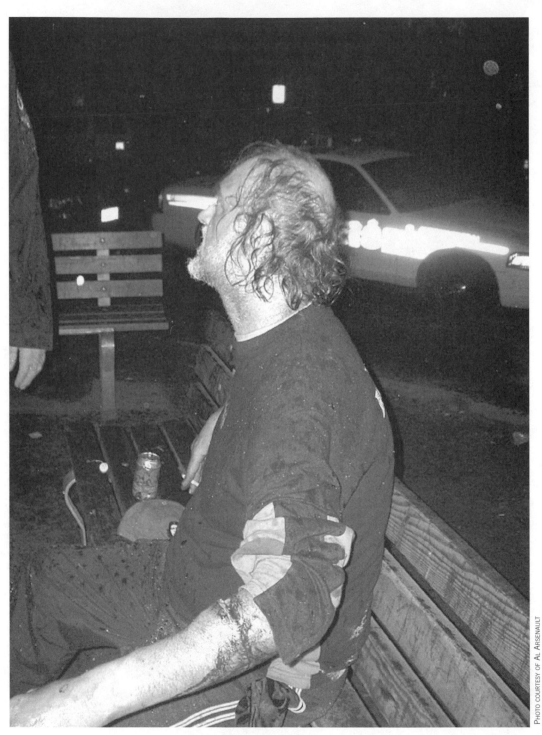

MACHETE ATTACK VICTIM.

CHAPTER 7

Nine Rules to Live By

"On May 17, 1792, Deputy Sheriff Isaac Smith with the New York City Sheriff's Office investigated a disturbance at a colonial inn owned by Levi Hunt, located in what is now the Bronx. The victim deputy was shot with one of two flintlock pistols carried by John Ryer, an unruly drunk, whom the officer was attempting to arrest. Although Ryer fled north into Canada, he was shortly located, arrested, and extradited to New York, where he was tried and hanged for the murder on October 2, 1793. This scenario describes what is now believed to have been the first law enforcement officer feloniously killed in the line of duty in the United States." [1]

– Federal Bureau of Investigation

While the tactics you might employ to defend yourself from the various pointy objects and blunt implements you might be facing will vary, certain principles remain the same. I consider these principles critical items to remember to help keep you safe, affectionately calling them my nine rules to live by. All this information has been discussed in greater detail somewhere else in this work yet I feel that that it is important enough to be collected in one place for emphasis. Since you have seen this before in one fashion or another, however, I'll be brief:

Rules:
- Don't get hit.
- Pain is your friend.
- Weapons are ubiquitous.
- Always assume they are armed.
- Bad guys cheat to win, so should you.
- Understand how weapons work.
- Expect the unexpected.
- Yell for help.
- Check for bleeding.

1) Rule Number One is, "Don't get hit"

"I don't care how tough you are, a knife in the guts will mess up your day. In light of this, I fight like a mongoose against the cobra. Unlike a king snake, which is immune to the rattlesnake's venom, the mongoose could be killed by the cobra's bite. One hit and it's all over for Mr. Mongy. Therefore, when the cobra strikes, the mongoose dodges. Then, once it is off the line of danger, the mongoose strikes and kills the snake. That's how something that isn't immune to snake venom can survive hunting snakes, and that's how you can survive a street situation." [2]

– Marc MacYoung

The first person to be forcefully struck is at a severe disadvantage in any fight. This is especially true in armed confrontations. If possible, withdraw before the first blow is thrown. Awareness, avoidance, and de-escalation are paramount. Never start a fight and always do your best to avoid situations that are likely to lead to violence. If things do go bad and weapons are involved, your best tactic may simply be to run away. If you do have to engage an armed aggressor in combat, end the fight as quickly as possible to increase your chance of survival.

Not getting hit means that if you cannot avoid a violent encounter altogether you must deal with the immediate threat expeditiously and do so in a manner that facilitates your ability to escape further harm. Getting off line is an important principle of weapons defense. It makes you much harder to hit. Doing so in a manner that precludes continuance of the attack or at least affords you the opportunity to counterattack is paramount. Use movement to control the fight, removing options and initiative from your attacker's arsenal.

2) Pain is Your Friend

"Focus on the offensive. Ignore the pain... Adrenaline pours into your system, adrenaline being the magical substance that doctors in emergency rooms inject into cardiac arrest patients to bring the dead back to life. It puts your pain tolerance through the roof... Remember that the control of fear and the commitment to ignore pain are the keys to your positive, aggressive response in a street survival situation." [3]

– Massad Ayoob

Okay, so you've blown rule number one. The next most important thing to remember is if it hurts, you are still alive. According to Massad Ayoob, a seasoned street fighter will usually beat a karate expert who has never been in a real fight. In order to survive, a practitioner must be prepared to ignore the pain while mercilessly counterattacking their assailant. Embrace your pain and fear to urge you on. Refuse to give up. Think about who you are fighting for beyond yourself—your family and friends. What will happen to them if you do not survive? If I can be clocked in the head with a bat and continue to fight so can you.

If one's heart is truly in a fight, strikes to non-vital areas can have little effect. Loren Christensen, a retired military policeman, civilian law enforcement officer, and martial artist who has survived a ton of violent confrontations wrote, "I've had to fight guys even after they have been shot and they still fought like maniacs. I know of two occasions where suspects had been shot in their hearts and they fought the officers for several seconds before they crumpled dead to the ground… I saw two cases of people shot in the head—one person took five rounds—and they were still running around screaming and putting up a fuss." In the heat of battle, it is very, very difficult to stop a determined combatant.

There is plenty of time to deal with pain after a battle is concluded. During the fight either do your best to ignore it completely or, if you are unsuccessful, use your pain as a reminder that you are still alive, still in the fight. Never stop until you have disabled your opponent and have escaped to a safe location. Then, and only then, can you afford to worry about how much it hurts.

---

3) Weapons Are Ubiquitous

"There are more and more fights taking place where a weapon was brought to use before, during, or after the confrontation. Especially knives. Always be aware and prepared for a weapon in a street fight at any time." [4]

– Darren Laur

The vast majority of aggressors carry weapons because it takes very little skill or special training to use one effectively. Be prepared for an armed confrontation. If someone is willing to pull a knife at a stadium in front of 78,000 potential witnesses, imagine what he would be willing do in a smoky bar or a dark alley. Expect to face an armed attacker.

Even if a fight initially begins with fists and feet that is no guarantee that someone will not pull a weapon at some point during the confrontation, especially if they feel that they are about to lose. Be especially cautious if you face up to someone who leaves the scene then later returns. There are thousands of cases each year, for example, where the loser of a bar fight subsequently retrieves a weapon from his or her vehicle then returns to seek retribution against the winner.

4) Always Assume They Are Armed

"I have stated for years that the only assumption I make in a fight is that the person I am dealing with may have a concealed weapon that I don't see." [5]

— Darren Laur

Awareness is your first line of defense. Scan everyone that approaches you, especially if his or her hands are not in plain sight or you sense a potential confrontation. Look everywhere, but pay particular attention to the hands and waistline. A man wearing a fanny pack is frequently concealing a firearm within it, especially when there is a cord or tab sticking out from between the zippers. Almost anyone can conceal a weapon beneath a loose t-shirt. Real knife fighters never show their blade until they have already cut you with it. Even if you do not see a weapon in an adversary's hands never assume that he or she does not have access to one.

To go a step further, unless you have personally searched an individual or he/she is fully unclothed and you can see every part of his or her anatomy, you must always assume that person has a weapon at his or her disposal—hidden in a sleeve, hanging around their neck, stuffed inside a boot, strapped to their hip, tucked in a pocket, or otherwise available. Since almost anything can be used as an improvised tool, be wary of anything within an attacker's reach as well.

5) Bad Guys Cheat to Win; So Should You

"In prison the knife is an assassin's weapon and victims are taken by surprise. Wardens who are assaulted are attacked without warning, with no chance of meeting the assault on equal terms. Policemen who are knifed have fractions of a second to respond, as the weapon is employed at very short range as a surprise attack. People who are mugged with knives usually don't see it coming until way too late. If you still imagine that these scenarios are duels then your wheel's spinning, but your hamster's dead." [6]

— Lloyd De Jongh

No one wants a fair fight, least of all criminals who are looking to make a quick profit at your expense. Armed assaults are assassination attempts. Since weapons tend to tilt the odds in the bad guy's favor, your training should prepare you to even things back up. Do anything you have to in order to survive. Unlike a tournament competition, there are no rules in a street fight. Do not stop until your attacker has been disabled and/or you can safely get away.

Never underestimate an enemy. In a brawl, anyone is capable of just about anything—sucker punching, hair pulling, eye gouging, and spitting are commonplace. Joint manipulations and vital area attacks are all fair game. Stamping on an attacker's foot, throwing dirt in their eye, striking them in the groin, or deploying a makeshift weapon are all acceptable tactics when your life is on the line. Never forget that anyone who attacks you thinks that he or she can win and has almost certainly done so before. He or she may not look especially dangerous but your attacker absolutely always has a bag of dirty tricks to use against you.

Once someone has assaulted you, never believe anything they say. A bad guy (or gal) is by definition bad. They will lie, cheat, manipulate, prevaricate, confuse, extort, bamboozle, and do anything else they can think of to trick you off guard and ultimately defeat you. You cannot afford to fall for your opponent's dirty tricks in a real fight. There are no rules, pauses, time outs, or do-overs. Street fighting is a no-holds-barred contest for survival, a situation that must be approached seriously.

6) Understand How Weapons Work

"Most of them (criminals) are looking for victims, not challenges. They will not continue an assault if confronted by a confident, determined opponent armed with a sharp knife and the knowledge to use it effectively." [7]

– *Michael Janich*

Just like empty-hand techniques, every weapon has strengths and weaknesses. Understand how they work and use this knowledge to your advantage. Mass weapons, projectile weapons, and edged weapons all have different and unique properties. Even within a single weapon family, for example, single-edged blades are typically used differently than double-edged ones. Strive to learn techniques that can stop a person from drawing their weapon or otherwise putting it into play effectively.

Miyamoto Musashi, arguably the greatest warrior who ever lived, was a strong advocate of mastering your own form first, then learning a little about every other martial style you might reasonably be expected to encounter. The more familiar you are with how various weapons and martial styles work the better your chances of countering them effectively on the street. A life or death struggle is hardly an environment conducive to learning. It is far better to make mistakes within the relatively friendly confines of a training hall.

7) Expect the Unexpected

"Officers who have faced cold steel report that they were surprised when the suspect attacked them with a knife because it was the furthest thing from their thoughts… Remember that most knife attacks are going to happen when the suspect is literally on top of you." [8]

— Loren Christensen

Anyone who is attacking you has probably ambushed someone successfully before. He or she will use that experience in an attempt to injure or kill you. Actual combat almost never resembles drills in the *dojo*. Remember the kid who threw a bat at me? Remain flexible letting the unique characteristics of a fight determine your reaction. Because every confrontation is different, it is important to ensure that your bag of tricks is deep enough to pull out a proper response.

Never underestimate an opponent. This advice is nothing new, of course, but warrants emphasis nevertheless. In his groundbreaking 1617 treatise, *The Schoole of the Noble and Worthy Science of Defence*, Joseph Swetnam wrote,

"For he that is well instructed in the perfect skill with his weapon although but small of stature, and weake of strength, may with a little moving of his foote or suddain turning of his hand, or with the quick agility of his body kill and bring to the ground the tall and strongest man that is."

There is no time for analysis in a fight. We must let our training take over and guide us safely through the danger. *Zanshin* in Japanese means "continuing mind." It is a state of enhanced awareness that should exist just before, during, and after combat. A practitioner in this state will become hyper-aware of his or her surroundings and be prepared for anything. In Western terms, when a person reaches *zanshin*, his or her brain has achieved an alpha wave state. This person is in the zone. Regardless of how you describe this condition, however, the key point is that we must be focused on the "now," reacting to whatever our opponent does without thinking too much. Flexibility is key.

8) Yell for Help

"How do you call for help successfully today when the tendency is for passers-by to cross to the other side of the road in case you are (a) part of the TV Candid Camera team, (b) going go make them look foolish anyway, (c) going to get them killed? Use everything. Screams, whispers, shouts…" [9]

– Anthony Greenbank

As mentioned previously, the word "help" is overused and often ignored, yet you really do need to get people's attention if you are attacked by an armed assailant. Yelling "Fire!" is a good strategy, but screaming, something along the lines of, "Oh my god, don't kill me with that knife" is even better in many cases. Not only may this tactic have a better chance of attracting the attention of a possible rescuer than generally yelling for help, but it also demonstrates for potential witnesses that you are, indeed, in reasonable fear for your life should you end up killing your attacker in self-defense. Screaming "fire," on the other hand, could be perceived as an irrational fear by passers-by. It may get their attention, but it is not as good in court.

We live in a litigious, legalistic society; one in which information is ubiquitous and media judgment hasty and frequently severe. Creating witnesses, therefore, becomes nearly as important for your well-being as defeating your opponent's weapon is for your survival. Beware of what you say and do. Always assume that your actions will be captured on videotape and reviewed before a judge or jury. Since a fundamental tenet of judicious countervailing force under the law is fear for one's life, your actions must demonstrate appropriate trepidation and true jeopardy before you take violent measures in self-defense.

Attracting attention to your plight not only helps justify your actions in the eyes of the law, but it also helps eliminate the privacy that most law breakers desire while they commit their crimes. While yelling for help may or may not spur a rescuer to intervene, there is very little down side in highlighting your peril.

9) Check for Bleeding

"If you have been injured, your first priority is medical assistance. You may have to care for yourself. If you've been stabbed or shot, your most immediate concern is hemorrhage and the traumatic shock that results from it." [10]

– Massad Ayoob

If a weapon is involved you may be seriously injured without even knowing it. As soon as a fight is concluded, check yourself over and attend to any medical needs before doing anything else. To protect yourself legally it is often a good idea to attend to your attacker's injuries too.

Twirling a sword at a demo a while ago I felt a slight tug on my pant leg but thought nothing of it until one of the kids yelled, "Ooh, you're bleeding." I still have a scar from where the tip of my sword passed through two layers of my canvas *gi* to leave a 1 ½ inch-long gash in my leg, yet I felt no pain until much later. You do not always immediately feel pain from a razor-sharp weapon. Imagine how badly you could be sliced up while under the analgesic effects of an adrenaline rush. Under such circumstances, exsanguination (bleeding to death) is a distinct possibility.

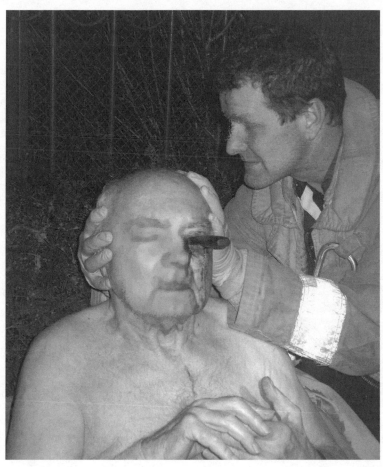

VIOLENT CRIME VICTIM. KNIFE IN EYE.

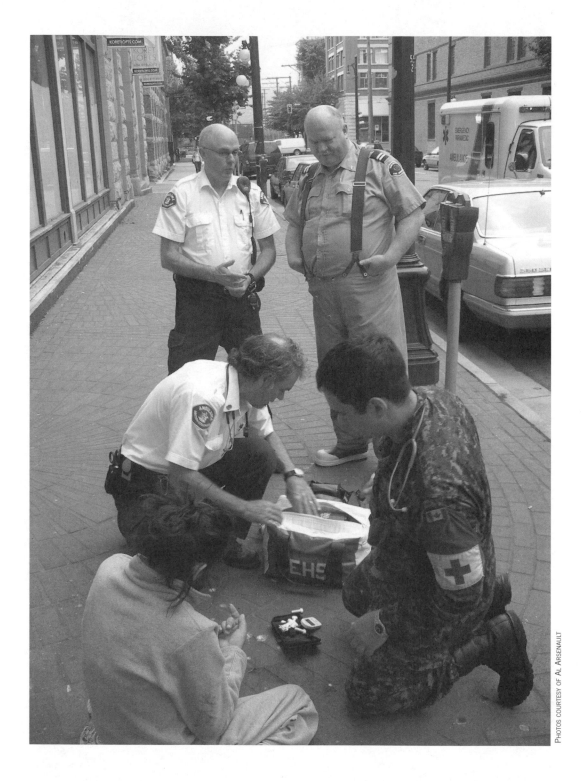

CHAPTER 8

Aftermath of Violence

"Winners have aftermaths too… the person you injured is quite likely to sue you. One friend of mine, an accomplished martial artist, shattered a man's jaw in a brawl; he wound up paying $5,000 to an orthodontist for putting the man's teeth back together. Even if the clown who sues you loses in court you still lose in your pocketbook. It can cost you thousands to mount even a minimal civil court defense…" [1]

– Massad Ayoob

Once you survive an armed conflict, there are a host of other consequences to address, including medical triage, legal issues, managing witnesses, dealing with the press, interacting with law enforcement, and dealing with psychological trauma. Your first order of business is survival. If you have been injured during a fight you may have to take care of yourself until professional help can arrive.

First and foremost, you need to make a mental commitment to live. Your attitude plays a large part of your ability to survive. The next most immediate concern will likely be hemorrhage and/or traumatic shock caused by an attacker's weapon. Control your breathing. Try to stay calm and rational when you are injured. Panic will not do anything but kill you faster as it raises your blood pressure increasing the impact of shock and hemorrhaging. If you are still in the grip of an adrenaline rush from your fight or flight reflex, the pain will be significantly dampened. Take advantage of this time to call for help and begin treating your wounds.

Medical Triage

"Calling for help is often the most important action you can take to help the person in need of aid. If the person is unconscious, call 9-1-1 or your local emergency number immediately. Sometimes a conscious person will tell you not to call 9-1-1, and you may not be sure what to do. Call anyway if the person becomes unconscious, is bleeding severely, has injuries to the head, neck, or back, or has possible broken bones…" [2]

– American Red Cross

Many martial arts students must receive first aid certification as part of their advancement testing requirements, typically somewhere in the upper *kyu* (colored belt) ranks. The Red Cross provides relatively inexpensive, comprehensive first aid and CPR classes throughout the world so access to quality training is rarely a problem. I wholeheartedly approve of this approach. If you have learned how to break someone, you ought to know how to fix him or her as well. Once you have received training, it is a good idea to carry a first aid kit in your vehicle. Be sure to include rubber gloves to protect yourself from blood-borne pathogens (such as hepatitis B, hepatitis C, or HIV/AIDS) if you have to treat others as well.

If you or another person with you has been injured in a fight, controlling bleeding must be your first priority. The Red Cross promulgates a check, call, care approach. Discern the safety of the scene and the condition of the victim first then call 9-1-1 (or the local emergency number), notifying them of the emergency so that they can dispatch an ambulance and professional help. The faster the paramedics get there, the better the victim's chances of survival. Only after these first two steps have been completed do you begin to care for the injury victim.

Once you have taken care of your own life-threatening injuries you will also want to treat your opponent. Remember that your goal in applying countervailing force is to keep yourself safe from harm. If your adversary is disabled and no longer a threat, it is both prudent and humane to try to keep him from dying from his wounds. Whenever possible, wash your hands before and after dealing with another person's injuries, even when you wear disposable gloves.

Controlling Bleeding

Heavy bleeding is controlled first through direct, firm pressure on the injury site, preferably through a gauze pad or sterile dressing. If it is a limb, it will bleed less if it is elevated so that the wound is above the heart. If hemorrhage persists, use pressure points. Only in the worst cases when emergency services will not be available for an extended period of time should you consider use of a tourniquet, which if improperly used could cause gangrene or death. The Red Cross has dropped tourniquet techniques from their curriculum, as they are rarely needed and dangerous to apply.

If you are the one who is injured and think that you might pass out, especially if you are bleeding heavily or it is very cold, you have to get help immediately. If you do not, it will most likely prove fatal. Take a moment to gather your wits and locate the nearest cell phone, payphone, or source of friendly human beings. If you are alone and bleeding badly and there is no phone readily available, you will need to decide whether to stay or attempt to go for help. Physical activity will make your heart race faster, increasing blood loss. You are likely to get dizzy and collapse, thereby losing your pressure hold on the wound, and causing even more blood flow.

Uncontrolled hemorrhage will cause you to exsanguinate (bleed to death).

If there is a reasonable chance that a rescuer will happen along soon, you may be better off dressing your wounds to the extent you can then putting yourself in "shock position" to wait for assistance. This is done by lying on your back with your legs elevated on something or with your legs bent sharply and your toes locked against a wall or similar object to keep them in position if you pass out. Wrap some garment around you to help keep yourself warm. This position helps ensure that as much blood as possible will remain available to your vital organs.

One of the most street-proven trauma dressings is a sanitary napkin or a box of Kleenex, something that ought to be in your first aid kit in addition to regular gauze pads and bandages. Key first aid methods for stopping heavy bleeding include:

- Cover the wound with a sterile dressing such as a gauze pad. If the dressing becomes soaked with blood, apply additional layers over the top of it without removing the original dressing.
- Apply direct pressure to the wound. If bleeding does not stop through a combination of dressings and pressure, you may have to apply direct pressure to a nearby artery to slow the flow of blood. On the arm, the best point is along the inside of the upper arm between the shoulder and elbow. On the leg, the best point is at the crease at the front of the hip in the groin area.
- Elevate the wound above the level of the heart if possible. If you suspect head, neck, or back injuries or broken bones, however, or it may be prudent to remain in place. Moving may increase severity of the damage.
- Imbedded objects should never be removed before you get to the hospital. Doing so may increase hemorrhaging and severely reduce your chances of survival.[3] Bulky dressings should be placed around the object and it should be bandaged in place to support it.
- Severed body parts, if any, should be wrapped in a sterile dressing, placed in a plastic bag, and covered with ice or cold water sufficient to keep the part cool without freezing. Limbs preserved in this manner can frequently be reattached at the hospital. On the other hand, freezing the severed part will cause irreversible damage.

Head, Neck, and Back Injuries

Head, neck, and back injuries are serious. Do not move the victim unless absolutely necessary. If you do need to move the person, be careful to support the injured area, avoiding any twisting, bending, or other contortions that could cause additional damage. If the person becomes unconscious, you will need to maintain a clear airway and possibly perform rescue breathing or cardio-pulmonary resuscitation.

Chest Wounds

Large chest wounds can cause a lung to collapse, a dangerous situation. Cover the wound with a sterile dressing or clean cloth and bandage it in place. If bubbles begin forming around a wound of significant size (open area that is greater than about an inch in diameter), cover that area with plastic or similar material that does not allow air to pass through. Tape the dressing in place, leaving one corner open to allow air to escape with exhalation.

Most normal stab and bullet injuries will not cause a sucking chest wound because the hole from the wound is smaller than the opening in the trachea and will not cause negative pressure which inhibits breathing. If you seal a wound that does not need it, you run the risk of tension pnuemothorax, which can cause a complete cardio respiratory arrest and subsequent death. If advanced medical care is readily available it is generally more important transport the victim to the hospital quickly than it is to seal off the wound with anything more than a breathable sterile dressing.

Abdominal Injuries

For abdominal injuries, try to keep the victim lying down with his/her knees bent if possible. If organs are exposed, do not apply pressure to the organs or push them back inside. Remove any clothing from around the wound. Apply moist, sterile dressings or clean cloth loosely over the wound. Keep the dressing moist with clean, warm water. Place a cloth over the dressing to keep the organs warm.

Broken Bones

Broken bones should usually be splinted to keep the injured part from moving and increasing the damage. There is a variety of ways to create an effective splint. The method you choose will be based in part on what materials you have available, the position you find the injury, its location on the body, and a variety of other factors. The most important thing is to pad and immobilize the injury to the extent possible.

Anatomic splints affix the injured body part to a convenient uninjured one such as tying one leg to the other. A soft splint can be made from a towel, blanket, jacket, or similar material. A rigid splint can be made from boards, rolled magazines, and similar materials.

Infection

If you have been injured by a weapon that breaks the skin, infection is a possibility even after medical treatment. If the wound area becomes red or swollen, throbs with pain, discharges pus, or develops red streaks contact medical personnel immediately. If you begin to develop a fever, it may also be a sign of infection. Seek direction from your physician as to how to bandage your injury, how frequently to change the dressing, and how best to clean the wound to minimize the chances of infection.

Creating a Witness

"As frustrated as we get at what onlookers claim to have seen we have to keep in mind that people are always going to be, well, people. They perceive things based on a combination of what they see, what they think they see, what they want to see, and what they see through a mind filter of their life experiences up to that point." [4]

– *Loren Christensen*

Once you have taken care of any life-threatening injuries you will want to turn your attention to notifying the authorities, calling your attorney, contacting your spouse/significant other, and identifying any witnesses who may be able to testify about your actions and those of your opponent. Let us talk about witnesses first. These folks have first-hand knowledge of the incident and what transpired through direct observation. Since any witnesses must, by definition, be present at the scene during your violent encounter, you may have interaction with them before medical professionals or law enforcement officials arrive. Their perceptions may have substantial impact on what happens to you later on.

Those of you who routinely watch professional or college sports such as football or basketball have, no doubt, seen instances wherein one player fouls another who subsequently retaliates. In the vast majority of those cases, it is the second player that the referee observes committing the infraction. Consequently, the victim of the initial attack is ultimately penalized rather than the person who started the confrontation. It works that way in real life as well. Witnesses frequently see the retaliation rather than the person who initiates a fight. If they misinterpret what actually occurred that could be problematic.

So how do people misinterpret events? The general mindset and biases of each individual will color his or her perception, filtering what is actually observed through the lens of previous experiences, beliefs, and expectations. These biases are part of the human make-up, both intellectually as well as emotionally. Influences on how people will interpret what they see include their previous experience with and attitude about the subject matter, what is urgent and important to them at the time, the mental models through which they make sense of the world, any previous experience they might have had (or may have heard about) with the subject, and any outside issues that may distract their attention. Another compounding factor is critical-incident amnesia. The more traumatic the event is, the greater the chance of distorted perceptions among those who experience it.

Even when a person carefully observes an entire incident from start to finish, his or her perception is bound to be at least a little bit biased, inaccurate, and/or incomplete. Memory is not like a photograph or digital recording. What we commonly think of as memory is actually constructed from available bits of information placed in long-term storage. Since even those paying careful attention rarely observe everything that happens in a sudden, violent encounter, they unconsciously fill in any factual gaps with inferences. When all the elements are integrated into what makes sense as a whole they become what we commonly think of as memory.

To delve a little deeper, memory has three major components, encoding, storage, and retrieval (recall). It is virtually impossible to encode every single element of a situation we observe, store, and later retrieve it with complete accuracy. While you may remember what you ate for breakfast, for example, you will not remember the exact sensation of every bite, chew, and swallow. Furthermore, there are three distinct phases of memory—sensory, short-term, and long-term. Sensory memory is transitory, retained for only a few seconds at best. Short-term memory (or working memory) lasts no longer than a few minutes. These stores have limited capacity and duration. Select data that is transferred into long-term memory can be recalled for days, months, or years.

Since everything we sense is not automatically stored nor retrievable, certain gaps are inferred when we recall a memory, potentially creating divergence between perception and reality. Most of the time that is not a big deal but on occasion it can be critical, something I discovered in a psychology and the law class I took in college. This particular class was taught by Professor Lee Roy Beach. My favorite unit of the class was on eyewitness testimony. Dr. Beach told us about an interesting experiment he used to perform whenever he taught an introductory psychology course. The class he described was generally held in a huge auditorium in Kane Hall* at the University of Washington, where he introduced the subject of psychology to between 700 and 800 freshmen and sophomore students. Here is how the experiment went:

Dr. Beach began the first day of class in each session with an overview of the course curriculum. About halfway through this introduction he had an actor walk in late, approach the podium, and then instigate a shouting match with him. He "accidentally" left the microphone on but moved far enough away from it that the students could not hear every word that was said. The argument would be about grades from the previous quarter. After a minute or two, he would appear to calm the disaffected student down and the actor would leave the room.

Ten or fifteen minutes later as the class was underway another actor who looked completely different from the one who started the argument would enter the room.

*Cool name, huh? No relation to me, however.

While the first actor might be tall and blond, the second actor would be short and brunette. Both actors were always the same gender (usually male), but not necessarily the same ethnicity. They would also wear completely different clothes; say a brown leather jacket and jeans for one while the other chose slacks and a sport coat. This second actor would take a few steps through the door, just far enough to be seen by the class, pull out a handgun, shoot the professor several times (with blanks), then flee the room. As the stunned students watched, their teacher would crumple to the floor, apparently injured or dead.

After a moment of chaos, Professor Beach would stand back up, brush himself off, and explain that everyone had just participated in a psychology experiment. He asked them to take out a piece of paper and write down what they saw, and then explained that they would be told more about the experiment and its results sometime later in class. This not only gave him data to use for his research but also ensured a high level of attendance for the duration of the class as everyone wanted to know what had transpired but did not know when it would be explained.*

What the students observed was, of course, not entirely logical. After all, the person who "shot" the teacher was not the one who had previously argued with him. Despite that fact, over 90 percent of eyewitnesses consistently reported that they had seen a student argue with the teacher about grades, leave visibly upset, and return later with a gun to settle the disagreement violently. Only one student in ten realized that the murderer was a completely different person than the actor with the grading dispute. Roughly, three quarters of the students got the perpetrator's description wrong as well, combining elements of both actors' appearance and/or clothing.

The point of the experiment, of course, was to show the inherent fallibility of eyewitness accounts. Real-life violent events happen suddenly and traumatically. Regardless of what actually occurred, our minds try to draw logical connections between events we observe that appear to be connected in some way. Consequently, the "argument" must have led to the "murder." That makes complete sense even though it is not at all what was truly happening at the time. Memory is not always the same as truth.

In her book, *Witness for the Defense*, Dr. Elizabeth Loftus (a colleague of Dr. Beach) wrote, "Eyewitness testimony, which relies on the accuracy of the human memory, has an enormous impact on the outcome of a trial. Aside from a smoking pistol, nothing carries as much weight with a jury as the testimony of an actual witness. The memory of a witness is crucial not only in criminal cases but in civil cases as well. Implicit in the acceptance of this testimony as solid evidence is the assumption that the human mind is a precise recorder and storer of events... But, in fact, the human memory is far from perfect or permanent, and forgetfulness is a fact of life."

---

*Pretty sneaky, huh? Gotta watch out for those psychologists... Incidentally, he eventually had to stop doing this when an off-duty police officer pulled a real gun and almost returned fire. From that point on students watched the experiment on video tape when he chose to show it.

Some information is never transferred from short-term to long-term memory in the first place, hence inaccessible later on. Most people, for example do not remember details of their drive into work each day. They retain only unusual or interesting occurrences but not every detail. For information we do retain, we do not always get it right. Observations are not continuously complete or correct. Furthermore, memory is fallible and corrodes with time. Contradictory or interfering facts can distort a person's perception from reality, often without him or her even realizing it. As time goes by a person's memories can change, blending fact and fiction, until he is convinced that what he observed is something completely different from the actual truth.

As Dr. Loftus relates, "The danger of eyewitness testimony is clear: Anyone in the world can be convicted of a crime he or she did not commit, or deprived of an award that is due, based solely on the evidence of a witness who convinces a jury that his memory about what he saw is correct." Research indicates that mistaken eyewitness identification accounts for about half of wrongful convictions[5] in the United States. As forensic science progresses this danger becomes partially ameliorated, but eyewitness, misidentification is still a very real danger.

No matter how legal, moral, and ethical your behavior, you will get judged not only by the court of law but also in the court of public opinion, especially if your actions are recorded on video tape, described by reporters, or otherwise communicated by a news organization. Few reporters are naturally sympathetic to those who employ countervailing force, especially where a weapon was involved. Consequently, it is important to act in a manner that demonstrates to any who observe a violent encounter that you are the victim rather than the instigator of the attack.

Always act as if you are on video camera, even if no one else is around (that you know of). Assume anything you do will be interpreted in the most derogatory manner possible and very likely used against you in a court of law. Never forget that most witnesses' only exposure to violence is through movies, books, or television shows. The common person really does not understand the reality of the situation you are in and may judge you harshly because of his or her ignorance. After all, if Jackie Chan, Chuck Norris, Jet Li, and Bruce Lee can subdue a hundred heavily armed ninjas apiece without actually killing anyone, why can't you, a big bad black belt, handle common thug with a switchblade delicately?

A recent news search of the key words "police brutality" turned up 974 stories that were reported within 30 days of my investigation. Law enforcement officers are highly trained, following specific policies and procedures as they conduct their business yet they are frequently accused of overreacting and abusing the criminals, they arrest regardless of whether or not they stay within procedural specifications. How much more likely is the average martial artist, who has no policy or procedure to follow, to be similarly accused of wrongdoing?

So how else can you create a witness who is likely to interpret your just actions favorably? Start by acting afraid, verbally calling for help. This is something you are likely to want to do anyway on the chance that you can ward off your assailant or convince someone to intervene on your behalf. Shouting something along the lines of, "Oh my god, don't kill me with that knife!" is a pretty good indicator of peril. It clearly differentiates who the bad guy is and can help you justify countervailing force in a court of law. "Put down the weapon," "Please don't hurt me," "I don't want to fight you," and "Help, he's got a gun" all put you in a much better light than "Go ahead, make my day!" or "I'm gonna kill you sucker!" Think about various scenarios ahead of time so that you will have a better chance of articulating strategically.

It is pretty easy to shout something during a fight. The real challenge is finding words that put you in the best possible light and your assailant in the worst. It is easy to shout but hard to verbalize so you need to practice this. What you say before, during, and after a confrontation holds a lot of weight in convincing witnesses that you are on the side of the angels while you struggle to avoid becoming one. What you do has significant impact as well. Once you have evaded the initial attack and disarmed, disabled, or escaped your assailant, be wary of reengaging the enemy. It is not only dangerous physically but also puts you on dangerous ground perceptually.

If, for example, you have knocked your attacker to the ground then proceed to kick or pummel him, you will be seen as overreacting even in many cases where you are on sound tactical ground and merely being prudent. A far better tactic in this example would be to precede any further action with verbal commands such as, "stay down", "stop fighting me", "drop the weapon," or "don't make me hurt you."

Where you have the option, the use of open hand strikes, throws, and certain grappling techniques look less offensive than closed fists and are less likely to injure your hands (e.g., boxers fracture). Beware of chokes, however. While *judoka* and other grapplers understand that chokes are only truly dangerous if applied improperly, they have a bad reputation in the news media and are frowned upon by many law enforcement personnel (at least in the administration ranks, anyway).

Everyone knows that blows to the head and face can be fatal. Even minor wounds there can draw a lot of blood, something that looks bad to the casual observer. Open hand techniques are less likely to draw blood than closed hand contact. Where practicable, you might be better off striking an ankle or a knee instead of aiming for the opponent's head. While severely disabling, a knee strike is rarely considered excessively forceful.

Even though it is prudent to consider how your actions may look to an independent observer, never let the fear of prosecution keep you from surviving a violent encounter. Do whatever it takes to survive. If you can react in a manner that helps others realize with certainty that you are the good guy so much the better.

Interacting with Law Enforcement Personnel

"The person in custody must, prior to interrogation, be clearly informed that he has the right to remain silent, and that anything he says will be used against him in court; he must be clearly informed that he has the right to consult with a attorney and to have that attorney present during interrogation, and that, if he is indigent, an attorney will be provided at no cost to represent him." [6]

– U.S. Supreme Court (Miranda v. Arizona)

Imagine for a moment the following scenario: Awareness, avoidance, and de-escalation have all failed and you were forced to defend yourself from an armed aggressor. You exercised appropriate restraint, morally, legally, and ethically applying judicious force to avoid immanent and unavoidable death or grievous bodily harm. You have attended to your injuries and, perhaps, those of your attacker who is wounded or deceased and can no longer harm you. You have also notified law enforcement authorities of your situation. You are coming down off of the effects of adrenaline, tired, shaking, and hurting. Suddenly an officer arrives on the scene. So what might happen next?

Officers are there to ascertain the truth, gathering unbiased facts and evidence about what transpired. They are not there to hand you a medal for heroism under adversity even if you really did act heroically. If in their best judgment there is probable cause that you should be locked up because you committed a crime then that's exactly what will happen. Not exactly fair, but common enough nevertheless, especially if you used a weapon and there is not compelling evidence (e.g., witnesses, video tape) that you used it in self-defense. The way you interact with police officers when they arrive is critical to your continued well being. First and foremost, no matter how upset, injured, angry, insulted, or unsettled you are, never forget that your words and demeanor can significantly affect the tone of the entire encounter and affect the eventual outcome.

Whether or not you are arrested hinges on a concept known as "probable cause." Probable cause means that the responding officer has a reasonable belief that a crime has been committed and that you are the perpetrator. This belief can be based upon several factors including direct observation, professional expertise, circumstantial evidence, or factual information. Officers will make a decision based upon what, if anything, he/she saw during the incident, what he/she can infer about the incident based upon professional experience, physical evidence or other factors at the scene, statements from witnesses, victims, or suspects, available video surveillance, and other relevant data.

Approach the responding officer(s) positively. Cops are people too. They likely have the same emotional make-up that you do. Officers arriving on the scene will be encountering an unknown, potentially hostile environment, where one or more combatants were, and possibly still are, armed. Like any sane person, they will be concerned, cautious, and likely scared. Since they do not know exactly what transpired they also do not know who the good guy is and who the bad guy is yet.

A confrontational attitude will do you no good and may well guarantee that you will be arrested or possibly even shot. Even undercover officers have been killed on occasion by their uniformed counterparts when they failed to immediately follow directions and/or did not identify themselves properly. If you are training a weapon on a subdued attacker, for example, be sure to follow the officer's instructions without any hesitation. While the officer does not know whether or not you are the good guy, he/she knows with absolute certainty that you are armed and dangerous. Do not resist arrest for any reason. Similarly, do not interfere with an attempt to arrest anyone who is with you at the time. Attempting to flee, evade, or elude responding officers is almost certainly going to make you look guilty and result in a chase and subsequent detention.

Be respectful, courteous, obedient, and kind but remember that the officer(s) is not your friend. He or she is not your enemy, but not your friend either. The officer's job is to secure the environment, provide for aid, gather facts, and enforce the law. Consequently he or she will not necessarily be on your side no matter how prudently you acted, at least not until all the facts are known.

Control your emotions to the extent possible. Carefully and calmly explain what happened so that the responding officer(s) will know that you are the good guy. Retain your composure and conduct yourself in a mature manner at all times, avoiding any words or actions that may appear threatening or volatile. Never forget that police are trained interrogators. They will note your body language, speech patterns, and eye movements to help ascertain your probable guilt or innocence when deciding whether or not to make an arrest.

Say as little as possible. Here is an example of something you might say that should be relatively well received, "This was very traumatic experience. I think I'm in shock. I don't think I should say anything until I'm calmer. Can I please call [your attorney or contact person]…?"

Do not, under any circumstances, make any incriminating statements that may be used against you at a later time. Do not confess to any crime, even if you think you exercised poor judgment or are actually guilty. While there may be a fine balance between implying guilt through silence and being overly talkative, if you are going to err, err on the side of caution. You really do not have to say anything at all without an attorney present though it is generally prudent to identify yourself, state that the other person attacked you and that you were in imminent and unavoidable danger, fearing for your life. You may even wish to explain why you could not simply run away. If you used a weapon and have a concealed weapons permit, it is generally a good idea to let the officers know that as well.

The Fourth Amendment generally prohibits seizure of persons without a warrant. However, in some instances a warrant may not required. These instances can include felonies, misdemeanors, danger to the public and violent crimes. A fight probably qualifies for warrant-less arrest under any of these conditions. If you are arrested and taken into custody be sure to understand why.

You should always carry the phone number of an attorney you trust and of a person who can contact an attorney for you if your lawyer is not immediately available. Ask permission to telephone your attorney or contact person immediately after being booked into jail. Be polite and respectful to the jail guards. They can deny you phone access and generally make your life even more miserable if you act out inappropriately. In most jurisdictions you must be taken before an officer of the court (e.g., judge, magistrate) within 24 hours of your arrest. You should always secure counsel and have legal representation before this initial court appearance. If you cannot afford an attorney you can be represented by a public defender though that is generally not preferable.

Exercise Your Right to Remain Silent

Despite Miranda requirements, your fundamental rights and responsibilities may not always be clearly spelled out by the responding officers. You should keep in mind that conversations that precede an arrest and spontaneous statements are usually admissible in court. Remember that you have a Fifth Amendment right against self-incrimination and that it is often prudent to have an attorney present during any questioning.* Your priority should be to alleviate or minimize any potential charges against you, so be enormously cautious about what you say and do before you have a chance to talk to your attorney.

Never forget that anything you say can be used against you later on. While the Miranda rights must be given once you are placed in custody, they always apply. In any event, custody begins when a reasonable person feels they are not free to leave. Rightly assume that once the police arrive at the fight scene you are not free to leave unless specifically told so by the responding officer(s).

A court will generally give more weight to statements made during or soon after an incident, because events are very fresh in everyone's mind. The assumption is that those involved are still in the grip of the moment and generally have not had time to create a false story.

As mentioned previously, the mind fills in the holes of missing data. Filling in

---

*It is a good idea to consult with an attorney before any incident happens to get professional advice about what you should do or not do as an insurance policy against what might eventually occur.

the holes is a process of trial and error conducted by the mind until it finds a reasonable explanation given that individual mind's past experience. The same holds true for victims. They only know portions of what happened, seen through eyes otherwise busy calculating threats and defenses. Soon after the event, the effects of adrenaline and injury interfere with the process of distilling what happened. When forced to talk shortly after an incident the mind simply runs the trial and error process out loud. The result is frequently disjointed and may lead to contradictory statements that will be given great weight later on, even when you were trying to be completely truthful in the first place.

The real trick is to feel comfortable not having everything make perfect sense. There is no need to create a complete story. Be honest. Be brief. For example, "I was walking along minding my own business when bad guy jumps out and threatens me. I tried to get away. I tried to reason with him. It didn't work. When he attacked I defended myself." That's it. Repeat it over and over to all the questions and do not try to be more specific. You most likely will not be able to remember everything you said or did, nor everything the bad guy said or did. You also cannot know what was in bad guy's mind at the time of the incident. Never guess about such things. Be factual and pithy.

In any encounter there is always a metaphorical "his truth," "her truth," and the "real truth" somewhere in between. In the eyes of the law, it really does not matter what actually was. It only matters what can be proven. If you exercise your Constitutional right against self-incrimination, the fact that you did not speak cannot be used against you. It is almost always better to keep your mouth shut and be thought a liar than to open it and have to explain in court later on why you were not a liar.

If the officer(s) believe that there is probable cause to make an arrest you are not likely to talk yourself out of a trip to jail simply by telling a good story. Waxing long will only postpone your trip long enough for the officer at the scene to write down everything you say so that it can potentially be used against you later on.

Do not talk too much and do not try to make anything up. Simply act like what you are—a scared citizen who has just been in and survived a horrible situation. If you are going to talk at all, be honest, be contrite, and be brief. Think about what you are going to say before speaking. Know that everything you say is absolutely correct before you say it, and then remember what you said. Set things up such that you cannot easily contradict yourself later on.

No one at the scene, no one in jail, and no one other than your attorney is your friend when it comes to a violent encounter. Not even the responding officer(s). That's because everyone other than your attorney can be called to testify against you in a court of law. Other than your initial statement to police at the scene, do not talk about the incident without counsel.

Working with an Attorney

"Hiring a defense lawyer may well rank among the most important decisions a person can make. You will be relying on this person to protect your freedom, your family, and your reputation. This is not the time to cut corners or to skimp." [7]

– Laurie Shertz

A criminal defense attorney is a specialist who helps you navigate through the legal process, mapping a strategy to alleviate or minimize any charges against you. He or she acts as an advocate, your voice before the court. It is important, therefore, that you choose somebody who is highly qualified, motivated, and interested in handling your case. Knowledge, skill, and ability are important. Experience is essential. When interviewing potential lawyers, be sure to take note of their experience handling cases similar to yours, their attention to the details of your case, and their ability to explain what you should expect during a trial. A good attorney can articulate complex legal concepts in plain English.

As mentioned previously, you should already have an attorney in mind before you actually need one. Even if you already have someone on retainer, however, it is a good idea to prepare a summary of your case before meeting with him or her. This information will facilitate the conversation and make best use of your time as well as your lawyer's. Attorneys often charge by the hour after all. Even where they do not, the more prepared you are the better the interview will go. You will want to include details such as:

- When and where did the arrest occur?
- What are you accused of doing?
- What did you actually do before, during, and after the incident that led to your arrest?
- How many adversaries were involved and in what manner? Describe significant features such as their number, size, demeanor, activities, weapons, etc.
- Did you use a weapon? If so, what kind of weapon did you use and how was it obtained and deployed? Were you legally entitled to carry said weapon?
- Was anyone else involved?
- Were there any witnesses? If so, do you have names and contact information?

- What did you tell the police? Who were the arresting officers? How did they treat you?
- What is the case against you?
- Do you have a criminal history? If so, what have you been arrested and/or convicted of in the past?

Bring any other pertinent documentation you might have regarding your case. The information you bring to the initial consultation with your attorney can help him or her determine whether or not he or she can adequately represent you. Even if you already have a person in mind, he or she may not feel sufficiently qualified to handle the particular aspects of your case. Further, workload or other issues may preclude that person's ability to take on more work at the time you need it. In such cases, you may be referred to a more experienced or more available colleague.

Before selecting the attorney who will represent you, be sure to find out how much experience that person has in the specific area of criminal law that applies to your case. A DWI* specialist, for example, is probably not the person you want defending you against a murder or assault charge. Because a large number of cases are settled by plea bargain, be sure to specifically ask about the person's trial experience in addition to his or her general capability and proficiency in case you end up in front of a jury.

Find a lawyer with a long track record in the applicable field of law who has successfully worked on cases like yours in the recent past. In firms with multiple attorneys, different lawyers may represent different cases or different aspects of the same case. Be sure to meet the person who will actually be representing your case. If a team is likely to be involved, be sure to meet with each specialist before agreeing to anything. This reasonable request should be readily accommodated. After all, it is your welfare on the line. You are the paying customer.

Understand what and how you will be charged for the case. You will undoubtedly want to hire the best attorney you can possibly afford but you should always understand the pricing structure before signing any contract. For example, research work may include activities performed by clerks, investigators, or analysts in addition to the attorney who heads up your case. Expert witnesses may be retained as well. Understand how the fees for each aspect of the case will be handled and what options, if any, there are. Some attorneys quote flat fees while others charge by the hour. Some accept payment schedules while others require payment prior to performance of the service.

Ascertain how reliable, available, and responsive your prospective lawyer is likely to be. Most attorneys keep a running backlog of cases, managing multiple clients at the same time. Regardless, it is important that you be able to contact your attor-

---

*Driving While Intoxicated (DWI), or Driving Under the Influence (DUI) in some jurisdictions, is a crime committed by a person who operates a motor vehicle while impaired by alcohol or drugs.

ney whenever you need assistance throughout the legal process as well as whenever any new information about your case may arise. Understand your attorney's schedule and availability asking questions such as how often you will be able to meet with him or her. You may be relying on this person not only to defend you in a criminal court but also in any follow-on civil procedure as well.

Once you have selected someone to defend you, you will need to be patient and cooperate with him or her. Never forget that this person is literally your lifeline, protecting your freedom and reputation. While you are bound to be anxious and generally afraid, the justice system moves rather slowly at times.

Ask about the costs, benefits, and risks of pursuing any particular legal strategy. Cooperate with your defense attorney to help expedite the process by promptly providing information. Be willing to do some of your own legwork, gathering documents and information as requested. Keep a log of any questions you might have so that you can discuss them during regular consultations rather than contacting your attorney every time something pops into your head.

As your case progresses, your attorney will work with you to develop a plan for securing your freedom and restoring your reputation. Criminal defense strategies can include alibis, justifications, procedural defenses, and excuses. While the particulars of each case will be different, alibis and justifications are fairly common and are generally effective defense strategies. Procedural and excuse defenses can be challenging to prove in a court of law. There are a few other innovated defenses as well but they are unorthodox, fairly rare, and not generally effective.

An alibi is based upon a premise that the defendant is completely innocent, attempting to prove that he or she was in another place when the alleged act was committed and could not possibly, therefore, be guilty.

A justification is where the defendant admits that he or she committed the act but should not be held liable because of certain special or extenuating circumstances. A justification for murder, for example, is a legitimate claim of self-defense (which makes it not a murder in the eyes of the court).

A procedural defense attempts to prove that while the defendant broke the law he or she cannot be held criminally liable because the state violated a procedural rule. Examples include entrapment, prosecutorial misconduct, double jeopardy,[8] or denial of a speedy trial.

An excuse is an argument that the defendant was not liable for his or her actions at the time a law was broken. Examples include diminished capacity, duress, or insanity.

Other so called "innovative defenses" can include allegations of long term abuse, premenstrual syndrome, battered women's syndrome, urban survival syndrome, and other creative things that lawyers occasionally use to try to convince a jury to acquit a defendant.[9]

The Legal Process

"A jury consists of twelve persons chosen to decide who has the better lawyer." [10]

— *Robert Frost*

There is a difference between jail and prison, at least in the United States. Jail is generally considered a facility where inmates are locked up for a relatively short time such as awaiting trial or serving a short-term sentence, while prison denotes a place where inmates go to serve longer terms after having been convicted of a felony or other serious crime. Whenever you use countervailing force there is a reasonably chance that you will be arrested and spend at least a short time in jail. If you are convicted of a crime such as murder or aggravated assault, you may go to prison as well. Getting from one to the other requires a few steps along the legal process.

While things vary a bit by jurisdiction, the first step in the legal process is almost always an arrest. Arrest is when a suspect is apprehended by an authority figure such as a law enforcement officer or, in some cases, a civilian. If the crime is serious the suspect is usually brought to a jail (or possibly a police station) where he or she will be incarcerated pending an arraignment hearing (judicial bail determination). For less serious crimes, the police will usually issue a notice to appear specifying a time and date where a misdemeanor or infraction suspect has to go for his or her arraignment.

Shortly after being arrested, you will be booked. Booking is the process that creates an administrative record of those who were arrested. This usually involves taking photographs of the suspect, recording physical data, detailing the charges against the individual, and taking his or her fingerprints. Shortly after being booked there will usually be an administrative bail hearing. [11]

Bail is a form of property that is deposited or pledged to a court in order to persuade the judge to release a suspect from jail. Most can be released on bond, which is typically 10% of bail. If the suspect fails to return for trial, he or she will forfeit the bail. In the case of a bond, the person who put up the bond is liable for the entire amount if the suspect skips. In most cases bail money (less a handling fee) will be returned at the end of the trial if all court appearances are met, regardless of whether or not the suspect is found guilty. Bail can be denied for serious crimes such as murder, requiring the suspect to remain in jail until his or her trial.

Arraignment is a formal reading of a criminal complaint, in the presence of the defendant, to inform him or her of the charges. In response to arraignment, the accused is expected to enter a plea. Acceptable pleas vary from jurisdiction to jurisdiction, but they generally include guilty, not guilty, or a peremptory plea [12] which set out reasons why a trial cannot proceed. Some jurisdictions allow pleas of *nolo contendere** or "no contest" as well. This means that the defendant does not admit the charge and does not dispute it either. With this plea, a defendant agrees that the court may find him or her guilty of a crime without ever admitting to the act(s) he or she is charged with.

Even if a defendant pleads guilty, an evidentiary (or preliminary) hearing generally follows arraignment. The court does not have to accept a guilty plea. An evidentiary hearing is a proceeding, which follows the filing of a criminal complaint to determine whether and to what extent criminal charges and civil cause of actions will be heard by a court. Specific rules regarding the admissibility of evidence vary from jurisdiction to jurisdiction. The goal of this hearing is to ascertain whether or not the alleged crime occurred within the court's jurisdiction as well as whether or not there is probable cause[13] to believe that the defendant actually committed the alleged crime. Alternately, a grand jury may investigate the case in certain jurisdictions.

A grand jury is a panel of individuals that can be used to decide whether enough evidence exists to charge the defendant with a crime. Unlike the police, the grand jury has subpoena power to compel evidence and testimony. Everything said before the grand jury is kept secret. The rules of evidence are much more relaxed and therefore cannot be used in a criminal trial. Some states require the grand jury to decide whether charges may be filed while others allow the State's Attorney (prosecutor) to decide.

If the court (or grand jury) finds that there is probable cause to proceed, a formal charging instrument will be issued and a trial date will be set. The defendant and his or her council will get together to chart out a legal defense strategy while the prosecutor will similarly get his/her plan of prosecution together. If the court determines that there is no probable cause, the prosecution will generally cease and the suspect will be released.

The vast majority of criminal cases in the United States never get to trial. They are concluded by plea bargain, effectively a negotiated settlement agreed upon by both the defense and prosecution. The defendant typically pleads guilty (or *nolo contendere*)* to reduced charges to avoid the uncertainty of a trial wherein he or she may be acquitted but might also face a much more substantial penalty. Alternately the defendant may be offered a reduced sentence in exchange for testifying against another defendant and plead guilty for that reason. Either way, if the court finds probable cause to proceed and the defendant chooses not to accept a plea deal, the case will go to trial.

A trial is a test to ascertain whether or not something meets a given standard, in our case to see whether or not a defendant has broken a particular law or set of laws. In the United States, the Sixth Amendment to the Constitution guarantees every person accused of a felony the right to a trial by jury.[14] Many jurisdictions allow a jury

---

*The literal translation from Latin means "I do not wish to argue."

trial for misdemeanor crimes as well. A felony is typically a serious offense such as a murder, aggravated assault, arson, or rape carrying a potential penalty of more than one year in prison. A criminal offense carrying a lesser potential sentence is usually a misdemeanor.

Once the trial begins, the court will convene a panel of citizens from which a jury will be selected. During the *voir dire* process,[15] the judge and/or attorneys involved may question potential jurors to empanel those who will hear the case. Both the defense and prosecuting attorneys may request that certain members of the panel be removed from consideration through a peremptory strike. After any strikes, the court impanels a jury, administering an oath, and the trial can begin. In most jurisdictions, a felony jury trial has twelve jurors and one or more alternates.

In certain instances, your trial may be adjudicated before a judge rather than a jury. This is commonly called a bench trial. Bench trials are generally shorter than jury trials and are only used for crimes where the potential penalty involves imprisonment of less than a few months. The courts have interpreted the Constitutional prohibition of taking life and liberty such that "taking" means more than a few months when applied to the right to a trial by a jury of your peers. Most judges are not particularly sympathetic to criminal defendants, so you will likely want to opt for a jury trial whenever you have the option of doing so (though if the facts of the case are on your side, a bench trial may be your best bet). If faced with this option, your attorney can help you decide what to do given the unique aspects of your case. The bench trial process is essentially the same as that of a jury trial but the fact finder is different.

The next step in the trial process is the opening statements where the prosecution and defense attorneys lay out the fundamentals of their case. They then proceed into the heart of the trial. Prosecutors usually go first because they have the burden of proving beyond a reasonable doubt that the defendant committed the crime for which he or she has been accused. Evidence, including eyewitness testimony, expert witnesses, and scientific (forensic) evidence must be in accordance with the rules of evidence outlined by the court. Witnesses may be cross-examined or interrogated by the opposing side. Any disputes are handled through objections by the opposing party and rulings by the judge. After the prosecutor is finished, he or she will "rest."

The defense side is then permitted to present evidence under the same rules and procedures used by the prosecutor. The defendant is not required to do so, however, as the burden of proof rests solely with the prosecutor. Once their case has been made, the defense will then rest. There may then be a rebuttal by the prosecution, and sometimes a further rebuttal by the defense.

Once both parties have rested, the court will direct them to begin closing statements. Because the prosecutor bears the burden of proof, he or she is usually allowed to speak first and last with the defense presenting their closing arguments in between. The judge will then give the jury instructions about how they will adjudicate. The jury will then be directed to a private room where they will select a foreperson and decide whether the defendant committed the acts of which he or she was accused. Upon making a determination, they will inform the bailiff, who will inform the judge.

All parties will be recalled to the courtroom, where the judge will ask the jurors if they have reached a verdict. If the answer is "yes," the verdict will be read aloud. If the jury cannot reach a unanimous verdict after extended deliberations, the judge may declare a mistrial after which the case may later be retried. If a verdict is reached and the decision is "not guilty", the defendant will be released.[16] If the verdict is "guilty," the defendant will be sentenced for his or her crime(s). In criminal cases, the jury will also meet to determine the sentence for the crime. What follows is a mini-trial in which the prosecution and defense may present evidence of mitigating and aggravating circumstances.

Once a person is convicted of a crime, he or she can still challenge this ruling based upon certain legal grounds. Appellate courts will usually review cases where errors of law, fact, or due process may have taken place. While either party can file an appeal of a civil verdict, in criminal matters an appeal can only be filed by a convicted defendant due to the double jeopardy principle in most cases. The legal process is arduous, expensive, confusing, and severely consequential. It is important to retain professional counsel to help you through the process. A good attorney can be worth his or her weight in gold.

Dealing with the Press

"I can offer one paramount piece of advice. Meek-appearing journalists can turn rabid when they are lied to. Even the response of silence is better than a lack of candor. Duplicity will come back to haunt you." [17]

– John Entine

Dealing with the press is dangerous. Check with your attorney before accepting any interviews and be prepared to have him/her either coach you or handle questions in your stead. According to the Media Research Center, a watchdog organization, conservatives believe that mass media slants reports in favor of liberal positions on most issues. They have data on their web site showing that seventy eight percent of Americans surveyed agree, yet assert that many members of the media continue to deny a liberal bias. The reason that martial artists should care about this purported bias is that liberals generally favor gun control and generally oppose countervailing force.

Whether or not you believe that a bias exists, it is prudent to consider that if you speak with a reporter about a violent incident you were involved with you may well be dealing with a hostile audience. Reporters should be objective, of course, but that does not necessarily mean that they always are. It is important to understand what angle a story is likely to take. If the reporter is evasive, tread lightly. It may be useful to pull up copies of other stories the person has written or produced to get a feel for how you might be treated.

You may be excited to do an interview or get in front of the cameras, but it is very important to look before you leap into headlines. Never forget that your fifteen minutes of fame could easily be used against you in a court of law. It is generally considered taboo for a reporter to send you a copy of a story to review or approve, so do not expect to be able to do that regardless of how much you may want the opportunity to do so. Always get the reporter's business card and find out when and where the piece will appear so that you can view the end result however.

For on-camera interviews, ask for some warm-up questions so that you can compose yourself before you speak. If you can get a hold of the questions you will be asked ahead of time, you will have some time to think of answers that are meaningful and hard to be misinterpreted or taken out of context.

If it is an off-camera interview, take your time to answer, and then say what you feel. Be sure to check in with the reporter and understand whether or not he or she understood your message. If the person repeats back your quotes and paraphrases his/her understanding, you will have a chance to clear up any confusion.

Once the interview is published or the story is aired, you can call or e-mail the writer or editor and request a correction if you were misquoted or there is an egregious error. Better still; avoid talking to reporters altogether unless specifically advised by your attorney that it will help your case to do so.

Summary

"Criminal court is where bad people are on their best behavior. It's much more danger-ous for lawyers and judges in family court, where good people are at their worst." [18]

– *Richard Dooling*

Once you survive an armed conflict, there are a host of other consequences to address, including medical triage, legal issues, managing witnesses, dealing with the press, interacting with law enforcement, and dealing with psychological trauma. Your first order of business is survival. If you have been injured during a fight you may have to take care of yourself until professional help can arrive. First, you need to make a mental commitment to live. Your attitude plays a large part of your ability to survive. If you or another person with you has been injured in a fight, controlling bleeding must be your first priority.

Once you have taken care of any life-threatening injuries you will want to turn your attention to notifying the authorities, calling your attorney, contacting your spouse/significant other, and identifying any witnesses who may be able to testify about your actions and those of your opponent. It is extraordinarily important to act in a manner that demonstrates to any who observe a violent encounter that you are the victim rather than the instigator of the attack. Always act as if you are on video camera, even if no one else is around. Assume anything you do will be interpreted in the most derogatory manner possible and likely used against you in a court of law. Calculate your verbal response and physical actions to put you in the best possible light.

When the authorities arrive, approach the responding officers calmly and politely. A confrontational attitude will do you no good. Follow the officers' instructions without hesitation. Do not resist arrest for any reason. Similarly, do not interfere with an attempt to arrest anyone who is with you at the time.

Do not, under any circumstances, make any incriminating statements that may be used against you at a later time. Despite Miranda requirements, your fundamental rights and responsibilities may not always be clearly spelled out by the responding officers, especially in any conversations that precede an arrest. Remember that you have a Fifth Amendment right against self-incrimination and that it is often prudent to have an attorney present during any questioning. Your priority should be to alleviate or minimize any potential charges against you, so be enormously cautious about what you say and do.

The legal process is arduous, complicated, and expensive. It generally begins with an arrest followed by a booking, arraignment, evidentiary hearing, and trial. At times, an appeal will be necessary as well. Because your freedom, family, livelihood, and reputation are on the line, it is essential to have a highly skilled attorney to help you navigate the process. You should always carry the phone number of an attorney you can trust and of a person who can contact a lawyer for you if yours is not immediately available.

A criminal defense attorney is a specialist who helps you navigate through the legal process, mapping a strategy to alleviate or minimize any charges against you. He or she acts as an advocate, your voice before the court. It is important, therefore, that you choose somebody who is highly qualified, motivated, and interested in handling your case. Knowledge, skill, and ability are important. Experience is essential. When interviewing potential lawyers, be sure to take note of their experience handling cases similar to yours, their attention to the details of your case, and their ability to explain what you should expect during a trial.

Reporters should always be objective, yet that does not necessarily mean that they always are. Dealing with the press is dangerous. Check with your attorney before accepting any interviews and be prepared to have him/her either coach you or handle questions in your stead. While you may be excited to do an interview or get in front of the cameras, it is crucial to look before you leap into headlines. Never forget that your fifteen minutes of fame could subsequently be used against you in a court of law.

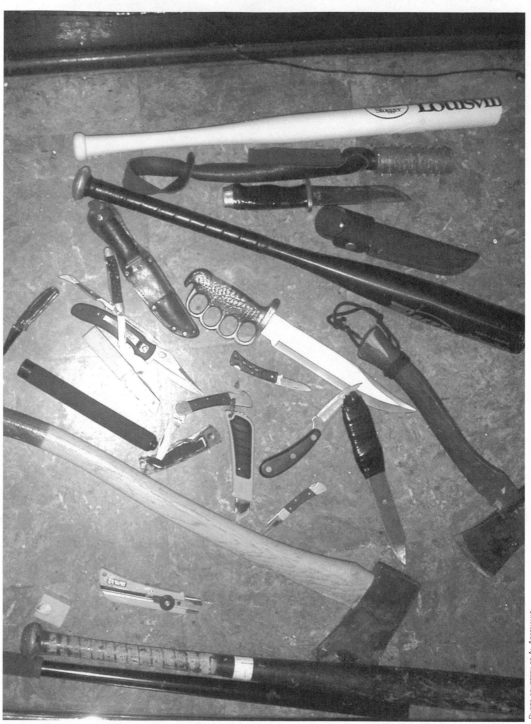

PHOTO COURTESY OF AL ARSENAULT

CHAPTER 9

Weapon Features/Functions

"Weapons can get long term ugly. Losing the fight, cops, hospitals, and revenge seekers all make the aftermath of weapon fighting a real pain in the ass... In case you hadn't noticed, there are a lot of guys in jail for a thing called murder. Jails are for the guys who lived. There are also a lot of people in graveyards for something called death. You may not always be the one swinging the bottle. If you've got a hot head, you'd better learn to control it before you get into this territory. With weapons there is no room for 'loose cannons on deck.' The people who live and stay free are the ones who think before they act." [1]

– Marc MacYoung

In this chapter, we will discuss the attributes of various weapons along with how they are generally used. Categories covered will include hand weapons, knives, swords, mass weapons, pole arms, multi-element weapons, projectiles, and unusual weapons. One could write an entire book about each type of weapon listed herein, so the sake of brevity I'll only hit the high points of how they are commonly used, covering certain strengths or weaknesses and important features of each category such as availability, effective range, carry-ability, conceal-ability, reliability, and commonality.

My goal is primarily to explain what each weapon can do as opposed to describing specific techniques for how to defeat them. There are simply too many variables to consider including any weapons you might have available, your skill level, fitness level, martial style, body type, predilections, fighting environment, and range considerations. The type and number of adversaries you face, their intent, disposition, size, and skill level also come into play. So do all the other things we have covered previously, of course, including the legal, ethical and moral issues that may temper your response. On the street, you must be flexible; relying on the knowledge you have gained herein along with the strategy and tactics of the martial art you practice to keep you safe.

Knowing how the various weapons work will give you a leg up on figuring out how best to deploy counter-weapons or, if they are unavailable, apply your empty-hand martial techniques to survive an armed confrontation. Clearly if we have to respond to an armed opponent it is vastly preferable to so when we ourselves are armed. When this is not possible, we can find empty-hand techniques to meet the threat.

Though it may not be obvious in your forms, unarmed applications found in *kata* can be used effectively against a weapon. What initially appears to be a defense against a punch or a kick, for instance, may also be useful for defense against an armed aggressor. To illustrate this I will show how movements from a karate *kata* are directly applicable to defense against a knife, particularly against a lunge thrust from a knife.

There are plenty of other defenses against a knife thrust that work just as well if not better than the example I will portray below. The reason for choosing this particular sequence is that it obviously mirrors the *kata* it comes from and does not rely on *okuden waza* (hidden applications) for success. I have also used a slightly modified version of this technique in real life to counter a knife thrust successfully so I can tell you that under the right circumstances it really is an effective procedure. I will demonstrate the *kata* first for clarity and then show the street application.

The following figures illustrate the opening sequence of *saifa kata*, a *Goju Ryu* karate form. Despite the fact that this example progression is explained as a series of numbered steps, it must be executed swiftly, smoothly, and without pause or it will not be effective:

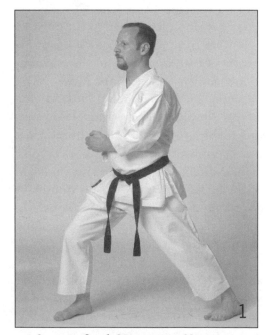

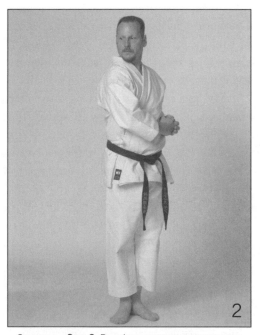

SAIFA KATA – **STEP 1:** SHIFT OFF-LINE ~ 30 DEGREES IN *ZENKUTSU DACHI* WITH LEFT HAND COVERING RIGHT.

SAIFA KATA – **STEP 2:** PIVOT/ELBOW STRIKE IN *MASUBI DACHI*.

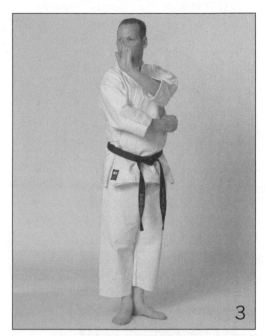

SAIFA KATA – **STEP 3:** PRESS BLOCK/GRAB.

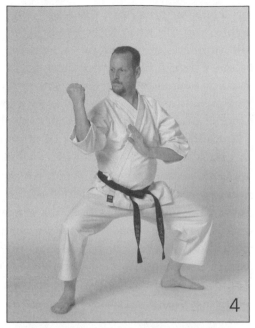

SAIFA KATA – **STEP 4:** DROP TO *SHIKO DACHI* AND BACKFIST STRIKE. NOTE THAT THE STRIKE IS NEARLY VERTICAL IMPLYING VERY CLOSE PROXIMITY TO THE OPPONENT.

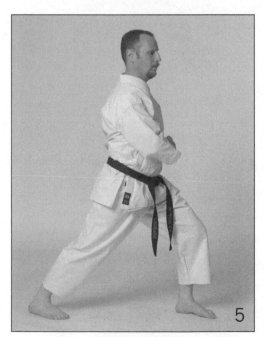

SAIFA KATA – **STEP 5:** REPEAT THE SAME SEQUENCE AGAIN TO THE OTHER SIDE, BEGINNING WITH A 30 DEGREE STEP IN *ZENKUTSU DACHI*.

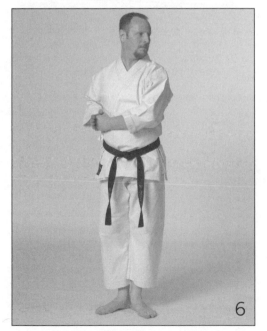

SAIFA KATA – **STEP 6:** PIVOT/ELBOW STRIKE.

Here is how this sequence can be applied on the street with very little modification. It is important to note that there is more than one correct interpretation of each movement of every *kata*. This is only one possibility, yet one that is realistic and simple enough that it can effectively be employed under combat stress conditions.

Because the attacker can move his weapon faster than you can move your whole body your hands must move first, something not obvious with these static pictures. These steps all happen as one continuous movement in practical application so the numbering is only here to align each movement with the *kata* sequence shown earlier.

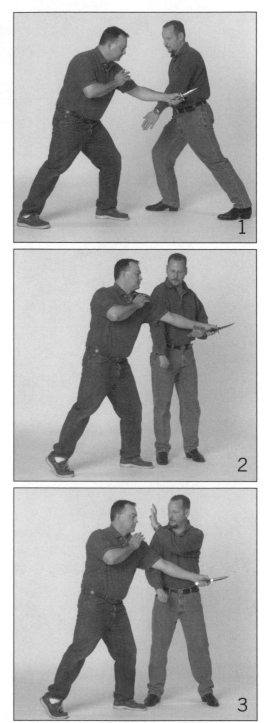

Saifa application – **Step 1**: Because the *kata* is initially performed to the right we will use a left-hand lunge thrust to defend against. It can be done to either side, of course. Reach out with your left hand to check or deflect the thrust while shifting off-line away from the weapon to your right ~ 30 degrees to your attacker's line of force. As you dodge the knife, you must remain close enough to your opponent to counterstrike before he can attack again, yet clear the weapon sufficiently to avoid being cut. It is a delicate balance.

Saifa application – **Step 2**: Deflect the opponent's knife arm with your own arm while pivoting, adding another level of safety to your dodge through a simultaneous combination of parrying, shifting, and deflecting. Your contact with the adversary's arm should be considered a strike, hopefully damaging his elbow in the best case scenario, but at least slowing his ability to evade your next technique or initiate another blow before you can react.

SAIFA APPLICATION – **STEP 3**: CAPTURE THE OPPONENT'S ARM TO PREVENT REDEPLOYMENT OF THE WEAPON. REACHING TOWARD YOUR OPPONENT, LATCHING ON NEAR THE ELBOW, THEN PULLING YOUR HAND BACK TOWARDS HIS WRIST GIVES YOU THE BEST OPPORTUNITY TO SOLIDLY CAPTURE AND CONTROL HIS LIMB WITHOUT BEING CUT. YOUR GRIP TIGHTENS AS YOUR ARM SLIDES TOWARD HIS WRIST. IF YOU CAN STRIKE HIM IN THE FACE WITH A PALM HEEL BEFORE LATCHING ONTO THE ARM SO MUCH THE BETTER. IF HE PULLS HIS KNIFE HAND BACK IN TO INITIATE ANOTHER STRIKE THIS JUST MAKES YOUR JOB EASIER.

SAIFA APPLICATION – **STEP 4**: DROP TO *SHIKO DACHI* AND COUNTERSTRIKE TO THE TEMPLE. NOTE THAT THE SIMULTANEOUS WEIGHT DROP AND ELBOW STRIKE TO THE UPPER ARM (WHICH HITS A PRESSURE POINT IF YOU DO IT RIGHT) FACILITATES THE BLOW. AT THE SAME TIME YOU ARE FINALIZING THE GRAB/PULL FROM STEP 3, SECURING THE WEAPON SAFELY AWAY FROM YOUR BODY WHILE KEEPING THE OPPONENT FROM ESCAPING YOUR STRIKE. IF YOU CONNECT SOLIDLY WITH THE BACKFIST YOU SHOULD STUN YOUR OPPONENT.

SAIFA APPLICATION – **STEP 5**: USE YOUR FREE ARM TO CAPTURE THE OPPONENT'S WEAPON, TAKING ADVANTAGE OF THE FACT THAT HE IS TEMPORARILY STUNNED FROM YOUR BACKFIST BLOW. NEVER LET GO OF A WEAPON YOU HAVE CAPTURED BEFORE SECURING IT WITH YOUR OTHER HAND. IF YOUR OPPONENT GETS THE BLADE BACK IN PLAY BEFORE YOUR NEXT MOVEMENT YOU WILL BE IN A LOT OF TROUBLE. FURTHERMORE, IF YOUR PREVIOUS TECHNIQUE DID NOT SUCCEED YOU WILL HAVE TO BAIL OUT AND TRY A DIFFERENT APPROACH. KEEPING A SOLID HOLD ON YOUR ADVERSARY'S WEAPON GIVES YOU AN ADVANTAGE NO MATTER WHAT YOU DO AND NOT MATTER HOW HE RESPONDS.

SAIFA APPLICATION – **STEP 6**: USE YOUR HIPS TO TURN YOUR WHOLE BODY, TWISTING AND RIPPING THE KNIFE AWAY FROM YOUR ADVERSARY. WHILE HE MIGHT BE ABLE TO FIGHT YOUR ARM STRENGTH, VERY FEW OPPONENTS WILL BE ABLE TO STOP THE POWER OF YOUR WHOLE BODY.

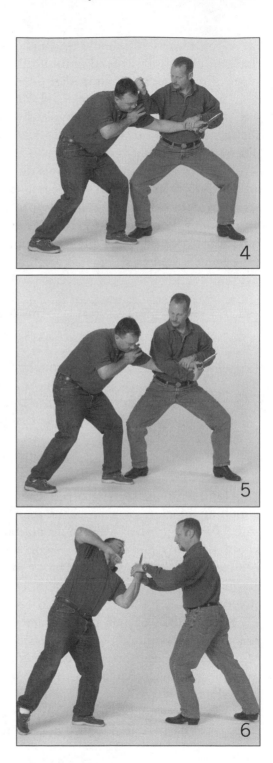

Upon review, you should find a plethora of techniques in your own martial style that can effectively be used against an armed attacker. It is far better to avoid these types of confrontations altogether or respond weapon against weapon, but on occasion, we do not have that luxury. Having set the stage, we will now proceed to cover some highlights of the various types of weapons you might be likely to encounter on the street. While this is not an all-inclusive list, it should have sufficient depth to be illuminating.

There are entire martial schools devoted to many of these weapon forms. If you are a practitioner of one of those arts, you will undoubtedly find that this material is far from comprehensive and is also, in some cases, divergent from what you have been taught. For street survival, however, style and form are far less important than function. After all, while any idiot can run you through with a pointy object most experienced *budoka* do not go around assaulting law abiding citizens with deadly weapons.

Hand Weapons

> *"The Viking ring has a helmet with a sharp, raised faceguard, creating a cutting surface that will peel long, narrow strips of hide from your attacker's face. The wolf's head, with its tiny fangs protruding from its open mouth, lacerates almost as well... At this writing, I know of no state or jurisdiction that considers any sort of ring to be a weapon, while virtually every state prohibits brass knuckles."* [2]
>
> – *Massad Ayoob*

Hand weapons add impetus to things that most people already know how to do, punching, blocking, grabbing, and so on. They are most effective in grappling, close, and short range where you would normally utilize empty-hand combat techniques. Hand weapons fall into two major subcategories—strike enhancers and control devices. The former make your blows more powerful while the latter help you apply grappling applications such as locks, chokes, or pressure point manipulations more effectively.

Strike enhancers are popular among certain criminal elements. For example, Kostas Nikolakopoulos, a Greek sports journalist suffered serious head injuries on May 14, 2005 after being beaten by four hooded men carrying brass knuckles and iron bars. Nikolakopoulos was on his way home in downtown Athens around 4:00 P.M. when he was attacked. Doctors reported that he would remain at Nikea hospital for at least two days. Fellow sports writer Philipos Syrigos, another sports journalist, was similarly beaten by two hooded men the previous October.

There is a fair amount of commonality in the way devices within the two subcategories (strike enhancers and control devices) are used which makes them easy and generally reliable to employ even when adrenalized. Hand weapons are generally small, easy to carry, readily available, and not horribly expensive nor particularly difficult to use. Some, such as fighting rings, are easy to disguise unless you know what to look for. Others such as brass knuckles or *kubatons* are more obvious and take slightly longer to deploy if they are not already in or on your hand. Strike enhancers are easier to use and take less skill to use effectively than control devices.

Strike Enhancers

Strike enhancers can be fist-loads such as *yawara* sticks, brass knuckles, or sap gloves, which add solidity and power to a punch, or rippers such as keys, *shuko* (tiger claws), fighting rings, or car keys that slash or gouge. In either case they can help a person hit harder and cause more damage than can typically be done with the hand alone. They tend to either decrease the surface area of the strike facilitating better penetration and/or stabilize the fist to prevent your bones from breaking on impact. Highly trained martial artists probably do not need these items all that much, but in the hands of a regular person, they can become particularly dangerous.

Fighting rings are sneaky because they frequently do not look like weapons yet they have bumps, ridges, spikes, or even blades sticking out that can be used to rip and tear an opponent's flesh. I've seen a 14-karat gold "crown of thorns" ring, a religiously significant icon for those of the Christian faith, where some of the thorns were raised enough to cause significant damage were it used to strike an opponent. Given its intended purpose, I would never have considered it a weapon had someone not pointed that application out. More common styles include eagle-heads with protruding beaks, Viking helmets with jutting horns, spiked skulls, or animal totems with raised or extruded surfaces. Many have medieval, Nordic, or Celtic designs. They are can be made of silver, gold, brass, stainless steel, or just about any type of metal and are popular among the biker, Goth, and counterculture crowds.

Since we punch with our knuckles, many martial artists might not even consider a ring a reasonable striking surface. A slight variation in technique, however, could easily make the ring come into contact with an opponent. A punch or backfist can rake the sharp parts across a person's face, drawing blood to distract, temporarily blind, or even severely damage the person struck. It can also damage the hand, especially the fingers next to the ring. The ring can also be reversed with the pointy side palm-ward to add impetus to slaps, grabs, or even certain types of traditional blocks. This is probably the most common usage.

Another subtle strike enhancer is a sap glove, generally recognizable by fancy stitching and extra thickness around the knuckles that hold lead or steel shot or a

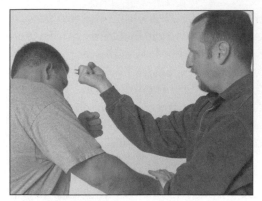

FIGHTING RING DEPLOYED WITH POINTS OUTWARD FOR A BACKFIST STRIKE. THE DESIGN OF THIS RING HAS MORE OBVIOUS MARTIAL APPLICATIONS THAN MANY OTHER STYLES YET IT MAKES AN EFFECTIVE EXAMPLE AS YOU CAN READILY SEE THE SPIKES.

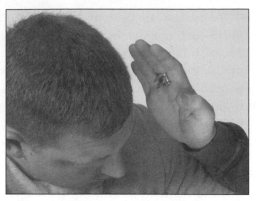

FIGHTING RING DEPLOYED WITH POINTS INWARD FOR A SLAP. THIS IS PROBABLY THE MOST COMMON APPLICATION.

similarly hard powdered substance in place. This padded area molds around the user's knuckles to protect them while the sap load adds weight and power to the punch. *Yawara* sticks do not look all that dangerous either, yet they can be used as fist-loads, blunt instruments, or control devices. That is a lot of utility out of a simple five- or six-inch wooden rod.

Other strike enhancers look like the weapons that they are. Brass knuckles are a good example, albeit a highly illegal one in most jurisdictions. There is no confusing this device with anything but what it is meant to be, a bludgeon. *Shuko* (tiger claws) are clearly dangerous in the right hands as are regular car keys that can be used similarly to rake an opponent's face or eyes. Anything with extruding spikes, ridges, or blades can mess you up pretty badly in a real fight.

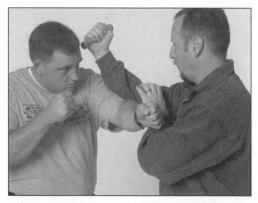

YAWARA STICK AUGMENTING A HAMMER FIST STRIKE TO TEMPLE.

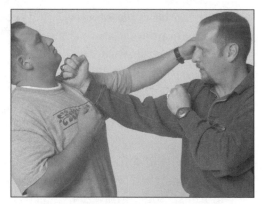

BRASS KNUCKLES AUGMENTING A PUNCH TO JAW.

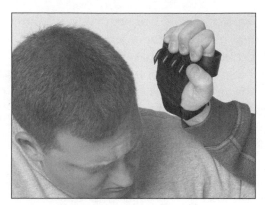

SHUKO (TIGER CLAW) ENHANCING A RAKE TO THE FACE.

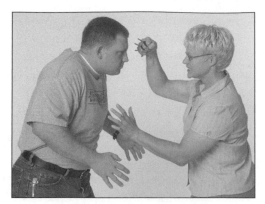

CAR KEYS AUGMENTING A RAKE TO THE EYES.

Control Devices

Control devices are frequently small tubes, items that are not generally big enough to cause the same level of damage as a larger mass weapon, but which can effectively be used to facilitate controlling or grappling techniques such as locks, arm bars, and pressure point manipulations. They can further be used to strike an opponent as well as to block or control certain other weapons such as knives, flashlights, or clubs. Common objects that fall into this category include *kubatons*, *mo gems*, *yawara* sticks, certain pens, and smaller flashlights.

A *kubaton* is generally a five or six inch long metal tube, about 5/8" in diameter. The *mo gem* is a longer, thicker version of the same thing, perhaps eight and a half inches long and about an inch wide. Most are made of metal such as aircraft aluminum. *Yawara* sticks, as previously mentioned are generally made of wood, roughly six inches long and an inch wide. They differ from the *mo gem* mostly in shape. There are metal, Grivory, and Zytel *yawara* commercially available too. A recognized martial arts weapon, they are legal in fewer jurisdictions than the thinner *kubaton* that frequently doubles as a key

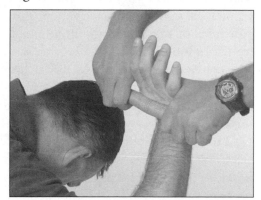

YAWARA AUGMENTED WRISTLOCK.

ring. As such, they are often unregulated. Asp even makes a *kubaton* that holds a pepper spray cartridge for a dual-purpose self-defense device.

An aluminum *karambit* trainer can make an excellent control device as well. Even flashlights can be used in this manner. A solidly built Surefire or similar brand flashlight has roughly the same dimensions as a *yawara* stick and can be used in the same manner without the inherent legal risk the more obvious weapon entails.

While you can certainly strike, jab, or thrust with these types of devices, they can also be used to provide added leverage for grappling and control techniques. They may be used to dig into joints, pressure points, or vital areas such as the trachea. They may be used to snag weapons or limbs (e.g., to facilitate disarming techniques).

Knives

"If one accepts the often-heard statement that most gunfights take place at a distance of about 5 feet, then most situations where you would need a gun can be adequately handled with a knife. Within its range (and, for a trained person who knows how to move, 5 feet is well within knife range), the edged weapon can actually be more destructive to the opponent than a gun. The knife never runs out of ammunition and it never jams. Some find a knife more intimidating to an opponent." [3]

– Massad Ayoob

Knives are very common murder weapons. In a case that shocked the nation, Jerry Branton Hobbs, 34, reportedly confessed to killing his eight-year-old daughter Laura and her nine-year-old best friend Krystal Tobias on May 8, 2005. He allegedly confessed his crime to police interrogators who interviewed him. According to published reports, he had anger management problems and led a violent life. In 1990, he was convicted of aggravated assault for stabbing a motorist who was screeching his tires in front of Hobbs' home. In 1996, he was convicted of domestic violence. In 1997, he was convicted of assault. In 2001, he was sentenced to probation for threatening neighbors with a running chain saw, ordered to attend an anger management class, and instructed to undergo substance abuse counseling. He refused to attend and served two years in prison for violating the terms of his probation.

Hobbs had reportedly grounded his daughter for stealing $40.00 from her mother's purse then flew into a rage when he discovered that she had snuck out of the house to play with her friend in a nearby park. He allegedly punched his daughter in the mouth and then stabbed her 20 times, including nine times to her neck and once to each eye. Police reports indicated that Laura's neck wounds were delivered with such force that the blade not only pierced her throat, but also went deep enough to strike her spinal cord. Krystal was reportedly stabbed eleven times, including four times to her neck. After killing the girls, Hobbs reportedly told police that he dragged their bodies an undetermined distance to the place where he pretended to discover them the next morning while searching for them.

Knives are deadly weapons. They are popular, easy to obtain and silent to operate. They are readily concealable, highly reliable, and do not take much special training to use to hurt somebody. They can be highly effective in grappling, close, and short ranges. With enough training, certain types of knives can be effectively utilized or accurately thrown even greater distances than that. It is generally a bad idea to let go of your weapon in combat, however.

Other pointy objects such as scissors, ice picks, and screwdrivers can be used in the same fashion as knives. For example, on March 26, 1984, 21-year-old Robert Conklin killed George Crooks, 28, with a screwdriver, and then dismembered the corpse in an attempt to cover up his crime. He was executed by lethal injection in Jackson, Georgia on July 12, 2005.

Knife Safety

This same information generally applies to swords and other sharp objects as well but I will only list it in one location for the sake of brevity. Knives, including kitchen, carving, and multi-tool varieties, are a frequent source of disabling injuries. Always treat any sharp object with respect and responsibility. Sharp objects in general and knives in particular should not be treated cavalierly.

Never touch a blade, save with great caution during the sharpening or cleaning process. Combat blades are usually crafted from high-carbon spring steel. While this material is durable and holds a good edge, it can rust quickly especially when exposed to oils from your fingers. If you press your fingers against a properly sharpened blade edge, it can severely injure you before you even realize that you have been cut. Furthermore, if you drop an edged weapon, do not attempt to catch it. Just get out of the way, letting it fall to the ground before you pick it up. It is difficult to check the instinctive reaction to grab a falling object, but sharp edges and gravity can do you a lot of harm.

Keep all knives sharpened and in good condition, using them for their intended purpose, cutting. A sharp knife is safer to use for carving and slicing applications because it is less likely to slip and cut you. Knives should not be used on anything that will dull or break them. Furthermore, blades do not hold up well to prying and twisting applications. If one breaks, it can severely injure you. Carry knives with exposed blades in sheath or container. Never leave a knife with an exposed edge on a table, bench, or floor where someone may accidentally encounter it.

Never sheath a blade without cleaning and drying it first as you can damage not only the knife but the sheath as well. Use caution when sheathing your blade, keeping your fingers away from the cutting surface. When closing a folding knife, use the palm of your hand so that you will not accidentally trap your fingers beneath the blade.

Common Grips

There is a plethora of ways to hold and deploy a knife. The most common ways to grip a blade include the natural grip, the saber grip, the Filipino grip, and the reverse grip. Each has inherent strengths as well as weaknesses.

With the natural grip, you simply wrap your whole hand around the handle of the weapon, like making a fist. The thumb curls around your fingers. The natural grip is effective for thrusting techniques. It can even be used for driving a blade through light armor such as a

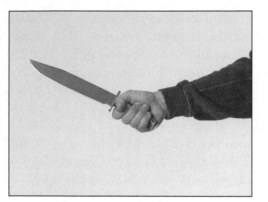

NATURAL GRIP. WRAP YOUR HAND AROUND THE HANDLE LIKE MAKING A FIST WITH THE THUMB CURLING AROUND YOUR FINGERS.

leather jacket or a ballistic vest.[4] You can also throw a regular punch with the blade sticking out, creating a planar attack. While this grip takes impact well, it is not as flexible as other styles in changing your blade edge direction quickly. If your knife does not have a cross-guard that prevents your hand from sliding onto the blade, this grip may be somewhat dangerous for thrusting, especially if you hit something solid.

With the saber grip, you wrap your hand around the handle as if you are shaking hands, and then press your thumb downward on top. The handle cants back a little more in your hand than the natural grip, facilitating lightning direction changes with the blade. The drawback of this style is that the handle is somewhat loose in your hands, making it easier to be dislodged. If your knife does not have a cross-guard that prevents your hand from sliding onto the blade, this grip can be somewhat dangerous for thrusting, especially if you hit something solid.

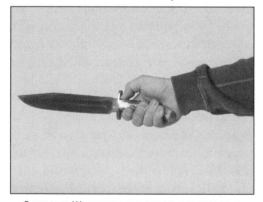

SABER GRIP. WRAP YOUR HAND AROUND THE HANDLE LIKE SHAKING HANDS, AND THEN PRESS YOUR THUMB DOWNWARD ON TOP.

The Filipino grip is very similar to the saber grip save that the thumb floats above the blade instead of pressing down onto it. This type of grip was popularized by certain styles of *escrima*, *kali*, and other Filipino fighting arts. To do it properly you wrap your last three fingers tightly around the handle with the index finger holding on more loosely. This grip is flexible for lightning fast direction changes, slashes, and thrusts. It has many of the benefits of the saber grip without the inherent danger of crunching your thumb or letting your hand slide onto the blade during a thrust. The thumb can also be used to help guide the blade to your target.

The reverse grip, sometimes called the oriental or ice-pick grip, holds the handle in your palm while the blade extends backward away from the thumb. It is typically used for surprise attacks, hiding the fact that the weapon exists until the last possible second. For single-edged knives, the sharp end should face away from your body. This grip position facilitates forward slashes, blocks, and reverse thrusts. It can also be used to punch with.

Types of Attack

Never forget that most knife attacks begin with surprise. You may not see the weapon until it cuts you so awareness and avoidance are paramount. Even a legal 2 ½ inch blade can kill if it is used against the proper vital target (e.g., artery, vital organ). According to Darren Laur, the typical depth of a stab wound in homicide

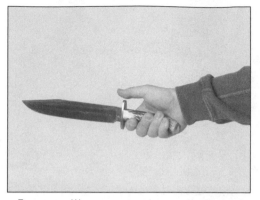

FILIPINO GRIP. WRAP YOUR HAND AROUND THE HANDLE LIKE SHAKING HANDS, LEAVING YOUR THUMB FLOATING ABOVE YOUR FIST.

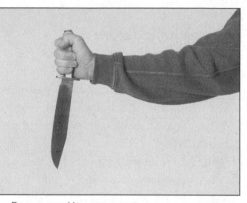

REVERSE GRIP. HOLD THE HANDLE IN YOUR PALM USING A NATURAL GRIP WITH THE BLADE EXTENDED BACKWARD AWAY FROM YOUR THUMB.

cases is only 1 to 1 ½ inches through the rib cage. Most edged weapon attack victims die from multiple wounds.

At the simplest level there are two kinds of attacks with a knife—cuts and thrusts. Cuts generally produce more bleeding while thrusts can cause more serious damage (depending on the target hit). Cuts can include slashes, chops, hacks, snap cuts, and vertical whips. Thrusts can include rakes, jabs, hooks, lunge (fencing-style) thrusts, and loops. Cuts and thrusts are often combined as an opponent can feint with a thrust then switch to a cut or vice versa with a simple flip of the wrist. In addition to the blade, it is important to realize that the pommel of a knife can be used for strikes, blocks, and even pressure point techniques.

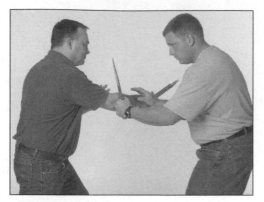

KNIFE THRUST (STAB). CUTS GENERALLY CAUSE MORE BLEEDING WHILE THRUSTS CAN CAUSE MORE SERIOUS DAMAGE. HERE THE LUNGE THRUST IS BLOCKED WITH INWARD SWEEP OF THE KNIFE.

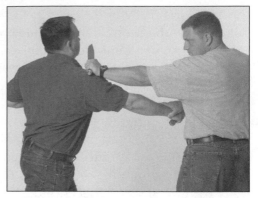

KNIFE CUT (SLASH). AFTER DEFLECTING THE OPPONENT'S THRUST, THE KNIFE HAND IS GRABBED AND A RIPOSTE SLASH GOES FOR THE THROAT.

Common Knife Targets

Common targets that have generally proven lethal or severely disabling in knife combat include the heart, subclavian artery (behind the collarbone), stomach, brachial artery, radial artery, carotid artery, femoral artery, axiliary artery, and kidneys. Thrusts are generally more damaging than slashes yet they also require you to move deeper into your opponent's target zone where he or she can easily reach you with his/her weapon. Consequently, other frequent targets include the hands, wrists, and elbows, which may be cut at somewhat less risk of riposte.

Single-Edged Knives

Single-edged knives have only one sharpened surface. This facilitates an ability use them as tools for carving, cooking, and other applications where you may wish to press on the back of the blade for leverage and stability. Not every single-edged knife is a tool, however. Probably the most famous single-edged fighting

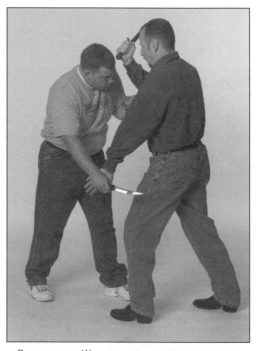

POMMEL STRIKE. WHILE THE BLADE OF A KNIFE IS PRIMARILY USED FOR ATTACKS AND DEFENSE, THE POMMEL CAN BE USED FOR STRIKES, BLOCKS, AND PRESSURE POINT MANIPULATIONS AS WELL. HERE IS A HAMMER FIST STRIKE USING THE POMMEL OF THE KNIFE. NOTE THAT THE OPPONENT'S BLADE IS DEFLECTED WITH THE OFF HAND COMMENSURATE WITH THE STRIKE. NEVER FORGET ABOUT YOUR FREE HAND WHEN HOLDING A WEAPON.

knife is the Bowie, designed by Colonel James "Jim" Bowie in the 1830s.

Other combat blades with a single sharpened edge include the Japanese *tanto* (sort of a shortened *wakizashi* blade), the Norse *scramasax*, the *skean dhu* (Scottish stocking knife), and the dirk. Single-edged blades excel at slicing, chopping, and slashing attacks but are not always as good at thrusting as double-edged daggers. Some single edged knives are balanced for throwing.

Double-Edged Knives

Double-edged knives are, for the most part, designed exclusively for combat. They are far better at stabbing than they are at slicing or cutting. Stilettos, most bayonets, daggers, rondels, push daggers, and many switchblades fall into this category. In general, the narrower the blade the more effective a stab will be and, conversely, the more ineffectual a slash. Some double-edged knives are balanced for throwing, though it is almost never a good idea to let go of your weapon during a real fight.

Fixed Blades vs. Folding Knives

Both single and double-edged knives can be found in fixed-blade or folding varieties. The strength of a folding knife is carry-ability. In most locations, blades less than 2 ½ or 3 inches in length are legal to carry concealed in your pocket. Most folding knives look more like tools than combat weapons though they can certainly be used for both purposes. A major weakness of folding knives is reliability, particularly

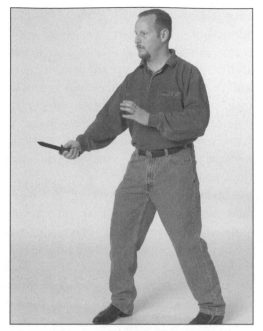

SINGLE-EDGE KNIFE. THIS IS A GLOCK KNIFE.

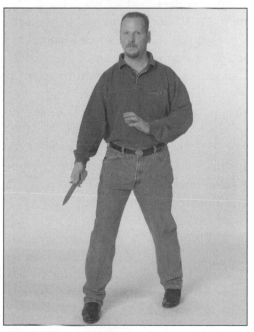

DOUBLE-EDGE KNIFE. THIS IS A HAND-MADE DAGGER.

as it relates to opening them under an adrenaline surge when fine motor control is lost. Another reliability issue is dependability of the locking mechanism. Only knives with a mechanical locking mechanism that secures the blade in an open position can be used effectively in combat. Blades without this feature will close unexpectedly, often cutting you rather than your opponent.

Similarly, if the locking mechanism fails in use, the blade may unexpectedly close. There are several varieties of these mechanisms including lever locks, axis locks, rolling locks, and liner locks. Because they have more moving parts than fixed blade knives (which do not have any moving parts), folders have more points of weakness where things can go wrong. Furthermore, folding blades are also usually slower to deploy than fixed blades because they must both be drawn and opened before they can be used rather than simply drawn.

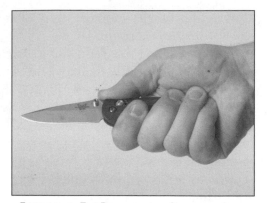

Folding knife. This Benchmade mini Griptillian uses an axis lock system that is very reliable and durable. When clipped it is secured blade upward, something that is frequently hard to find in many folders. I prefer this method as the draw is similar to that of a pistol. As the knife clears your pocket, you press downward on the thumb knob to flip the blade open. Commonality among weapons makes them more reliable under extreme stress/combat conditions.

In order to carry a fixed-blade knife you must have a sheath of some sort to put it in and something to secure the sheath to (e.g., belt, neck lanyard, or boot). Consequently, they tend to be more awkward to carry around than folding blades though they are generally easier and faster to deploy since they do not have to be opened once they are drawn. Beyond speed of deployment, the main strength of a fixed-blade knife is reliability since there are no working parts to fail. On the other hand, many fixed-blade knives exceed the legal length of a concealed weapon in many jurisdictions. They also look more like weapons than most folding knives do, something that makes them harder to explain in court.

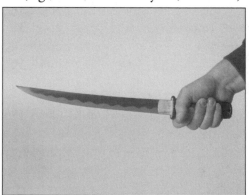

Fixed blade knife. This *tanto* is not only too big to conceal legally in most jurisdictions but also far too large to carry comfortably on a daily basis, hence impractical for self-defense in most environments. If you cannot legally and/or practically carry a weapon with you at all times the odds are good that it will not be available when you need it.

Specialty Blades

There is a variety of specialty blades available such as switchblades, *balisongs*, and *karambits*. Switchblades are folding knives that automatically spring open when a button is pushed. The blade either rotates open or thrusts straight out using a mechanical spring. The blades themselves can be single or double edged, though the latter are a bit more popular. Switchblades are not legal in most jurisdictions.

The *balisong* (or butterfly knife) is a form of folding knife with two handles that counter-rotate around the tang such that when closed the blade is concealed within grooves between the handles. *Balisong* in Tagálog (the main Filipino dialect) means "broken horn" as many of these knives were originally created from carved animal horns and recycled knife blades. They are popular with some because they can be quickly opened with one hand and appear impressive when flipped open and closed. Most *balisong* knives are inexpensively built and not horribly reliable in combat. They are frequently considered a thug weapon hence frowned upon in court even where they are legal.

The *karambit* is a sharply curved blade indigenous to the Indonesian Archipelago and certain regions of the Philippines. They are frequently double-edged. Many martial artists believe that the biomechanics of the weapon allow for more powerful cutting strokes, particularly against an attacker's limbs, than a traditional straight blade. *Karambits* can do a lot of damage even with a short cutting edge. Because they have an integral finger ring, they are difficult to disarm and may allow better control than a traditional straight blade knife with a conventional handle.

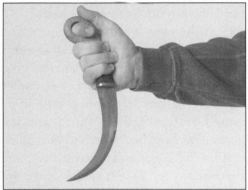

KARAMBIT KNIFE. THIS ONE WAS MADE IN THE PHILIPPINES. SMALLER VERSIONS SUCH AS THOSE MADE BY TARANI-STRIDER ARE MORE PRACTICAL (AND LEGAL) FOR SELF-DEFENSE CARRY.

Swords

"Swords, when at their rest,
Gleam with golden candlelight.
Bared, glare they anger." [5]

– Robin Ashley Smith

Less common for murder than knives, swords are formidable weapons even in untrained hands. For example, on April 17, 2005, Charles Barrett, a 58-year-old Kent (Washington) man, died from a sword stab to his abdomen. An unidentified 40-year-old man, reportedly the deceased's stepson-in-law, was ordered held on $750,000 bail in the Kent jail for investigation of second-degree murder. Apparently, Barrett called the suspect's apartment because he wanted his granddaughter to come over to his place to do some chores. The suspect became incensed because the call came during his weekend visitation with the 11-year-old girl. The argument escalated and the men decided to fight.

According to news reports, the two lived in apartment complexes close to each other and met about 7:00 P.M. The suspect took a sword with him, while Barrett carried a small bat. The suspect told police he decided not to fight and turned to leave, but that Barrett struck him with the bat before he could get away. He allegedly turned, unsheathed the sword, and stabbed Barrett. The suspect told police he did not realize how badly he had hurt Barrett, yet the suspect's girlfriend told detectives that he called her and asked her to provide an alibi for him. She allegedly went to the apartment they shared and watched as he washed the sword with bleach, reportedly saying, "I probably killed him."

The following morning, the suspect hid the sword in some woods. While he was gone, his girlfriend learned from television news that Barrett had died of his wounds. She called the suspect, who talked with his family and decided to turn himself in. The man called 9-1-1, told police where to find him, and then showed them where to find his sword in the woods.

A surprisingly large number of people today are skilled with swords. Fencing as you probably know is an Olympic sport with thousands of practitioners in various clubs throughout the world learning how to use foil, epee, and saber. *Kendo* and *iaido* are popular Japanese martial arts, where people can learn how to use wooden weapons such as *bokken* or *shinai* or live steel such as *katana* and *wakizashi* effectively. Practitioners of some forms of *kobudo*, *aikido*, Filipino *escrima*, *kali*, and many forms of Chinese *kung fu* learn blade techniques as well.

Similarly, historical reenactment groups have hundreds of thousands of members worldwide. The Society for Creative Anachronism (SCA) alone, for example, had just over 32,000 paid members in 2005 with many times that number of people attending their events annually. These types of groups practice both fencing with "light" weapons such as sabers or rapiers as well as "heavy" fighting with sword and shield techniques (e.g., broadsword) performed in medieval-style armor.

Swords, machetes, and similar long-bladed weapons are readily available and, with some notable exceptions at the high end of quality, not particularly expensive. Reliability is somewhat based upon materials and manufacturing methods as many popular blades are primarily designed for hanging on a wall rather than for use in actual combat. Regardless, even a $20 sword that breaks on the first strike can kill you. Most $40 machetes can hack you to pieces without significantly harming the blade as was tragically demonstrated in Rwanda a few years back.[6] Further, there are several well made, high-carbon spring steel blades available on the internet for under $200. I have even used one of them to cut brush and small trees for hours at a time without significantly damaging it.[7]

Swords are very popular recently because of movies such as *The Last Samurai, Lord of the Rings, Pirates of the Caribbean, The Mask of Zorro, Braveheart, Kill Bill,* and *Gladiator.* While a decent blade is easy to come by it is not horribly easy to haul around with you unless you are attending a renaissance fair or historical reenactment event.

Swords are neither generally legal nor practical to carry concealed for self-defense. They are, however, effective in short- to mid-range combat and can even be used in close or grappling range though not quite as efficiently. Even a cheap sword can cause massive damage if used properly, however. A major advantage that swords have over knives and other short weapons is their ability to kill from a distance. With good footwork and a modicum of training, a person with a sword can easily defeat a knife-wielder without ever stepping into his or her opponent's target zone.

Sword Components

While every sword is different they all share common characteristics. All swords have a blade and a handle (frequently called a grip). What differentiates them from knives is the length and, in most cases, the girth of the blade. Most have a pommel, which keeps your hand from slipping off the bottom and acts as a counterbalance along with a cross-guard, which protects your hand from your opponent's weapon during a parry while further preventing it from sliding onto your own blade during a thrust.

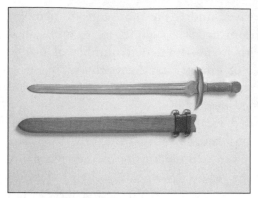

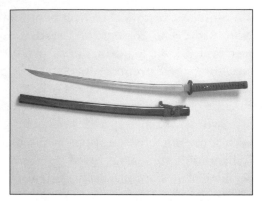

SWORD COMPONENTS (EUROPEAN BROADSWORD). THE HILT IS THE ENTIRE HANDLE, INCLUDING THE GROSS-GUARD, GRIP, AND POMMEL. THE BLADE IS THE SHARPENED PORTION, THE POINTY END OF WHICH IS CALLED THE TIP. THE TANG IS THE UNSHARPENED PORTION OF THE BLADE THAT EXTENDS THROUGH THE HILT ASSEMBLY. GROOVES IN THE SURFACE OF THE BLADE ARE CALLED FULLERS. THEY ARE DESIGNED TO LIGHTEN AND STRENGTHEN THE BLADE (AS CURVED SURFACES ARE STRUCTURALLY STRONGER THAN FLAT ONES). THE COMMON TERM "BLOOD GROOVE" IS INCORRECT. THE PROTECTIVE SHEATH THE SWORD IS CARRIED IN IS CALLED A SCABBARD. THIS IS A HANDMADE PIECE FROM MY COLLECTION.

SWORD COMPONENTS (JAPANESE *KATANA*). THE JAPANESE HAVE NAMES FOR EVEN MORE PORTIONS OF THE BLADE THAN THE EUROPEANS DO. TO KEEP THINGS SIMPLE, THE CROSS-GUARD IS CALLED THE *TSUBA*. THE HANDLE IS CALLED THE *TSUKA*. THE CUTTING EDGE IS CALLED THE *HA*, WHILE THE TIP OF THE BLADE IS CALLED THE *KISSAKI*. UNLIKE MOST EUROPEAN BLADES, THE CUTTING EDGE OF A *KATANA* BLADE IS EXTREMELY HARD WHILE THE BACK (*MUNE*) IS MUCH SOFTER. THE TEMPER LINE WHERE THE HARD AND SOFT PORTIONS MEET IS CALLED THE *HAMON*. THE SCABBARD IS CALLED A *SAYA*. THIS SWORD IS A PRODUCTION MODEL BUILT BY LAST LEGEND COMPETITION BLADES.

Common Types of Attack

In general, swords are primarily designed to be used with one hand or two, though some are balanced appropriately for use with either method. One-handed swords can be used solo or combined with shields, daggers, or other off-hand weapons. Most any type of sword can be used for thrusting, slashing, or combination attacks, though some are primarily designed for one type of attack or the other. The rapier and *gladius*, for example, are primarily thrusting weapons. The broadsword and *katana*, on the other hand, are primarily used for slashing attacks.

There are tons of ways to use a sword. Unlike a knife where targeting can be important, nearly any powerful blow from a full-sized sword can prove severely disabling or even fatal. While whole schools and systems are devoted to subtle nuances between different variations, fundamentally there are only two methods to hold a blade, one handed or two handed. Within that split, there are at the most basic level two major types of techniques—slashes and thrusts. There are further combinations and feints, of course, but in general, almost every blow fits into one of these two categories.

When using a traditional broadsword, for example, your primary attack will typically be a one-handed slash. The whole body is used to generate power for these types of blows, rotating the hips and upper body while the arm snaps the blade out

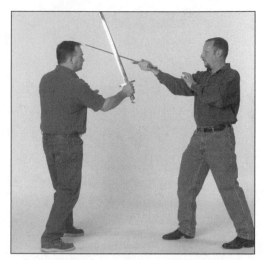

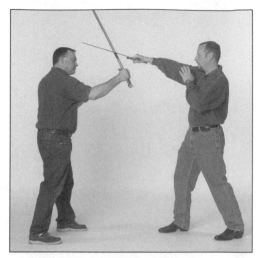

SWORD SLASH: AS THE BLADE MOVES INSIDE RIGHT TO LEFT TOWARD THE LEFT SIDE OF OPPONENT'S HEAD YOU WILL NOTE THAT THE PALM IS UP LIKE SERVING A BOWL OF SOUP. IF YOU STUDY KARATE YOU SHOULD RECOGNIZE THIS AS A *NAKINSHUTO UCHI* (INSIDE SWORD HAND STRIKE) TECHNIQUE.

SWORD SLASH: AS THE BLADE MOVES OUTSIDE LEFT TO RIGHT TOWARD THE RIGHT SIDE OF THE OPPONENT'S HEAD, YOU WILL NOTE THAT PALM IS DOWN. IF YOU STUDY KARATE YOU SHOULD RECOGNIZE THIS AS A *SOTOSHUTO UCHI* (OUTSIDE SWORD HAND STRIKE) TECHNIQUE.

toward your opponent. Conversely, if you use a sword with your arm and shoulder alone, you will tire quickly.

When I studied medieval fighting, we called the sword slash technique "serving the soup." Start with your arm up by the side of your head like a waiter holding a bowl of soup, and then swing it out in a shallow arc as if you were presenting food to a diner. For *karateka*, you will recognize this as a *nakinshuto uchi* (inside sword hand strike). Off-side techniques, which cross your body inside to outside, are done similarly but with the palm down rather than up. That would be *sotoshuto uchi* (outside sword hand) for *karateka*.

With a two-handed weapon, the slash is more of a push/pull technique. The hip is still involved, but not necessarily to as obvious of a degree. The lower arm pulls while the upper arm pushes to generate power. The weak-side arm is generally held on the bottom near the pommel. In general, the greater the separation between the hands the easier it is to add power to your blow using a pick-ax-style swing (push/pull). You can pivot your arms and/or shoulder to control your aim

Thrusts can be also be performed with a broadsword though certain weapons such as a rapier are, perhaps, better designed for that type of technique. One-handed thrusts are pretty easy to do. Such blows are generally performed while lunging forward and simultaneously thrusting the blade outward toward your opponent. With certain styles of swordplay, there is also a twisting movement so that the sword more or less screws into its target somewhat like a traditional karate punch (very similar to

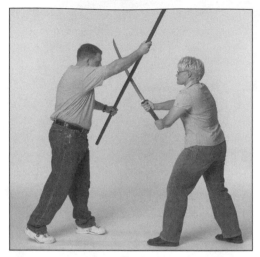

Two-handed sword slash. This diagonal blow toward the opponent's head uses a push/pull technique for power. The upper hand pushes while the lower hand pulls.

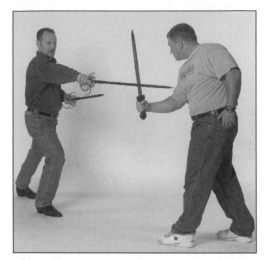

Sword thrust one-handed. This is a lunge thrust with a rapier. The weapon is another hand-made piece from my collection. The wavy edges are commonly called *flamberge*. This style of edge was common to certain types of rapiers, long swords, and great swords.

using a *sai* if you are familiar with how those work). Two-handed thrusts require a bit more coordination than one-handed thrusts and are a bit harder to disguise, though they can be more powerful.

Curved blades like those of the saber, *katana*, and *dao* generally have better cutting properties on a mass-to-mass basis than straight blades when used for slashing attacks. Light cavalry soldiers, for example, invariably carried curved swords rather than straight ones. Their preferred method of attack was a slash rather than a thrust.

Unless the horse was not moving,* a thrust that struck home too deeply could be torn from the rider's hand before the blade could be withdrawn. Furthermore,

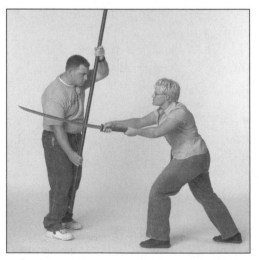

Sword thrust two-handed. Here a *katana* is used to demonstrate a two-handed thrust.

if a thrust from a moving horse missed, the rider would often have difficulty repositioning his mount to repeat the thrust. This was particularly important during skirmishes, the normal form of fighting for light troops. Heavy cavalry, which tended to charge en masse rather than dual one-on-one, usually carried heavier straight swords.

Unless you are into live-steel choreography, the odds of your fighting someone

*Which gives up one of the major advantages of having a mount in the first place.

sword to sword are pretty remote. If you ever do, however, you will need to know a little bit about how to block. Unlike what you see in Hollywood, never block another weapon with the edge of your own blade. Edge to edge contact invariably damages a sword (usually both swords), no matter how well made it is. Blocking should be done with the flat of the blade or with an off-hand weapon or shield. Your sword should be moving when it connects with your adversary's blade. In this manner, you can use the weight of the weapon along with its momentum to counter or deflect the energy of your opponent's attack.

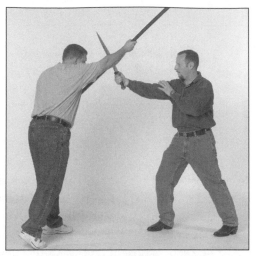

SINGLE-EDGED SWORD. HERE A NORSE-STYLE LONG *SAX* IS USED TO DEMONSTRATE A SLASHING ATTACK TOWARD THE HEAD. THIS BLADE IS THE FIRST SWORD I EVER MADE.

Single-Edged Blades

Single-edged swords include the falchion, *scramasax*, *grosse messer*, cutlass, saber, long *sax* (Norse shortsword), *machete*, *katana*, *borang* (Filipino shortsword), and *dao* (Chinese broadsword), among others. These weapons are generally used for slashing attacks. While devastating to the unarmored individual, certain types of swords, such as the medieval falchion or *grosse messer*, could even cleave through heavy armor with relative ease.

Double-Edged Blades

Double-edged swords include the broadsword, bastard sword, *spatha* (Roman cavalry sword), *gladius* (Roman shortsword), rapier, claymore, *sweihander* (German greatsword), and *jian* (Chinese straight sword), among others. They can be used to thrust and, if the blade is wide enough, slash as well.

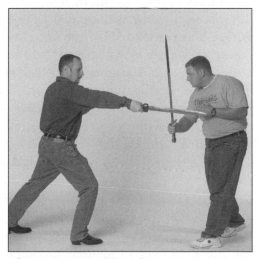

DOUBLE-EDGED SWORD. HERE A ROMAN *GLADIUS* IS USED TO STAB TOWARD THE OPPONENT'S STOMACH. THESE SHORT SWORDS ARE VERY EFFICIENT FOR THRUSTING. THIS IS ANOTHER HAND-MADE PIECE FROM MY COLLECTION. THE DEFENDER'S BLADE IS HAND-MADE AS WELL.

Mass Weapons

"If you hit somebody with anything heavy and hard enough to cause injury, you have just assaulted him with a deadly weapon; it doesn't matter whether you hit him with a blackjack or with the ashtray from your nightstand. In the eyes of the court, you will be justified only if you did so in self-defense." [8]

— Massad Ayoob

Mass weapons such as baseball bats are very dangerous.[9] For example on April 13, 2005 a 13-year-old pitcher whose baseball team, the Angels, had just lost for the first time that season was being teased at the concession stand when he allegedly pulled out a bat and clobbered his 15-year-old antagonist. He now faces a murder charge.

The teen, whose name was not released, is suspected of killing spectator Jeremy Rourke, 15, after the Tuesday night game. The suspect was the starting pitcher when his team was beaten for the first time in eight games by the Dodgers, a team that went into the game with a losing one and six record. Reports say that the two boys teased each other before the suspect pulled a bat from his bag and hit Rourke in the knees and then in the head.

Mass weapons are simply heavy objects such as a baseball bat that can be used to hit someone. They may be easiest to understand when broken into three subcategories: blunt instruments, extrusion weapons, and specialty weapons. Blunt instruments are simply heavy objects like a baseball bat or aluminum flashlight. Extrusion weapons have an extruding head such as an ax or pick that extends beyond the shaft. They are especially dangerous because even if you block the haft of the weapon the business end can still hit you. Specialty weapons are items that you can use to clobber someone with yet which require special skills to use optimally. Martial arts devices such as *tonfa*, *sai*, or *jutte* fit into this category.

These types of devices have been around for a long time. One of the most effective weapons of the late middle ages, for example, was the mace, a spiked, flanged, or weighted ball at the end of a short shaft. These instruments could crush and kill even through heavy armor and padding.

Mass weapons can be found just about anywhere, in the trunk of your car (tire iron, jack, or fire extinguisher), lying by the side of the road (e.g., board, stick, or rock), at the table where you eat (e.g., bottle, mug, or plate), or even at your desk (e.g., hole punch, stapler, or phone). Certain types of mass weapons such as tactical batons are designed for carry-ability and conceal-ability and are legal in many jurisdictions. Reliability varies widely among the various types of mass weapons. Collapsible batons, for example, have more moving parts and are more prone to breakage than solid batons or heavy pipes yet are generally much handier when you need them. Mass weapons are generally most effective at short to mid range, depending on the length of the device you employ and whether it requires one or two hands to wield effectively.

Blunt Instruments

Blunt instruments include things like clubs, canes, tactical batons, tire irons, pipes, wrenches, large flashlights, laptop computers, bottles, heavy mugs, blackjacks, chairs, shovels, or *arnis* sticks, and dumbbell weights to name a few. Mass weapons can frequently be swung like a sword or knife with one or both hands, though the weight of the weapon makes them a little less deft to maneuver. Blades generally work best on soft places (e.g., kidneys, throat) while blunt weapons work better on hard places (e.g., skull, joints). Because there is no sharp edge, they rely on blunt force trauma to injure an opponent.

A stout cane or short walking staff makes an excellent self-defense weapon, one that is legal just about everywhere. It can be wielded much like a sword with one or both hands, striking with either end as well as along the shaft. Furthermore, there are even martial arts specifically designed around combat canes, striking with the shaft as well as utilizing the hooked handle for grappling techniques.

Extrusion Weapons

Extrusion weapons can include hammers, hand axes, *kama* (sickles), rock picks, ice axes, and so on. They are typically

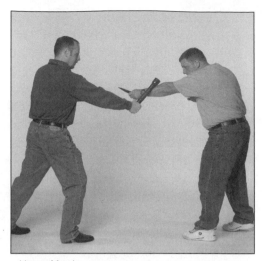

HERE A MAG-LITE FLASHLIGHT IS USED TO STRIKE A BLOW TO THE ARM OF A KNIFE WIELDING ASSAILANT. AIRCRAFT ALUMINUM FLASHLIGHTS ARE EXCELLENT MASS WEAPONS. DURABLE AND LEGAL TO OWN ANYWHERE, THEY CAN CAUSE ENORMOUS DAMAGE WHEN SWUNG WITH FORCE.

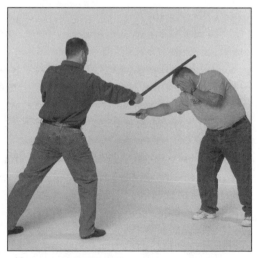

HERE A WALKING STICK CANE IS USED TO STRIKE A BLOW TO A KNIFE-WIELDING ASSAILANT. WITH GOOD FOOTWORK, THE RANGE BENEFIT OF THE WALKING STICK ALLOWS A COUNTERVAILING RESPONSE WELL OUTSIDE THE OPPONENT'S TARGET ZONE. I BUILT THIS CANE OUT OF PURPLEHEART WOOD. IT IS LIGHTWEIGHT AND DURABLE.

swung a little different from a sword in that momentum along with the weight of the weapon is used to deliver the blow. Hip and body alignment is still important yet arm strength is primarily used for aiming and redirecting rather than delivering the strike. These types of weapons are ergonomically designed to penetrate, causing serious damage if you are struck by one.

Because the head of the weapon extends beyond the shaft, it not only penetrates deeply but also is also difficult to block. To readily understand how powerful this design can be, try pounding a nail into a board with a large 2x4 board or a baseball bat. Try it again with a hammer. Even though the board or bat is more massive than a common claw hammer, the hammer delivers a lot more force where you need it with a lot less effort.

Specialty Weapons

Specialty weapons include items like *tonfa*, *sai*, and *jutte*. These devices can be used with a bit more finesse than most blunt instruments yet they take more training to employ effectively as well. Without special training, you can still hit someone with a specialty weapon, of course, yet you will not be able to make the most of its unique functionality.

The *tonfa* is an Okinawan martial arts weapon similar in size and shape to a modern side-handled police baton, which can be used offensively and defensively, to defeat an opponent's weapon. If you hold the handle and spin the long shaft toward an opponent, you can add significant momentum to your strike, well beyond

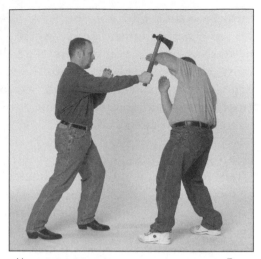

HERE AN AX STRIKE TOWARD THE HEAD IS INTERCEPTED. EVEN THOUGHT THE HAFT HAS BEEN STOPPED, IT IS IMPORTANT TO NOTE THAT THE HEAD OF THE AX EXTENDS BEYOND THE POINT OF IMPACT. IF YOU BLOCK AN EXTRUSION WEAPON INCORRECTLY, IT WILL HIT YOU ANYWAY.

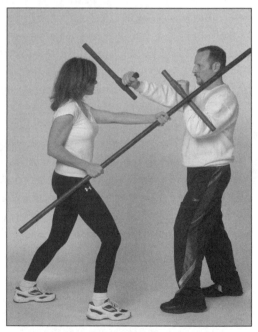

TONFA STRIKE AGAINST *BO*. NOTE THAT WHILE ONE *TONFA* CONTROLS THE OPPONENT'S WEAPON THE OTHER DELIVERS A POWERFUL COUNTERSTRIKE.

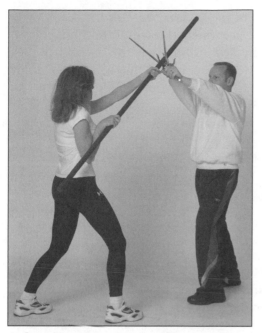

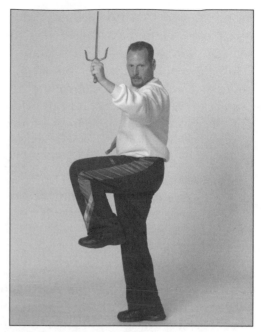

SAI CAN NOT ONLY BE USED TO STRIKE AN OPPONENT BUT ALSO TO TRAP HER WEAPON AS WELL. THIS ADDITIONAL FUNCTIONALITY REQUIRES A BIT OF TRAINING, HENCE ITS CATEGORIZATION AS A SPECIALTY WEAPON. HERE THE TINES (*TSUBA*) ARE USED TO CAPTURE THE OPPONENT'S *BO* STAFF. I BUILT THE *BO* FROM LAMINATED PURPLEHEART WOOD. IT HAS HELD UP TO FOUR YEARS OF STEADY USE WITHOUT BREAKING.

SAI CAN ALSO BE THROWN EFFECTIVELY. THIS MOVEMENT IS FROM *NICHO SAI KATA* WHERE ONE APPLICATION IS TO STOP AN OPPONENT WHO IS ATTEMPTING TO RUN AWAY. THE THROWN WEAPON MAY STRIKE THE LOWER LEG, INJURING THE ENEMY, AND/OR PINNING HIS FOOT OR ANKLE TO THE GROUND. *KOBUDO* PRACTITIONERS OFTEN CARRIED THREE *SAI* AT A TIME SO THAT ONE COULD BE THROWN AT AN ENEMY.

what can generally be created with a straight baton. The knob of the handle can also be used as a striking surface, as can both ends.

In skilled hands, *tonfa* can also be used for trapping and locking weapons or limbs. Defensively, when holding the handle, the shaft of the *tonfa* can protect the forearm and hand and elbow from blows, while the knob of the handle can protect against blows to the thumb. Unlike the police nightstick, *tonfa* are traditionally wielded in pairs.

The *sai* is another traditional Okinawan martial arts weapon. It has recently been popularized in movies such as *The Mummy Returns*, *Mortal Kombat*, and *Elektra*. Effectively an unsharpened dagger with an extended, upswept cross-guard, *sai* can be used not only to strike but also to trap and even break enemy weapons. Swung outward or held along the side of the arm the *sai* can be used to block most any weapon too.

Used as a truncheon, the *sai* is capable of powerful crushing blows with the side of the central shaft or it can be used like a blade by stabbing with the point. The base of the handle can be used to strike with too. Traditionally *sai* were most often carried in threes, two at the side with a third tucked in the back of the belt for throwing or to act as a backup. In skilled hands, *sai* can be accurately thrown 20 to 30 feet.

The *jutte* is a specialized weapon used by law enforcement officers during the Edo period in feudal Japan. Similar to the *sai*, it had a protruding prong that could be used to ensnare an opponent's weapon. Unlike the *sai*, it generally had only one protrusion rather than two. It can be used to deliver crushing blows to an opponent as well as for joint manipulation or pressure point techniques.

Pole Arms

"Throughout history, mankind has come up with all sorts of ways to poke somebody's ass without getting theirs too close." [10]

– Marc MacYoung

Pole arms are simply long shafts you can hurt someone with without having to get too close to them making yourself vulnerable in return. A good example of a pole weapon is a spear, a long wooden rod that has either been sharpened at one end or has a pointy metal or stone head attached to it. While spears were once the ultimate weapon of battle during the dark and middle ages due to their range and penetrating power, they have not completely fallen by the wayside of history. For example, on December 23, 1986, William Basemore, 23, allegedly murdered 68-year-old security guard George Weiss, stabbing him eight times in the chest with a spear, and then slicing his throat with a knife to ensure his demise. A more common pole arm you might encounter on the street, however, is a common walking staff or pool cue.

The major strength of pole arms is their reach, fully effective to long range. With a bit of training they can be used successfully at short and mid range as well. They are not particularly useful at close or grappling range, however, as a certain amount of space is necessary to develop enough momentum for the weapon to work well.* Clearly, a pole weapon is not something you can carry around concealed yet in certain environments, you might well have a walking stick, pool cue, pitchfork, length of pipe, or similar device readily at hand. They do have a significant range advantage over most concealable devices (save for projectile weapons of course).

Because they are used a bit differently, I find it useful to break pole arms into three categories: long weapons, pointed long weapons, and bladed long weapons. The primary difference is that the latter two have a potentially deadly implement mounted on one end that can cause more damage than the shaft alone. The weight and balance of the weapon is also affected by whatever is mounted on the top leading to small differences in how they are commonly used.

---

*Nothing is absolute, however. For example, there are standing grappling techniques for the *bo* staff. Without proper training it is difficult to execute these applications though.

Long Weapons

Long weapons include walking sticks, pool cues, *ueku* (oar), *bo* staffs, and similar implements. The most common way to use these weapons is like a quarterstaff or *bo*, striking along the length of the weapon or with either end. Because you can attack unexpectedly with the top or bottom of the weapon and strike from almost any angle, long weapons can be very effective in combat, particularly against anything shorter or lighter weight.

While there are several schools of thought about how to hold and deploy a *bo* staff I'm partial to the Matayoshi *kobudo* approach. The grip is done with one hand facing up and one hand facing down, each held about one third of the distance from either end. Power is typically generated using a push/pull technique, though you can also grip only one end and use a baseball bat-style swing as well. As the staff is extended in a traditional strike, the back portion rests alongside the trailing arm, protecting it from counterattack.

As with any weapon, blocks require momentum and stance integrity. Thrusts can be intercepted by posting the back end of the staff against your side and curling the front in a manner similar to a standard *chudan uke* chest block. Slashing attacks are generally met force-to-force at a ninety-degree angle. This can be done either by moving the staff toward the incoming weapon with both hands or by rotating the bottom portion of the staff upward pressing outward in a circular pattern.

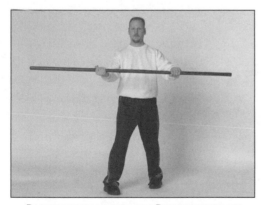

Bo staff starting hand position. Begin by gripping the staff in even thirds with one palm up and one palm down.

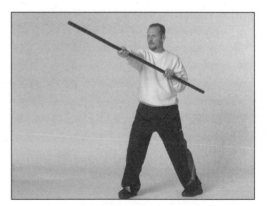

Bo staff basic strike. Note that the back end of the staff rests alongside the trailing arm. Some schools draw the back of the *bo* up under the arm to hold it securely but I prefer this method, as I believe that it provides better protection.

Pointed Long Weapons

Pointed long weapons include spears, pikes, lances, bayonets, *yari* (Japanese spear), pike awls, javelins, harpoons, *nunti bo* (hooked spear), tridents, tiger forks (Chinese trident),* pitchforks, and *pila* (ancient Roman javelin). While the shaft can be used to strike with similar to a *bo* staff, the point can be used to stab with as well. The strength of these pointed weapons is in the thrust where the head can easily penetrate deep into an opponent. Certain pointed long weapons such as light spears and javelins are

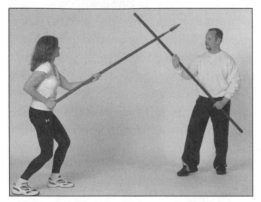

Bo staff *CHUDAN KAKE UKE* (MIDDLE BLOCK), INTERCEPTING A SPEAR THRUST. THIS TECHNIQUE ALLOWS YOU TO SIMULTANEOUSLY CONTROL AND DEFLECT THE OPPONENT'S WEAPON.

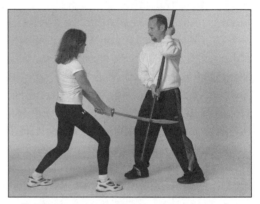

Bo staff *GEDAN HARAI UKE* (DOWNWARD SWEEPING BLOCK) TO INTERCEPT A LEG SLASH FROM A SWORD. NOTE THAT THE TECHNIQUE IS SOMEWHAT SAFER IF YOU STEP BACKWARD TO MOVE YOUR LEG FURTHER AWAY FROM THE ATTACK.

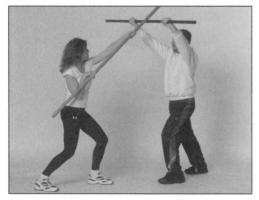

Bo staff *JODAN UKE* (HEAD BLOCK) INTERCEPTING A DOWNWARD STRIKE FROM THE OPPONENT'S *BO* TO THE HEAD USING A TRADITIONAL BLOCK. MOMENTUM IS GAINED BY PUNCHING UPWARD WITH BOTH HANDS TO MEET THE OPPONENT'S FORCE.

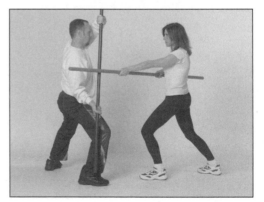

Bo staff *CHUDAN YOKO UKE* (MIDDLE SIDE BLOCK) INTERCEPTING A BLOW TO THE SIDE WITH A REVERSE GRIP. IT IS HARD TO TELL FROM THIS STATIC PICTURE BUT THIS BLOCK IS PERFORMED BY ROTATING THE BOTTOM PORTION OF THE *BO* UPWARD AND MOVING IT OUTWARD CIRCULARLY.

Nunti bo, tridents, and tiger forks could also be classified as specialty weapons since they can be used for disarms and other advanced techniques with a little training.

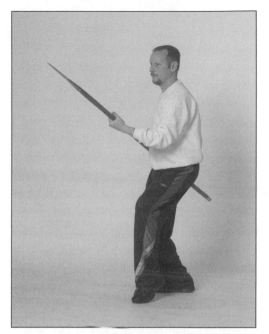

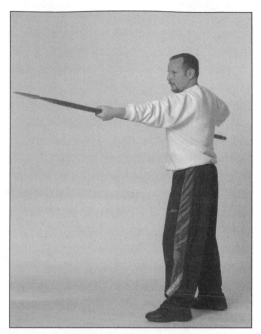

SPEAR *TSUKI* (STRIKE) STEP 1: SET IN *NEKO ASHI DACHI* (CAT STANCE) FROM BLOCKING POSITION. YOU CAN USE MOST ANY STANCE BUT *NEKO* FACILITATES SPRINGING FORWARD INTO ACTION.

SPEAR *TSUKI* (STRIKE) STEP 2: SHIFT FORWARD AND STRIKE SIMULTANEOUSLY. NOTE THAT WHILE THE ARMS EXTEND, THE HANDS REMAIN FIXED WHERE THEY WERE ORIGINALLY HOLDING THE SPEAR AT EVEN THIRDS.

designed primarily for throwing while others are designed primarily for ground fighting. Lugged spears, bayonets, and pikes, for example, cannot be thrown effectively.

There are two major types of thrusts with a pointed long weapon. To use Japanese terminology, these are *tsuki* (strike) and *nuki* (thrust). The difference is primarily in the hand position. For a *tsuki* attack, the hands remain fixed in place on the weapon. For the *nuki* attack, the leading hand loosely grips the weapon so that it can be slid forward in a pool cue-style movement. This covers greater distance than the *tsuki*. In either case, the pointed tip of the weapon is the primary striking surface.

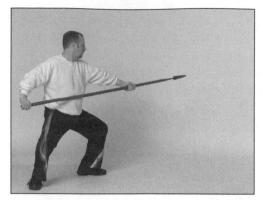

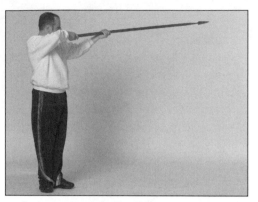

SPEAR *NUKI* (THRUST) – STEP 1: SET IN *SHIKO DACHI* (STRADDLE STANCE). AGAIN MOST ANY STANCE CAN BE USED BUT *SHIKO DACHI* FACILITATES SHIFTING YOUR WHOLE BODY WEIGHT BEHIND THE FOLLOW-ON STRIKE AND MAY SOMEWHAT DISGUISE YOUR INTENTION BY BLOCKING YOUR OPPONENT'S VIEW OF YOUR REARWARD HAND AS YOU SLIDE IT TOWARD THE END OF THE SHAFT PRIOR TO INITIATING YOUR THRUST.

SPEAR *NUKI* (THRUST) – STEP 2: STEP UP SLIDING YOUR BACK LEG TOWARD YOUR FRONT LEG WHILE THRUSTING SIMULTANEOUSLY. NOTE THAT THE FRONT HAND REMAINS STATIC WHILE THE BACK HAND SLIDES THE SPEAR FORWARD LIKE SHOOTING POOL.

Bladed Long Weapons

Bladed long weapons include pole axes, *kuwa* (hoe), halberds, hockey sticks, *kwan dao* (Chinese halberd), glaives, and *naginata*. While the shaft can be used to strike with similar to a *bo* staff, the blade can be used to slash with as well. Certain configurations can also be used to thrust if there is a point in addition to the blade. Many of these types of weapons were developed to defeat heavily armored opponents during feudal times. They were effective primarily because they caused tremendous damage yet were relatively cheap to produce and easy to operate with minimal training.

Multi-Element Weapons

"On the continent of Asia, in Japan, and in many other Indonesian countries, flexible chain weapons were used extensively during ancient times, but their use peaked during the 1600s and 1700s. The Chinese employed various types of chain and cord-connected flails against warriors mounted on horseback, as well as shorter versions where several sections of weighted chains were attached to one handle." [11]

— Sid Campbell

Multi-element weapons include pliable devices such as whips or chains as well as composite devices such as *nunchaku* or *sansetsu kon bo* (three-sectional staff). They use momentum to cause damage to an opponent and can be effective offensive

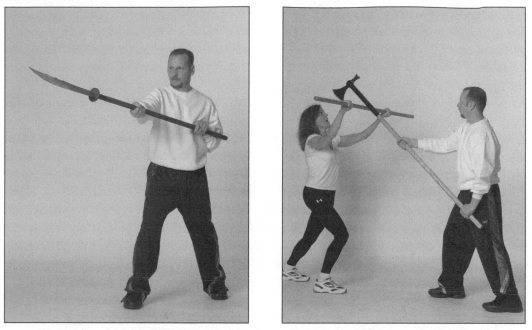

HALBERD (GLAIVE) SLASH ATTACK (ANGULAR).

POLE AX SLASH ATTACK (DOWNWARD). LIKE A SHORTER EXTRUSION WEAPON, THE HEAD EXTENDS BEYOND THE SHAFT.

weapons in skilled hands. They have good range characteristics and can be very challenging to block yet must be moving in order to cause damage hence may become difficult to control after an initial strike. In unskilled hands, they can become as much a danger to the wielder as to the opponent. Depending upon which weapon you choose, they can be effectively used in short to mid or even long range.

While common as a martial arts practice weapon, *nunchaku* are illegal to carry on the street in most jurisdictions. *Sansetsu kon* are generally too big to conceal though some are manufactured to be disguised as a solid staff. Other multi-element weapons that can readily be concealed include belts or chains.

Despite the fact that they are frequently illegal, *nunchaku* are common enough nevertheless. For example, a Berwick (Maine) man, Kenneth Jones, had a rough 32nd birthday. He allegedly refused to stop when pulled over for a speeding violation, leading police on a high speed chase until his tires were punctured by a spike mat. Abandoning his 1988 Chevrolet Nova at a Portsmouth traffic circle, he fled a short distance on foot, and then threatened the officers with *nunchaku* sticks before being subdued with a Taser and arrested. He was subsequently arraigned at the Strafford County Jail on five charges, including criminal threatening with a deadly weapon, speeding, disobeying a police officer, reckless conduct, and resisting arrest. Officers reported that the arraignment was held at the jail because Jones was reported to be combative and not fit to appear in court.

A friend of mine who works in a jail recently discovered that one of the inmates had built a set of *nunchaku* sticks out of tightly rolled magazines with a toothpaste/water mixture between the pages. This impromptu weapon was so solid that it took the corner off a table when he tested it.

Pliable Weapons

No book on self-defense could truly be complete without a section on whips and chains. Pliable weapons are pretty much any non-rigid material that you can use offensively or defensively such as whips, chains, *suruchin* (weighted chains), ropes, bolas, belts, *sjambok* (South African whip), car antennas, or even laptop power cords. Lighter weight weapons such as belts are most effective when used defensively to distract, harass, or deflect an attacker.

Belts are really not all that good as an offensive weapon, especially after initial contact, unless equipped with a substantial buckle. Heavier devices such as chains, on the other hand, can cause serious damage. They can not only be swung as a momentum weapon but can also be wrapped around the hand to add impetus to a traditional strike in a fashion similar to brass knuckles. *Suruchin*, bolas, and similar weapons can be thrown to entangle an opponent's legs. *Sjambok*, bullwhips, and other heavy whips can easily pop out an eye or strip the flesh from a victim. The handle end can also be used as a bludgeon.

Composite Weapons

Composite weapons such as *nunchaku*, *sansetsu kon bo*, flails, and lashing staffs (pole flail) are even more dangerous than pliable weapons since they combine the momentum of an articulated part with a solid striking surface. *Sansetsu kon*, for example, is both a short range weapon and long flexible whip, designed as defense against spears and other long weapons. The *sam-jit-gwun** is particularly suited to striking around an enemy's shield as feudal Chinese soldiers discovered the hard way. Even shorter *nunchaku* can cause serious crushing damage to an opponent.

---

*Chinese term for the three-sectional staff. I use this word rather than *sansetsu kon bo* because the feudal Japanese did not use shields.

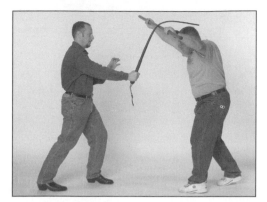

PLIABLE WEAPONS SUCH AS THIS *SJAMBOK* CAN BE USED OFFENSIVELY OR DEFENSIVELY. WHIP-TYPE WEAPONS CAN GENERATE A LOT OF POWER WITH A SIMPLE FLICK OF THE WRIST.

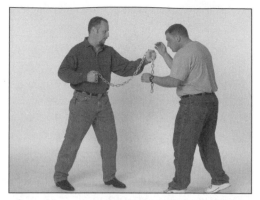

CHAIN CAN NOT ONLY BE USED LIKE A WHIP BUT CAN ALSO BE WRAPPED AROUND THE HAND TO ACT AS A FIST LOAD DEVICE.

Medieval flails and lashing staffs were similarly suited to crushing through armor, even around a shield. The weakness of many of these weapons is the difficulty in using them to block an opponent's weapon. Because they must be constantly moving, they are difficult to control when a sudden direction change is required to intercept an opponent's attack. Unlike *nunchaku* or *sansetsu kon* where the practitioner can readily stop the weapon for a static defense, flails are not particularly well suited to such techniques.

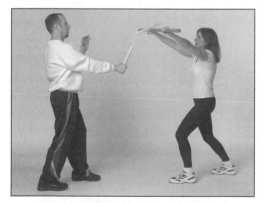

COMPOSITE WEAPONS SUCH AS THIS *NUNCHAKU* ARE VERY DANGEROUS AS THEY COMBINE WHIPPING MOMENTUM WITH A SOLID STRIKING SURFACE. HERE THE *NUNCHAKU* ARE USED AGAINST A *BO* STAFF.

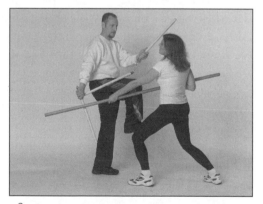

SANSETSU KON BO BLOCKING A *BO* STRIKE TO LEG AND SIMULTANEOUSLY USED TO COUNTERATTACK TO THE HEAD. ARTICULATION IN THIS WEAPON FACILITATES TECHNIQUES THAT A STANDARD *BO* STAFF CANNOT BE USED TO PERFORM.

Projectile Weapons

"Hitler, Mussolini, Stalin, Mao, Idi Amin, Castro, Pol Pot. All these monsters began by confiscating private arms, then literally soaking the earth with the blood of tens and tens of millions of their people. Ah, the joys of gun control." [12]

– *Charlton Heston*

Projectile weapons, particularly firearms are common murder weapons throughout the world but especially in the United States. In a highly publicized case Mark Hacking, a 28-year-old Utah man recently pled guilty to killing his wife Lori in July 2004, admitting that he shot her in the head with a .22 caliber rifle as she slept, then dumped her body in a trash bin. Volunteers scouring a landfill discovered her decomposed remains about three months later. Hacking had initially reported his wife missing to police, saying she had not returned from her regular morning jog at a nearby Salt Lake City park. The news made headlines nationally, prompting thousands of volunteers to participate in a weeklong search for the former stockbroker's assistant.

Mark Hacking was hospitalized after suffering a nervous breakdown when he confessed to his brothers that he killed his wife and they reported his confession to the authorities. His motivation was reportedly that she had discovered he had been lying about attending medical school, his career plans, and their future together. She apparently became aware of his lies after contacting school administrators in North Carolina, where her husband claimed he was enrolled for medical school. Hacking had also lied about graduating from the University of Utah.

Hacking, a hospital orderly, pled guilty to first-degree murder for the death of his wife. He was also charged with obstructing justice by disposing of the body, the gun, and a bloody mattress, but those charges were dropped as part of the plea deal. Prosecutors were unable to determine if Lori Hacking was five weeks' pregnant, as she had told friends. That meant that her husband could not be charged with a capital crime.

While bullets are the most common form of projectile weapon, anything sent through the air with force can be considered a projectile, including hot coffee, rocks, balls, bottles, arrows, darts, and certain types of spears, knives, and axes. Depending upon the type of projectile employed, these weapons can be effectively used anywhere in close to extreme range. Major subcategories include liquids, thrown objects, bows, and firearms.

Liquids

Hot coffee, boiling water, and other scalding liquids can make excellent improvised weapons, distracting or even disabling an opponent. For example, on April 27,

2005 a man who had allegedly robbed 21 beauty salons in Manhattan, Brooklyn, Queens, and the Bronx since March 4th finally met his match, a 41-year-old salon owner armed with a kettle of boiling water. After the robber pulled a gun and began collecting money and jewelry from customers, Andree Crawford and her younger sister, Sylvie Liehi, 31, decided to fight back. Spotting a kettle of water used for dipping client's hair as part of the braiding process, Crawford asked her sister in French if she should do something.

"She said yes, and I threw the hot water on him," Crawford told reporters after the incident. "He said, 'Oh, that's how you want to do it?' And he starts fighting with me." Her sister hit him with a stool, while Crawford swung a chair. The robber dropped his gun and fled. Police recovered a blank-firing starter pistol at the scene. The robber stopped briefly at the Kings County Hospital Center emergency room, but left shortly thereafter when he realized that there was a long waiting list.

Flammable liquids can also be used as weapons for good or evil. For example, Charles Rothenberg (a.k.a. Charley Charles) was convicted in 1983 of severely burning his 6-year-old son David and sentenced to 13 years in prison for attempted murder, arson and other charges. He drove the boy to a motel in the Southern California suburb of Buena Park and gave him a sleeping pill, then doused him with kerosene, set him afire and left the room. The boy miraculously survived. Suffering third-degree burns over 90 percent of his body, he lost his fingers, ears, nose, and genitals during the heinous attack. Rothenberg was released for good behavior after serving only 6 ½ years. Sentencing guidelines were later increased.

Chemical sprays, fire extinguishers, Molotov cocktails, and other liquids can be used offensively or defensively as well. Certain liquids are even designed specifically for self defense purposes. Self-defense sprays, which contain natural or chemical irritants, are commonly used and fairly popular due to their relatively high efficiency, ease of use, low price, and carry-ability. They are designed to temporarily distract or disable an assailant by affecting the eyes and mucous membranes.

While generally effective, they do not work all the time and can even become detrimental to a person who uses them. Here is why: some people are not very susceptible to chemical irritants. Alcohol and drugs can further reduce a person's receptivity to these types of irritants as can glasses or even contact lenses. Further, the use of a defense spray may enrage an attacker if it does not stop him or her, increasing the severity of the attack. If the spray does not stop your opponent, it may also affect you as you try to grapple with him or her. Chemical sprays are also slippery and may make the fighting terrain more hazardous and/or make grappling techniques more difficult to perform successfully.

It is also dangerous for you to use self-defense sprays in tight spaces such as bedrooms or vehicle interiors because of the likelihood of getting the irritant on yourself. In addition, the canisters have been known to leak. These sprays are also sensitive to weather conditions and other environmental characteristics. Wind and rain may reduce a spray's range and effectiveness. When discharged into a strong wind, for example, it may even blow back onto you.

Having said all that, they are a relatively safe and sane way to slow down an attacker and facilitate your ability to get away successfully. Most sprays come in small (typically 2 to 7 ounce) aluminum or plastic containers, though they are also available as pens, *kubaton*, and other assorted disguises including jogging weights,* cell phones, and pagers. Models that contain a safety catch to avoid accidental discharge are best. These containers hold the irritant along with a propellant† so that it can be sprayed roughly five to fifteen feet. Depending on the container, you can typically get 8 to 10 one-second bursts per bottle. There are foaming, fogging, narrow, and wide-spray varieties. There are several common types of irritants available, CN, CS, and OC being the most common. OC is recommended.

CN (chloracetophenone) is an eye, throat, and skin irritant. It is commonly called "tear gas" and is frequently deployed by military and law enforcement agencies as a riot control agent (though many have moved exclusively to OC). CN causes a flow of tears when sprayed, but the irritant is relatively mild. It typically does not exert a strong influence on most people with effects usually measured in minutes. It is also ineffective against dogs, drunks and many drug-affected individuals. It reacts with water (including sweat) and is, therefore, more effective on scared/nervous people.

CS (ortho-chlorobenzalmalononitrile) is a double-action chemical agent that irritates both the eyes and the respiratory tract. It is generally more effective than CN. CS is a white crystalline substance that has been used for many years by civilians in Germany, Russia, and other countries, but is pretty much restricted to law enforcement in the United States. Because CS is a teratogen that can cause malformations of an embryo or fetus so is not recommended for common use. Similar to CN, CS is not very effective on dogs, drunken or drug-affected people, and reacts with water (including sweat).

OC (oleoresin capsicum), or pepper spray, is a derivative of cayenne pepper. OC is a much more efficient inflammatory agent than CN or CS. It causes an intense burning sensation, temporary blindness, restricted breathing, and disorientation on most people.‡ Unlike CN and CS, the effect of OC can last from 15 to 60 minutes depending on the concentration and environment in which it is used. A natural substance, it is also much more effective on dogs, drunken, and drug-affected individuals yet is pretty innocuous in comparison with the chemical irritants.[13] Of the three common types of self-defense sprays OC is the most effective.

Self-defense sprays such as OC are prohibited in certain jurisdictions so be sure to check the law before carrying one. For example, in the UK where it is classed as

---

*Typically five-pound weights that wrap around your hand you can wear as you jog.
†And sometimes other additives that increase the solution's viscosity.
‡Determined attackers can still fight blind so be cautious.

an offensive weapon, the sale and possession of pepper spray is illegal. In Washington, DC, pepper spray must be registered with the police. Pepper spray is also prohibited on airlines.

If you plan to carry a self-defense spray, be sure to practice with it. Classes are available from several training institutions where you can not only get hands-on instruction, but also get sprayed with the substance (typically OC) so that you will understand how it works. Many manufacturers sell an inert substance that operates similarly so that you can get used to disabling the safety and discharging the spray without having to think about it too much. Such practice is invaluable should you ever need to deploy the spray in an adrenalized state. Since they are not very expensive, I recommend buying two containers and spraying a "live" stream a few times at a safe outdoor location too. Do not attempt to do this if you have not already felt the affects of the spray in a safe training environment with readily available medical personnel first though.

Thrown Weapons

You can throw just about anything at another person with sufficient force to injure them. For example, on June 6, 2005, Academy Award winning actor Russell Crowe threw a telephone at concierge Nestor Estrada in a fit of pique at the Mercer hotel where he was staying in New York. Estrada, 28, was struck in the face, requiring stitches and Crowe was subsequently charged with assault in the second degree and criminal possession of a weapon in the fourth degree. He pled guilty to third degree assault on November 18, 2005.

According to published reports Crowe told police that he was frustrated because the phone did not work correctly and that he really did not mean to hit the hotel employee, aiming at the wall rather then the person. He later discussed the event on "The Late Show with David Letterman" telling the host that the incident was "possibly the most shameful situation I've ever got myself in my life. In addition, I have done some pretty dumb things in my life. Therefore, to actually make a new number one is spectacularly stupid. Hopefully at some stage I'll be able to apologize directly to Nestor." Discussing the incident Crowe told *The Daily Telegraph*, an Australian newspaper. "I'm at the bottom of a well. I can't communicate how dark my life is right now."

If you throw a weapon at someone in a street fight, you are no longer armed and they may be able to throw it back at you. On the other hand, the distraction you cause may give you time to respond more effectively. Typical thrown weapons can include rocks, bottles, certain knives, keys, money clips, some axes, baseballs, darts, and on occasion, telephones.

Bow Weapons

Bows have been used throughout the ages for hunting, sport, and warfare. Archery has been an Olympic sport since 1900 and bow hunting remains popular today. Bows can also be used for more nefarious purposes. For example, on April 18, 2003 eight law enforcement officers shot Shaun Gilman to death after he rammed a patrol car and led them on a brief chase through downtown Denver (Colorado). According to published reports Gilman, 20, allegedly pointed a loaded crossbow at police just before they opened fire.

There are several types of bows available today. Popular designs can be made of solid wood (e.g., English longbow), laminated wood (e.g., Japanese *yumi*), or composite materials.* The most common

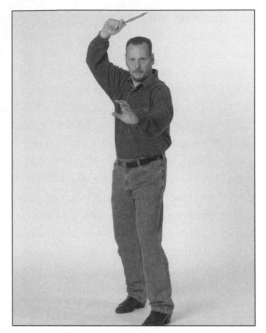

THROWING A KNIFE. THIS PARTICULAR BLADE IS DESIGNED FOR THROWING.

model today is a probably the compound bow, a modern recurve† design coupled with pulleys for mechanical advantage and consistent draw weight. Crossbows are also popular. They are much easier than a traditional bow to aim and fire accurately without much training, though they generally take longer to reload and have a much lower rate of fire.

There are many ways to shoot a traditional bow but the most common approach is to hold the weapon in the hand opposite your dominant eye. Right eye-dominant people, for example, would hold the bow in their left hand while standing with their left side facing the target. Sighting towards the target with the right eye, they would handle the arrow and bowstring with the right hand. The bow-side shoulder is generally aligned with the target such that you draw and fire across your body using the back muscles as well as the arms/shoulders. The common stance is similar to *heiko dachi* (natural stance with feet parallel, shoulder width apart).

To load, the bow is pointed toward the ground and the shaft of the arrow is placed on an arrow rest attached to the bow. The bowstring is then placed into the notch at the back of the arrow. When nocking (setting the arrow on the string) a three-vaned arrow, the most common variety, the single vane points away from the bow. This vane is often colored differently from the other two fletches (vanes) to make it readily identifiable. The bowstring and arrow are usually held with three fin-

*Such as laminated wood, plastic, and fiberglass.
†Ends that curve away from the archer.

gers. When using a sight, the index finger is placed above the arrow and the next two fingers below. The string is usually placed in either the first or second joint of the fingers.

The bow is then raised and drawn such that the string hand moves toward the face while the bow arm is pushed outward toward the target. Some archers anchor the string hand while pushing the bow outward. At the end of the draw, the string should rest lightly at an anchor point, which must be consistent from shot to shot for best accuracy. The anchor point is typically alongside the chin. Some competitors use the tip of the nose and the tip of the chin to get two consistent points of reference. The elbow of the bow arm should be rotated outward a little so that the bowstring does not scrape along the inside of the wrist or catch on a sleeve when released. Many archers wear a bracer (armguard) along their bow arm to protect against clothing entanglement and string burns. The bow should always remain vertical throughout the shot. To fire, the arrow is released by relaxing the fingers of the drawing hand.

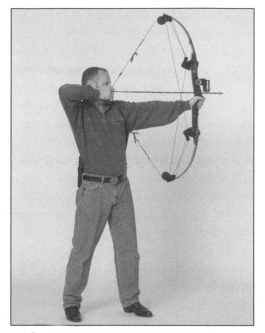

Bow held in firing position with arrow anchored alongside the jaw. Consistency of the anchor point selected is very important for overall accuracy, ensuring that variations in draw length and other variables will not affect your shot. Traditional Japanese *kyudo* archers anchor their shots by their right ear.

Arrows are frequently used for hunting and can be quite deadly when used on humans as well. A non-lethal hit with an arrow or quarrel (crossbow bolt) can be even more traumatic than a similar injury from a bullet in many instances. There is both physiological and psychological damage as you are not only injured but can also see the projectile sticking out of you. Certain types of arrowheads (e.g., barbed) can only be removed surgically as they are designed to cause further damage if moved. Many arrows and bolts are capable of penetrating soft body armor.

Firearms

Colonel Jeff Cooper wrote, "Remember the first rule of gun fighting… have a gun." Firearms are frequently used for self-defense. Case in point: on May 29, 2005 a 64-year old Indialantic (Florida) woman, Judith Kuntz, was awakened by the sound of breaking glass. Confronted by an intruder entering her bedroom, she fired her revolver from about a distance of about 10 feet killing Jason Lewis Preston, 33. The case was treated as a lawful shooting according to published reports. Agent Lou Heyn of the Brevard County Sheriff's Office told reporters, "The bottom line is that when somebody enters your home like that, it's self defense. Breaking into the house obviously shows some intent."

Modern firearms can generally be classified as handguns, rifles, or shotguns. Most handguns are readily concealable and maneuverable, hence practical for self-defense, especially on the street. Rifles are primarily used for military, sporting, and hunting purposes, too unwieldy for many self-defense applications since they cannot legally be carried around concealed and a majority of gunfights take place at fairly close range. Shotguns as well as handguns are popular for home defense.

Because guns are extremely dangerous, gun safety is essential. If you learn nothing else about firearms, at least learn how to handle them safely even if you never intend to do so. It is best to assume that all guns are loaded, even if you have removed the magazine (or opened the cylinder) and checked the chamber yourself. Never point the muzzle of a gun at anything you are not willing to shoot even if you believe that the weapon is unloaded. Keep you finger off the trigger until you are ready to pull it. Be sure not only of your target, but also what is in front, back, and to the sides of it before firing.

In my opinion, even toy guns should not be treated as toys. I never let my son point anything that even remotely looks like a gun, including a water pistol, at another human being. It is far too dangerous for everyone involved. I have nearly been shot by accident more than once. Further, as stated earlier I have come close to killing a kid who pointed a realistic-looking cap gun at me before realizing that it was not actually a threat. Trust me, these are experiences you really do not want to have! If you have children, you should never let them handle any gun, even a BB or pellet gun, without adult supervision.

Never let anyone you are with mix alcohol or drugs and guns. If you own a firearm, it is imperative that you know the safety rules and follow them at all times. Even if you do not own a weapon, the chances are good that you will come across one at some point in your life. The Sporting Arms and Ammunition Manufacturers Institute has published a great set of rules they call the "Ten Commandments of Gun Safety." The following advice is based upon their list:

1. Always keep the muzzle pointed in a safe direction. Loaded or unloaded, never aim a weapon at a person unless you are in a situation where you may legitimately kill in self-defense. "Unloaded" weapons have a habit of killing careless people.

2. Guns should be unloaded when not actually in use. I personally define "use" as not only range practice but also self-defense carry.[14] If my primary weapon is not holstered on my hip, it either is in use or locked in a quick-release safe to facilitate rapid deployment. My remaining guns are always unloaded and locked in a regular gun safe when not in use. I have owned firearms all my adult life and have never had an accidental discharge using this procedure.

3. Do not rely on your gun's mechanical "safety" device. Some firearms do not come with a mechanical safety (e.g., revolver) and even when they do, such devices do not always work. Treat every gun as if it can fire at any time, whether or not your finger is actually on the trigger. See rule number one and keep the muzzle pointed in a safe direction at all times.

4. Be sure of your target and what is beyond it. Even if you legitimately fire in self defense, your bullet may either miss an attacker or travel through him or her into an innocent bystander.[15] Be cognizant of everything around your target before pulling the trigger. This is especially true when hunting or otherwise using a scope, which restricts your peripheral vision.

5. Use correct ammunition. Know your gun's specifications and follow them. I lost a brand new rifle when an improperly hand-reloaded cartridge exploded in the breach and damaged the chamber. I was very, very lucky that no one was hurt. If you carry a backup weapon, it should either use the exact same ammunition as your primary gun or something completely different such that it is impossible to insert the wrong magazine accidentally during a violent confrontation.[16]

6. If your gun fails to fire when the trigger is pulled, handle it with extreme care. Keep the muzzle pointed in a safe direction. Unless you are in the middle of a gunfight wait a few moments to be sure the round is really not going to go off then exercise extreme caution when removing the cartridge from the gun. Learn and practice proper procedures for dealing with jams, misfires, and other common firearm failures so that you will instinctively know what to do when something goes awry.[17]

7. Wear eye and ear protection when shooting. Clearly, this is not always possible in self-defense situations on the street yet safety gear should be worn whenever you visit a range. Wearing sunglasses or protective eyewear is a good way to keep spent brass out of your eye on the street as can holding the weapon firmly in proper vertical fashion whenever you use it.[18]

8. Be sure the barrel is clear of obstructions before shooting. If you have a misfire, be sure to check the barrel to ensure that the bullet is not trapped inside. Even when the cartridge is removed, the bullet may still be in the

barrel. Anything that clogs the barrel can cause your gun to catastrophical-ly fail or even explode when another round is fired. Use proper ammuni-tion and learn emergency procedures to handle any misfires that occur dur-ing a gunfight.

9. Do not alter or modify your gun unless you have proper tools and train-ing. All modifications should only be performed by highly skilled person-nel as they can affect the safety and/or reliability of the weapon. Have your gun serviced regularly. Be sure you are properly trained to conduct routine cleaning and preventative maintenance.

10. Learn the mechanical and handling characteristics of the firearm you are using. Before carrying a gun on the street, you should be supremely con-fident in your weapon and comfortable using it. Do not use any firearm that you have not had proper instruction in handling. Be sure that the self-defense ammunition you wish to carry feeds and fires properly in your weapon. Hollow points, for example, feed differently than solid ball ammunition in certain guns, potentially leading to jams or other failures.[19]

Types of firearm weapons

There is a plethora of firearms out there. Because fully automatic weapons are generally illegal, I will focus on some common guns you are more likely to encounter on the street: semi-automatic pistols, revolvers, shotguns, bolt-action rifles, lever-action rifles, and semi-automatic rifles. Other handguns include derringers and sin-gle-shot pistols though statistics show that you are far less likely to encounter these types of guns on the street. While it may only take one accurate shot to win, maga-zine capacity can be an issue in self-defense situations.

Arguably, the most popular weapon on the street is the semi-automatic pistol. These pistols use the recoil or gas energy of spent rounds to automatically load another cartridge into the chamber. Magazine fed, the weapon fires one round each time you pull the trigger until the ammunition supply is exhausted. These pistols can carry large amounts of ammunition and can be reloaded quickly by changing the magazine.

In general semi-automatics fall into the categories of single action (e.g., colt 1911), single action/double action (e.g., Sig P-220), and double action only (e.g., Ruger P95). Single action handguns require an external hammer to be pulled back manually before the first shot. Subsequent shots re-cock the hammer when the slide retracts. They are sometimes carried "cocked and locked" with the hammer locked back in the ready position via a mechanical safety device.

Single/double action handguns have a longer first-shot trigger pull, which cocks the hammer, then a shorter single-action style trigger pull on subsequent shots as slide retraction prepares the weapon for the next shot. Some shooters prefer this type as it is harder to discharge the weapon accidentally when adrenalized though the difference between first- and second-shot trigger pulls can also throw off your aim. Double-action-only handguns have a long trigger pull on every shot much like a double-action revolver.

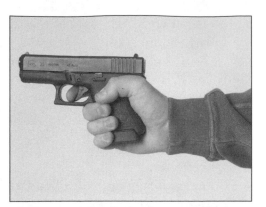

With nearly every type of semi-automatic, the slide locks back in the open position after all bullets in the magazine have been expended so that you know that the weapon is empty. This function can fail, of course, but it is supposed to work that way every time.

Another popular handheld weapon is the revolver. Revolvers are generally more mechanically reliable than semi-automatics yet hold less ammunition, take longer to reload, and are frequently bulkier to carry. Revolvers come in two basic types, single action (e.g., old west-style revolver) and double action (e.g., modern style weapons). The grip and frame shapes of these two types are generally a little different. Functionally, the single action's hammer must be cocked before the weapon can be fired. Cocking the hammer also causes the cylinder to rotate, bringing a fresh cartridge into firing position. In the double-action version, all these actions take place simultaneously with the trigger pull.

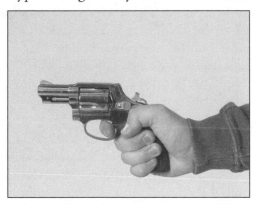

REVOLVER. THIS IS A TAURUS J-FRAME REVOLVER IN .357 MAGNUM CALIBER. IT HOLDS FIVE ROUNDS IN THE CYLINDER.

Shotguns are smooth-bore weapons that fire shells containing lots of small shot or special solid slug rounds. Because of shot spread in the typical pellet load which can hit a target that might otherwise be missed by a single bullet, these weapons can be dangerous even in untrained hands. The choke of the weapon, the gauge of the barrel, and the type of shot used determines the width and breadth of the shot spread.

There are several varieties including double-barrel (two barrels side by side), over and under (two barrels stacked one atop the other), pump action, and semi-automatic. Most jurisdictions require a minimum barrel length of at least 18 inches and prohibit law-abiding citizens from carrying these weapons concealed. Consequently, they are more frequently used for home or business defense rather than street carry.

Rifles are long guns with rifled (internally grooved) barrels that spin the bullet for stability and accuracy as it leaves the weapon. Bolt-action rifles are popular for hunting. Each time the weapon is fired the bolt must be pulled back by hand to mechanically extract the spent shell and load a new cartridge. Many are equipped with an optical scope to facilitate accuracy in distance shots.

Lever action rifles were common in the Old West and remain popular for hunting today. The lever allows a new bullet to be chambered more quickly than most bolt action varieties. The magazine capacity is typically larger as well. They frequently do not use a scope, relying on adjustable iron sights for accuracy.

Semi-automatic rifles are not generally legal for most hunting applications. They are more typically used for sport, defen-

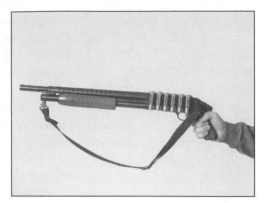

PUMP ACTION SHOTGUN. THIS IS A MOSSBERG 500 SHOT-GUN IN PISTOL GRIP CONFIGURATION WITH AN 18" BARREL. IN THIS CONFIGURATION IT CAN BE FIRED ONE- OR TWO-HANDED. THIS WEAPON COMES IN A KIT THAT ALSO INCLUDES A 28" BARREL AND TRADITIONAL STOCK SO THAT IT CAN EASILY BE RECONFIGURED FOR HUNTING AS WELL AS FOR SELF-DEFENSE.

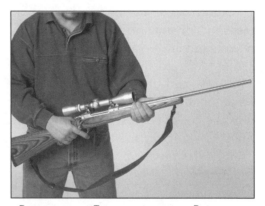

BOLT-ACTION RIFLE. THIS IS A STAINLESS STEEL RUGER MODEL 70 IN 30-06 CALIBER. THIS IS ONE OF THE MOST POPULAR ALL-AROUND HUNTING GUNS AVAILABLE.

sive, and military purposes. Magazine fed, the weapon fires one round each time you pull the trigger until the ammunition is exhausted. These rifles can carry large amounts of ammunition and can be reloaded quickly by changing the magazine. Carbines are semi-automatic rifles that have been chambered for use pistol ammunition (e.g., 9mm). They are typically shorter and lighter than rifles.

Common shooting stances

In order to accurately hit the target, shooters have a variety of stances to work with. For handguns, the most commonly used stances are the Weaver, Chapman (or modified Weaver), isosceles (or tripod), and one-arm stances. Each position has strengths and weaknesses. You will want to select the most appropriate stance to your specific tactical situation.

In the 1950s, L.A. County deputy sheriff Jack Weaver developed a shooting stance that still bears his name today. The Weaver stance is a two-handed hold, which utilizes isometric tension as the basis for controlling recoil and allowing faster follow-up shots. Since Jack Weaver demonstrated its effectiveness at the International Practical Shooting Confederation (IPSC) competitions,[20] his stance became widely emulated. It was much more accurate and controlled recoil better than the common one-hand stances of the time. To perform this stance properly, you push with your strong arm and pull with your weak arm keeping your elbows bent downwards to control muzzle lift. A thumb-on-thumb grip places the heel of the support hand well below the axis of recoil and protects your weak-hand thumb from being hit by the slide as spent cartridges are ejected if you are using a semi-automatic pistol.[21] Feet are in a boxer's stance with the gun foot to the rear.

This stance does not always hold up

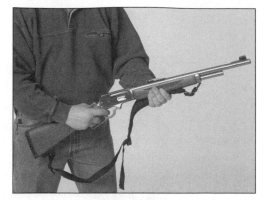

LEVER-ACTION RIFLE. THIS IS A LEVER-ACTION MARLIN 45-70 CALIBER RIFLE. IT IS COMMONLY USED AS A "BRUSH GUN" FOR HUNTING IN HEAVILY WOODED AREAS WHERE SCOPES ARE NOT PRACTICAL.

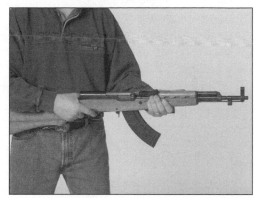

SEMI-AUTOMATIC RIFLE. THIS IS AN SKS SEMI-AUTOMATIC RIFLE. IT USES 7.62 X 39 MM CARTRIDGES.

well under extreme stress as fine motor skills are lost and the dominant hand tends to overpower the weaker one throwing off your aim. Because you aim across your body, if you are cross-eye dominant (e.g., right-handed but left-eyed) you will have to rotate your head to bring your chin or cheek to the shooting arm bicep in order to get your dominant eye lined up with the sights. If you wear body armor, the side seam (a weakness on many models) may be vulnerable. Conversely, you present a smaller target than standing face onto the opponent.

The Chapman stance, named for IPSC champion Ray Chapman, is very similar to the Weaver stance save that the strong arm is straight with only the weak arm bent. You take a narrowly bladed boxer's stance with gun side foot to the rear, lock the gun arm out, and use the support arm to pull the gun arm back into your shoulder (sort of like pretending it is a rifle stock). With your gun arm elbow locked, the limb is

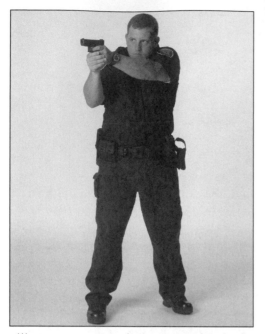

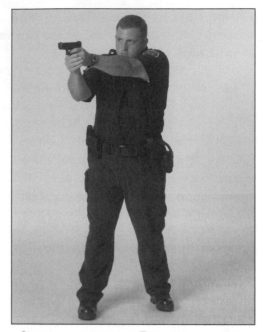

WEAVER STANCE WITH PISTOL. ISOMETRIC TENSION (PUSH/PULL) CONTROLS THE RECOIL. NOTE THE THUMB ON THUMB GRIP PROTECTS YOUR OFF-HAND THUMB FROM THE SLIDE.

CHAPMAN STANCE WITH PISTOL. THIS IS MY FAVORITE SHOOTING STANCE. THE GUN ARM ELBOW IS LOCKED, LIMB FULLY EXTENDED. THIS PROHIBITS YOUR STRONG HAND FROM OVERPOWERING YOUR WEAK ARM UNDER STRESS, A DISADVANTAGE OF THE WEAVER STANCE. THE SUPPORT ARM PULLS BACKWARD TOWARD THE SHOULDER.

fully extended. This prohibits your strong hand from overpowering your weak arm under stress, a disadvantage of the Weaver stances this was adapted from.

Like the Weaver stance, if you are cross-eye dominant you will have to rotate your head to bring your chin or cheek to the shooting arm bicep in order to get your dominant eye lined up with the sights. If you wear body armor, the side seam may be vulnerable. Conversely, you present a smaller target than standing face onto the opponent.

While the Weaver and Chapman stances use isometric (push/pull) tension to control recoil, the isosceles stance uses static contraction of the hands, arms, and wrists to passively absorb recoil with the whole body. This stance was popularized by gun guru Massad Ayoob in the early 1980s. He called it the Stressfire Isosceles stance. It is arguably the easiest and most accurate stance to perform under combat stress.

Both arms are braced behind the handgun with the elbows at natural extension forming a tripod with the gun centered over the midline of your body. This allows two pivot points at both shoulders. Shoulders are relaxed and down. Muscles and tendons of both forearms, the elbow joints, wrists, and hands are set in a medium to firm stat-

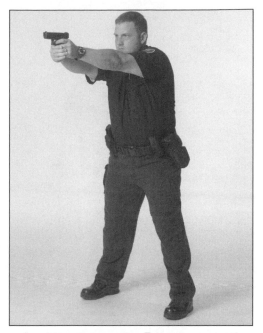

ISOSCELES STANCE WITH PISTOL. THIS STANCE IS NATURAL AND ACCURATE FOR MANY SHOOTERS, ESPECIALLY UNDER COMBAT STRESS.

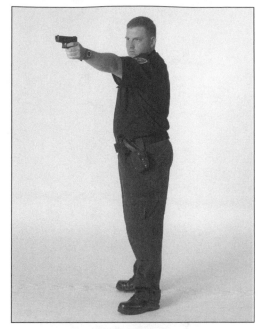

CLASSICAL ONE ARM STANCE WITH ARM EXTENDED. WHILE YOU DO NOT HAVE TO STAND SIDEWAYS TO THE TARGET, COMPETITION SHOOTERS FREQUENTLY STAND THIS WAY.

ic contraction, depending on the amount of recoil you expect. The rest of the body is relaxed. Stability is achieved by shifting the center of gravity forward and keeping your hands close to the same height as your shoulders in order to keep your arms from pivoting up with the recoil.

The shooting grip places the heel of the support hand close to bore-line, which decreases the leverage the gun has in recoil as well as putting the tendons of the support hand and wrist in a straight line, resulting in a bio-mechanically strong grip. Both wrists are locked. If you wear body armor, your most heavily protected side will face the opponent. Conversely, you provide a wider target profile for return fire.

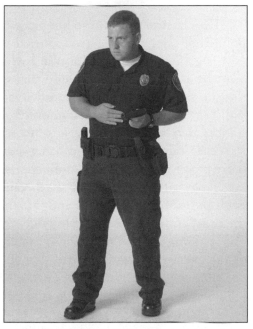

POINT SHOOTING. ONE ARM STANCE CLOSE-IN, FIRING FROM THE HIP.

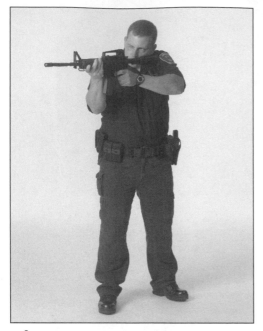

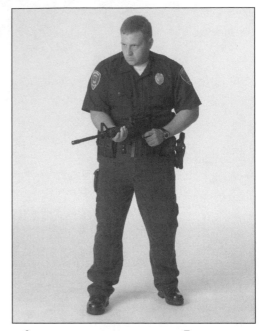

STANDING STANCE, TRADITIONAL SHOULDERING WITH RIFLE. FROM HERE, YOU CAN EASILY PIVOT TO ACQUIRE YOUR TARGET.

STANDING STANCE, HIP FIRING WITH RIFLE. THIS IS NEITHER PREFERABLE NOR PARTICULARLY ACCURATE (SINCE YOU CANNOT USE THE SIGHTS), THOUGH IT MAY BE REQUIRED IN CERTAIN SELF-DEFENSE SITUATIONS.

The classical one-arm stance places you sideways to the target, though any type of point shooting with one unsupported hand can fall into this category. The dominant arm is generally extended outward while you stand upright and relaxed. Your head must be as straight as possible so that you can sight directly down your arm through the gun sights to the target. Another variation is a close-in stance where you draw and fire from the hip. This is commonly called point shooting. All the various one-hand stances are less stable, hence less inherently accurate, than the Weaver, Chapman, or Isosceles stances because the firing arm is unsupported. Any unsupported stance is more prone to recoil either spoiling or slowing a second shot than a supported stance.

Long arms are generally fired standing, sitting, kneeling, crouching, or prone. Each position has strengths and weaknesses. Like handguns, you will want to select the most appropriate stance to your specific tactical situation.

Standing is not a particularly stable long arm stance given the weight and length of the average shotgun or rifle. The longer you hold your weapon on target in this position the more muscle fatigue will affect your aim. The most common way to hold a long gun while standing is to begin by placing your feet about shoulder width apart, standing roughly 90 degrees to your target. Raise the rifle butt tightly against your dominant arm shoulder, holding it in place by reverse pressure from your weak

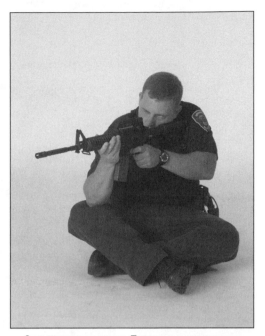

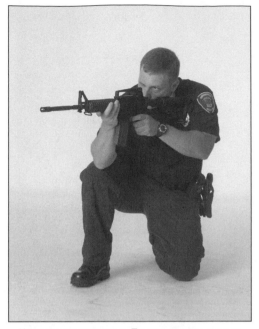

SITTING STANCE WITH RIFLE. THE SUPPORT ARM RESTS ON YOUR UPRAISED WEAK-SIDE KNEE FOR ADDED STABILITY.

KNEELING STANCE WITH RIFLE. THE SUPPORT ARM RESTS ON YOUR UPRAISED WEAK-SIDE KNEE FOR ADDED STABILITY.

hand held on the stock. Press your chin down on the cheek piece of the rifle to lock everything solid, bringing the centerline of your scope or sights in line with the center of your body. Weapons can also be hip-fired from a standing stance too, though it is neither preferable nor especially accurate to do so as you cannot see the sights to align them with your target.

If you use a scope, make sure that your eye is not too close to the rear lens so that recoil will not drive it into your face. The trigger finger should be placed on the trigger, and the rest of the trigger hand can be wrapped around the pistol grip of the weapon (base of the stock), though little if any force should be exerted to support the weight of the weapon with your shooting hand as it may throw off your aim. From this position the weapon can easily pivot, covering at least 60 degrees to either side of your centerline as you move to acquire your target.

While sitting can be a stable and accurate stance, it is not used all that often in the field either for hunting or for self-defense. Begin by sitting on the ground at roughly 90 degrees to your target. Bring the weak side foot close to the weak side of your body, bending the knee so that it rises up towards your face. The strong side foot can either be curled towards the weak side of your body behind the weak foot or it can stick out in front of the body with the knee slightly raised. Either way, it

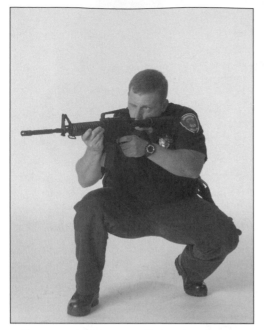

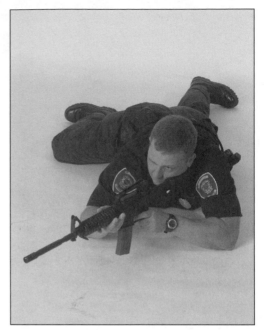

CROUCHING STANCE WITH RIFLE. SINCE ONLY THE BALLS OF YOUR FEET ARE IN FIRM CONTACT WITH THE GROUND YOU MUST LEAN FORWARD A LITTLE TO AVOID BEING OVERBALANCED BY THE RECOIL. THIS IS TYPICALLY A TRANSITIONAL STANCE NECESSITATED BY MOVEMENT UNDER FIRE.

PRONE STANCE WITH RIFLE. THE WEIGHT OF THE WEAPON AND YOUR BODY RESTS ON YOUR ELBOWS. THIS IS A VERY STABLE AND ACCURATE STANCE, WHICH ALSO MINIMIZES YOUR PROFILE FOR ANY RETURN FIRE. NOTE THAT THE BACK FOOT LIES FLAT SO THAT THE HEEL IS NOT STICKING UP WHERE IT CAN BE EASILY HIT BY INCOMING FIRE.

supports the stance. The gun is then shouldered traditionally with the weak side elbow resting on your upraised knee to support the weight of the weapon and provide added stability.

Kneeling stance may be performed low or high. The low kneel is similar to a sitting stance save that the weak side knee is raised with the strong side knee on the ground at roughly 90 degrees. The major difference between sitting and kneeling is whether or not you are actually sitting on the ground or supporting your weight on your feet and knees alone. The support arm rests on your upraised knee for added stability. With the high kneel both feet are parallel. It is somewhat less stable but facilitates rapid movement.

A crouching stance is typically only used when the standing or sitting stances are impractical such as when an obstacle is in the way of a standing shot and there is no time to take a sitting position. It is slightly more stable than a standing position due to a lower center of gravity, but not as stable as a sitting position. It is not horribly ergonomic either, so you will not want to use it for any extended period of time. Crouch down on your haunches with both knees out in front of you. Shoulder the rifle traditionally as in all other stances. Only the balls of your feet will be in firm contact with the ground so you must lean forward a little to avoid being overbalanced by the recoil. As with standing, you cannot rest an elbow on your knees.

The prone stance is very accurate and stable. You can drop into it from a standing position to make yourself a smaller target for enemy fire though you need to make sure you keep the barrel clear of debris when doing so. You can also use it from a combat crawl. Lie flat on the ground with the weapon out in front of you. Your target should ideally be a little to your weak side so that your body and the weapon do not form a straight line. The weak side elbow should be placed in front of the body, with the strong side elbow closer in. The weight of the weapon and upper body should rest on both your elbows. Once again, the weapon is shouldered traditionally.

Breathing and trigger pull

Breathing is important in every martial art, including gun fighting. Do not forget to breathe, especially as you move. If possible, it is best to fire while holding your breath after exhalation so that your muscles are relaxed and oxygenated. The second best approach is to fire during slow, controlled exhalation. Firing on inhalation, on the other hand, almost always throws off your aim to some degree. Try to take a deep breath, let part of it out, and then commence your trigger pull. This is not easy when you are adrenalized, running, or diving for cover, so it is an act that must be practiced repeatedly until it becomes second nature.[22]

The trigger should be squeezed rather than pulled, applying steady, consistent pressure until the weapon discharges. Jerking the trigger is bad because it inevitably pulls your weapon off target. Dry fire practice can help smooth your trigger pull. Be sure to use snap caps or make sure that it will not damage your weapon to do this type of exercise and follow all other safety rules to ensure that the weapon is unloaded, pointed in safe direction, and so on. If you are having trouble telling whether or not you are keeping the gun steady, you might try placing a dime on the barrel just behind the front sight. If you jerk the weapon, the dime will fall off, highlighting your error. For a harder challenge, you can substitute a marble or ball bearing for the coin.

Ammunition

Assuming correct shot placement, stopping power, ability to control your weapon, and carry-ability are the three main concerns with defensive weaponry. You must be able to stop one or more determined attackers before they can harm you, controlling recoil and accurately delivering multiple shots as necessary. You will want a weapon that is easily carried and fits your lifestyle. After all, if you do not have it with you in an emergency, your weapon cannot do anything to protect you.

Self-defense experts often say that your choice of caliber must precede your choice of weapon, since the delivery system is only as good as the projectile it uses. I suggest that you choose a bullet, which is generally available and inexpensive enough that you can afford to practice with it in addition to the aforementioned criteria. Because handguns are most commonly carried on the street, I will focus on handgun ammunition for this section. The most popular handgun self-defense rounds are the .45 ACP, .40 S&W, 9mm Parabellum, .357 magnum, and .38 special. Most shooting ranges will let you rent weapons so that you can try various sizes and styles before you buy.

Regardless of what you choose, however, reliable ammunition is essential. When storing your ammo, be sure to keep it in a cool, dry place. Heat, humidity, and moisture can damage ammunition, making it unreliable. Storing it in the trunk of your car, under your kitchen sink, in a garage, or in a damp basement can shorten its effective life span. Immediately replace any ammunition that has been exposed to liquids such as water or oil, or that has been dented or damaged in any way. This applies to both the casing and the bullet.

While properly stored ammunition has a pretty long shelf life, the rounds in your gun generally do not. Oils from your body or from cleaning or protective fluids can seep into the cartridges rendering the primer inoperable. Because of this hazard, be sure to rotate your ammunition on a regular basis. Self-defense rounds are expensive. I use my biannual rotation as an opportunity to practice with the good stuff at the gun range. Unless you are an expert re-loader, always purchase new factory rounds for self defense.

Firearms expert Massad Ayoob reviews shooting reports and autopsy results from all around the country every year. While laboratory results reported by ammunition manufacturers are interesting, I think that his real-world insight is especially useful. The following recommendations are based upon his March 2002 *Guns Magazine* article, "Duty Loads: Today's Best," as well as a bit of my own personal experience and observations.

.45 ACP

I really like the .45 ACP caliber for self-defense. Ammunition is readily available, reasonably priced,* and allowed at every range I have visited.[23] In standard pressure loads, Federal's 230-grain jacketed hollow point (JHP) Hydrashock has been around the longest of the self-defense rounds. Ayoob reports that it has "an unblemished record for high likelihood of stopping a gunfight with one or two chest hits." I have found that standard practice hardball ammunition has similar recoil and firing characteristics as the more expensive Hydrashock allowing me to practice relatively inexpensively. Be sure to fire enough of the more expensive rounds to ensure that they will feed reliably in your weapon—probably four or five full magazine's worth.

---

*Unless compared to .22 anyway... Some of the exotic calibers can get very expensive.

Another combat effective round is Winchester's 185-grain Silvertip, which has a bit lighter recoil and is somewhat less likely to travel through a target into an innocent bystander. Gun guru John Farnam[24] highly recommends Core-Bon's .45 ACP DPX round, which has good penetration and performs well in ballistic gelatin tests.[25] I have not seen any after action reports on it, however.

For home defense, I personally favor MagSafe's pre-fragmented rounds since they are hard-hitting in laboratory tests yet are pretty much guaranteed not to over-penetrate. I have had them recommended by several defensive handgun instructors over the years. I should point out, however, that I have (thank God!) never had to use one in self defense. I have also never seen them endorsed by Mr. Ayoob. They are expensive which may be a factor.

.40 S&W

The .40 S&W caliber bullet is effectively a 10 mm short (sort of like a .380 caliber is a 9 mm short). It has pretty good stopping power without the excessive recoil and potential over-penetration of a 10 mm handgun. This caliber is also popular because it works well in smaller frame semi-automatics, which have a higher magazine capacity than the larger .45's. I have found it a comfortable caliber to use on the range. Ayoob recommends the 155-grain Winchester Silvertip, 165-grain Black Hills EXP (available only to police), or the 135-grain Black Hills Pro-Load Tactical (for civilians).

9 mm Parabellum

While still relatively popular, many police and federal law enforcement agencies are moving away from this caliber due to its comparable ineffectiveness on the street. I have found it challenging for pin shooting competitions[26] and moved to the larger .45ACP that does not require the same degree of pinpoint accuracy to knock over the target successfully. Most ammunition in this caliber is relatively inexpensive and cheap surplus rounds are often available for practice.[27] Ayoob recommends 115-grain JHP from Pro-Load Tactical or Federal 9BP for self defense.

.357 Magnum

.357 magnums have a lot of stopping power with moderate to heavy recoil but tend to over-penetrate on occasion. A small j-frame .357 is easily concealable, almost exactly the same size as a .38 special but with much better stopping power. They can also fire the same bullets if you want cheaper practice rounds or find you cannot tolerate the recoil. Ayoob recommends a 125-grain Remington or Federal semi-jacketed hollow point. Once again, I have heard good things about MagSafe's products in this caliber but have no personal experience and have not seen them endorsed by Mr. Ayoob.

.38 Special

I have found that .38 specials tend to be easily concealable, imminently controllable, and comfortable to shoot. In fact, I frequently practice with my j-frame .357 using the cheaper .38 special rounds for general target shooting. Most gun experts I have talked to state that this is the minimum sized round they would recommend for self-defense. Ayoob recommends a Remington 158-grain +P lead semi-wadcutter hollow point (LSWCHP) for self-defense.

Non-Lethal Projectiles

The U.S. Department of Defense policy defines non-lethal weapons as "weapon systems that are explicitly designed and primarily employed so as to incapacitate personnel or material, while minimizing fatalities, permanent injury to personnel, and undesired damage to property and the environment." These include Tasers, rubber bullets, bean bag rounds, nets, and similar projectiles.

It is important to note that Department of Defense policy does not require or expect non-lethal weapons "to have a zero probability of producing fatalities or permanent injuries." Rather, non-lethal weapons are intended to significantly reduce the probability of such fatalities or injuries as compared with traditional military weapons, which achieve their effects through the physical damage, or destruction of targets. Just because a weapon is not supposed to be lethal does not guarantee that it will not be. Consequently, prudence must be exercised when discharging these devices just as it is required with all other types of weapons.

Tasers are a good example of a non-lethal projectile device, one that is popular with law enforcement and security personnel. These devices utilize compressed nitrogen to project two small probes up to 25 feet[28] at a speed of around 160 feet per second. These probes are connected to the Taser device by thin insulated wires. An electrical signal is transmitted through the wires to where the probes make contact with the body or clothing resulting in a near immediate loss of the victim's neuromuscular control and the ability to perform coordinated action for the duration of the impulse. While Taser devices are generally effective, they do not always stop a determined attacker. They do, however, have a higher one-shot stop percentage than bullets.

For example, sheriff's deputies in Lynwood, California were forced to shoot a man armed with a pair of knives and scissors on May 30, 2005 when their Taser failed to stop him and he continued to advance in a threatening manner. The officers were waved down by a man who said he had been stabbed by the suspect just prior to the incident. The man, whose name was not released in the news report, died at the scene. It is also possible for a victim to sweep block, breaking the wires before neuromuscular control is lost though this is rare.

Unusual Weapons

"Probably the most underutilized weapon for street survival is the dog. It is imperative that your dog look like he means business. This means something of the size of a German shepherd or Rottweiler. After all, deterrence is the best defense of all." [29]

— Eugene Sockut

Almost anything can be used as a weapon. This section is a catch-all for these and all the other odd things you might encounter on the street that do not fit nicely into the previous sections, including bodily fluids, animals, vehicles, and explosives. And there is some really odd stuff out there. For example, when Jared Gipson, 24, allegedly tried to rob Blalock's Beauty College on June 15, 2005, he was bludgeoned by 20 women armed with, among other things, curling irons. Beaten into submission, he was held until police arrived. He came in wielding a revolver and left in handcuffs, crying, bleeding, and covered in urine. Sharon Blalock, owner of the Shreveport (Louisiana) school, told reporters that she could not be prouder of her students and employees, saying "They just whooped the hell out of him."

Another wacky example is the case of 17-year-old Matthew Haefele, a Kansas high school student who was charged with battery, a misdemeanor offense, for intentionally vomiting on his Spanish teacher on May 23, 2005. On a more serious note, people have been strangled, mauled, suffocated, poisoned (e.g., anthrax, bromethalin),[30] run over, gassed (e.g., mustard gas, sarin),[31] set on fire, blown up, and killed in all sorts of horrific ways by truly odd implements of death. For example, while movie bad guys have been known to terrorize co-eds with a chainsaw, that sort of thing has happened on occasion in real life as well. On February 22, 2005 a 40-year-old Wilkes-Barre (Pennsylvania) man, William Henkle, was shot and killed by police after he ignored pepper spray and officers' commands and attacked a state trooper with a chain saw. Henkle who allegedly had 20 or 21 alcoholic drinks in his system and a blood-alcohol level of 0.495 percent (six times the legal limit) struck Trooper Michael Hartzel in the shoulder, lower back, and buttocks with the chainsaw before state and local officers who had surrounded him opened fire. Feeling no pain, he had to be shot 17 times before becoming incapacitated.

There is no way to concisely cover all the various unusual weapons in existence but for the sake of brevity, we will briefly explore bodily fluids, animals, vehicles, and explosives.

Bodily Fluids

Blood-borne pathogens such as HIV/AIDS, Hepatitis C, and TB can be used as weapons through syringes, rape scenarios, spittle, or open wounds. For example, on January 25, 2005 a 42-year-old shoplifter, Richard Kadlec Jr., allegedly stabbed a Bartell Drugs employee in Bellevue, Washington with the needle of a syringe. One of the store employees noticed a pinprick wound after a parking lot scuffle between the suspect, a security guard, and the store manager. After the fight, the suspect was chased from Bellevue into Seattle but eluded police. He escaped in a green 1996 Chevrolet Monte Carlo coupe, but was arrested eight hours later outside the Muckleshoot Casino in Auburn (Washington).

Kadlec was allegedly trying to make off with a little over $900 in cold medicine containing psuedoephedrine, the active ingredient used in making the illicit drug methamphetamine, when he was caught by store personnel. At the time, state law limited the sale of these medicines to three boxes per person per day. According to police, Kadlec was able to sell half the medicine, worth about $460, for $55 before his arrest.

Any time you are bled on, bit, spit on, or otherwise come into contact with an opponent's bodily fluids during a confrontation it is important to be tested and treated by medical personnel. Do not take such contact lightly as you could have been exposed to something life threatening.* Get the source of the contaminants tested if feasible, describe what happened, and let the professionals sort out the proper treatment and testing regimen.

Animal Attacks

In some areas, you are more likely to be attacked by a dog than you are to be attacked by a person. For example, a 79-year-old woman out for her morning walk was mauled by two dogs in south Thurston County (Washington) on May 16, 2005. Janet McCarthy was taken to Providence Centralia Hospital, where she was reported in stable condition after receiving bite wounds on her hands, head, and chest. The two dogs, a Rottweiler and a Rottweiler-pit bull mix, had reportedly been running loose and growling at people for some time before the attack. When he could not regain control of his pet, the owner of one of the dogs frantically called 9-1-1 while a neighbor struck the dogs with a 2 x 4 board, saving the victim's life. The owners of both animals later agreed that they should be put down for the good of the community.

There are two important lessons in this story. One is that animal attacks can be just as dangerous as any other type of weapon. The second is that quick thinking and use of impromptu counter-weapons can save your life from animals just as it can from people.

---

*Yet another reason why awareness and avoidance are so critical. Even a routine fistfight could expose you to bloodborne pathogens.

Dogs frequently attack on their own volition yet there is almost always a warning that precedes the assault. If a threatening dog is simply mean-spirited, you may be able to ward it off with a sharp command so long as you show no fear. Similar to a *kiai* (spirit shout), yell "no" as loudly as you can. The animal may not understand the language but it will certainly decipher your intent and demeanor. You may also be able to throw rocks or other objects to keep the animal away. If it attacks anyway, you may need to resort to kicks, punches, or even weapons to defend yourself. For example, you may be able to dislocate the animal's jaw or break some ribs with a solid kick. You can even apply choke holds to animals. If you have a family veterinarian, he or she may be willing to show you how to safely restrain a large dog in this manner.

Dogs instinctively go for your throat, genitals, extended limb(s), or even your face so they can be dangerous. If a dog bites you on the arm or leg it is generally not a good idea to yank your limb out of its mouth as this may only increase the damage. You are usually better off pushing back toward the rear of the animal's mouth to weaken the grip while counterattacking.

Dogs are very sensitive to self-defense sprays in most cases. Painful strikes to the nose or ribs may drive off a feral animal. Guard or attack animals are a wholly different breed altogether. They are trained to ignore pain. You will undoubtedly need to use a weapon to fend off one of these animals. Running from one of these beasts is almost certainly futile unless you can quickly scale a fence or similar obstacle. Dobermans, for example, can reach short duration speeds in excess of 40 MPH when they charge.

Mass weapons such as flashlights or batons can also be effective against these animals. A good target is above the snout, an inch or two above where you can imagine an invisible X drawn from right ear to left eye and left ear to right eye. A solid blow to that location will stun or kill most breeds.

In addition to spontaneous incidents, dog attacks can be instigated by an animal's owner as well. If someone orders his or her full-sized dog to attack you, you are dealing with a potentially deadly weapon regardless of whether or not the animal has been trained. Do not confuse the weapon with the wielder, however. The immediate threat is from the dog so you will have to deal with that first. Only attack the owner if he joins into the fray. With rare exceptions you cannot lawfully kill an unarmed person no matter how aggressive he or she is, so once you have dealt physically with the animal you will most likely want to use your attorney to deal with the owner rather than doing anything that places you on precarious legal grounds yourself.

If you were bitten during a violent animal encounter, you may need to be treated for rabies, tetanus, or other diseases after the incident. If you have to shoot a vicious animal, especially a feral one, try to aim for the body if you can safely do so. Doctors will need brain tissue samples to analyze whether or not it was infected with rabies.

Like any weapon, animals can be used in good ways too, of course. For example, on April 11, 2005 a dog saved his owner from a fake trooper. News reports stated that the victim had pulled over at the Highway 385 rest area in western South Dakota to let her dog out. She told authorities that as she started to leave, a man pulled up in a car that resembled a highway patrol vehicle, telling her he that was working as a special officer and needed to see papers for her dog.

Sensing something was wrong, the woman tried to get away, but the man grabbed her before she could do so. That is when her dog bit him, allowing her to escape. Fall River County Sheriff Jeff Tarrell later told reporters that the woman was lucky to have had her dog with her. "At that time in the morning at a rest stop, who knows what his intentions are," Tarrell said. "Thank God for that dog."

Vehicles

On April 21, 2005, a grocery store clerk was seriously injured and will probably be crippled for life after being run over by a shoplifter in the parking lot of the QFC store where he worked. The clerk and another store employee were on a break just before 4:30 A.M. when they saw a silver sedan pull into the parking lot with three men inside, according to a Seattle police report. Two of the men got out of the sedan and went into the store. As one of them started to leave, the clerk noticed a bulge in the man's jacket and asked what he had. The man promptly ran off, leaving his companion inside the store.

At first, the clerk gave chase, but stopped as the suspected shoplifter got into the passenger side of the sedan and the driver pulled away. Initially, the driver seemed to be leaving, but he suddenly circled back, sped up, and slammed into the clerk. He then backed up and ran over him again. The night manager told police he could see the car dragging the clerk. The vehicle, a stolen silver Honda Accord, then sped away.

The clerk was taken to Harborview Medical Center. The three men were reportedly all in their early 20s. The suspected shoplifter appeared to be Latino and was wearing a puffy yellow jacket and had a cream-colored bandana. No arrests were reported.

Vehicles can cause significant damage to a human being, especially when moving with any significant speed. Be cautious about pursuing a person in a vehicle if you are on foot. It is far better to jot down the license number and call the police. If someone does rush you with a car, you may be able to dodge around obstacles or run into a building to escape. As a last resort you may also be able to shoulder roll over the hood to lessen the impact as you are hit though that takes great timing and a bit of luck to pull this type of thing off successfully.

Vehicles can also be used to deliver explosive charges. Potential car bombs can often be identified by mismatched or precariously hung license plates, an extra heavy load in the back, or attempts to park in an inappropriate spot.

Bombs and Improvised Explosive Devices (IEDs)

On June 20, 2005, a camouflage clad man armed with a hand grenade and wearing a large yellow backpack on his chest was shot and killed in the lobby of the federal courthouse in downtown Seattle (Washington). He entered the building around noon and allegedly began making threats. Law enforcement officers opened fire when the 52-year-old suspect, Perry L. Manley, made aggressive movements after a 25 minute standoff during which they tried to talk him into surrendering his weapon.

Manley was shot twice, once in the chin with a rifle and once in the cheek with a shotgun. He died instantly, collapsing with the grenade still clutched in his hand. The Seattle police bomb squad was summoned to the scene to examine the suspect's grenade, discovering after the fact that it was inert. The backpack reportedly contained a cutting board, perhaps carried as a crude form of body armor, some papers, and a living will.

While this particular hand grenade turned out to be inert, live explosives are frequently used throughout the world to cause death and destruction. Oddly enough, movers found a live grenade stuck in the bottom of a couch in Selma, Alabama on July 7, 2005. According to the FBI Bomb Data Center, six pounds of explosives (cigar box) has a fragmentation range of 832 feet. Forty pounds of explosives (briefcase) has a fragmentation range of 1,129 feet. One hundred and sixty pounds of explosives (suitcase) has a fragmentation range of 1,792 feet. You can imagine how devastating a truck bomb twenty times that size could be. No matter how well trained a martial artist you are; you cannot fight a bullet or a bomb with your hands and feet and expect to win. The best defense is awareness, becoming conscious of and avoiding dangerous situations before it is too late.

Awareness can be used to protect not only yourself, but to save others around you as well. In his groundbreaking book, *The Gift of Fear*, Gavin DeBecker[32] wrote, "Before the courageous FBI raid, before the arrest, long before the news conference, there is a regular American citizen who sees something that seems suspicious, listens to intuition, and has the character to risk being wrong or seeming foolish when making the call to authorities." This concept includes awareness of your environment as well as awareness of timing. When environment and timing converge, your level of alertness should be at its highest.

Awareness of environment includes listening to your intuition and being aware of what is going on around you. Identify and report suspicious unattended vehicles, luggage, or packages in high traffic areas. Monitor irregular activity, such as when someone leaves a large package in a trashcan across from a government building or other strategic location and report anything suspicious to the proper authorities. For example, on January 23, 2005 a young boy playing in the village of Barangay

Malisbong, an Abu Sayyaf stronghold in the Philippines, discovered a powerful explosive device concealed in a two-liter plastic soy-sauce container packed with shrapnel and rigged to a timing device. He reported his discovery to the authorities who disarmed the weapon and subsequently arrested two terrorist suspects. Similar devices were retrieved unexploded from a packed public market in Midsayap and the Cotabato City Cathedral the next day.

Awareness of timing has to do with the time of day during which attacks are most likely to occur. Terrorists try to time attacks to inflict maximum casualties—typically during "rush hour." For example, the April 19, 1995, Oklahoma City bombing and the September 11, 2001, attacks all took place during the workday when and where the highest number of potential victims congregated. Similarly, the London subway and bus bombings on July 7, 2005 and the Madrid train bombings on March 11, 2004 also took place during peak traffic hours. A crowded mall in daytime is much more likely to be hit than the same location late at night or just before closing. Conversely, a dance club is more likely to be hit late at night once a sizeable crowd has gathered then during the day. Awareness of timing in the United States can also include Department of Homeland Security threat level indicators (e.g., yellow, orange, red) that help predict likely attacks. The U.S. State Department also issues travel restrictions and warnings when they sense hazardous conditions in other countries.

Where environment and timing converge, it is prudent to take extra precautions by avoiding good places to hide explosives (e.g., unsecured trash cans, mailboxes) near likely targets to the extent practicable. You do not want to walk around in a state of constant paranoia, yet you should take prudent precautions and avoid clearly dangerous situations.

A football game was played at the stadium where I work a couple of weeks after the 9/11 attacks. Right before that game, stadium officials got word that a local TV station was trying to plant a fake bomb in an unattended backpack to test the security. They were, of course, hoping to catch us unprepared and point out holes in our security. While we had always swept the stadium before each game, including a pass with bomb-sniffing dogs, extra diligence was taken due to a combination of the recent attacks and word of this so-called test. No such backpack was planted nor found at that time, but the incident was considered a good training opportunity.

This event led to drills in which suspicious packages were randomly left unattended to keep the event staff on our toes. Occasionally a timer would be set and left inside a package so that if it was not discovered expeditiously (that is, before the timer went off), it would simulate having already exploded. Similar drills can be duplicated in a *dojo* to help increase practitioners' levels of awareness.

While awareness can help you avoid terrorist attacks altogether, it can also help you thwart one before it can be pulled off successfully. Because the trained martial artist is far better prepared than the average citizen to take action in these cases, we should be prepared to intervene when necessary. Prudent application of countervailing force can be very effective even when dealing with suicide bombers.

For example, on March 8, 2002 a Palestinian youth in his 20s walked into the crowded Caffit coffee house in Jerusalem and asked for a glass of water. This was nothing unusual as that particular part of town was a popular hangout for Palestinian teenagers, many of whom frequented the café. What was unusual, however, was the fact that he was carrying a large black school bag, appeared nervous, and was sweating profusely.

An astute waiter, Shlomi Harel, became concerned by the youth's behavior, noticed a suspicious wire leading from the backpack, and took immediate action. Pushing the youth outside, Harel and a security guard who also worked in the building snatched the bomb from the assailant's hands, yanked the wire from the detonator, wrestled him to the ground, and held him until police could arrive. Their quick action averted what Police Chief Mickey Levy said would have been, "a major disaster."

Another type of IED discovered in the United States is a homemade hand grenade manufactured from a tennis ball. The tennis balls are apparently cut and filled with a combination of strike anywhere match heads and buckshot and then sealed with duct tape. When the ball is thrown against an object, the compression of the rubber allows the match heads to ignite. The resulting gaseous chain reaction causes the ball to explode expelling the shrapnel. These balls can easily cause injury to anyone struck directly or blow out a car window, adding to the shrapnel. Once filled and armed, however, tennis ball grenades are fairly unstable, detonating from very little pressure. They can frequently be identified by the duct tape seal.

Summary

"There is an old saying: 'Leave one's yard and find seven enemies.' No matter how skilled one is in the martial arts, he will find himself unprepared if encountered off-guard. Ideally, then, one should constantly be in a state of preparedness." [33]

– Hironori Otsuka

There is a plethora of deadly objects out there that you may encounter on the street. Knowing how they work can give you a leg up on protecting yourself from harm. Major categories include hand weapons, knives, swords, mass weapons, pole arms, multi-element weapons, projectiles, and unusual weapons.

Hand Weapons

Hand weapons add impetus to things that most people already know how to do, punching, blocking, grabbing, and so on. They are most effective in grappling, close, and short range where you would normally utilize empty-hand combat techniques. Hand weapons fall into two major subcategories: strike enhancers and control devices. The former make your blows more powerful while the latter help you apply grappling applications such as locks, chokes, or pressure point manipulations more effectively.

Knives

Knives are popular weapons, easy to obtain and silent to operate. They are readily concealable, highly reliable, and do not take much special training to use to hurt somebody, especially in grappling, close, and short ranges. At the simplest level, there are two kinds of attacks with a knife: cuts and thrusts. Cuts generally produce more bleeding while thrusts can cause more serious damage. The most effective knife attacks use the element of surprise to ambush a victim.

Swords

Swords are long-bladed weapons that can be used effectively for offensive or defensive techniques, especially in short- to mid-range combat. There is nothing scarier to most people than three feet of razor sharp steel in the hands of someone who knows how to use it effectively. Even a cheap sword can cause massive damage if used properly. Unlike a knife where targeting can be important, nearly any powerful blow from a full-sized sword can prove severely disabling or even fatal.

A major advantage that swords have over knives and other short weapons is their ability to kill from a distance. With good footwork and a modicum of training a person with a sword can easily defeat a knife-wielder without ever stepping into his/her opponent's target zone. Most any type of sword can be used for thrusting, slashing, or combination attacks.

Mass Weapons

Mass weapons are simply heavy objects that can be used to hit someone, typically from short to mid range. They can be found just about anywhere, in the trunk of your car (tire iron, jack, or fire extinguisher), lying by the side of the road (e.g., board, stick, or rock), at the table where you eat (e.g., bottle, mug, or plate), or even at your desk (e.g., hole punch, stapler, or phone). They may be easiest to understand when broken into three subcategories: blunt instruments, extrusion weapons, and specialty weapons.

Blunt instruments are simply heavy objects such as pipes or baseball bats. Extrusion weapons have an extruding head such as an ax or pick that extends beyond the shaft. They are especially dangerous because even if you block the shaft the business end can still hit you. Specialty weapons require special skills to use optimally, primarily martial arts devices such as *tonfa* or *sai*. Certain types of mass weapons such as tactical batons are designed for carry-ability and conceal-ability and are legal in many jurisdictions.

Pole Arms

Pole arms are long shafts you can use to strike someone, particularly at longer ranges. Clearly not something you would carry concealed or have available at every location, pole arms such as walking staffs, hockey sticks, or pool cues are available in certain environments. They have a significant range advantage over most concealable devices save for projectile weapons.

Because they are used a bit differently, I find it useful to break pole arms into three categories: long weapons, pointed long weapons, and bladed long weapons. The primary difference is that the latter two have a potentially deadly implement mounted on one end that can cause more damage than the shaft alone. The weight and balance of the weapon is also affected by whatever is mounted on the top.

Multi-Element Weapons

Multi-element weapons include pliable devices such as whips or chains as well as composite items such as *nunchaku* or *sansetsu kon bo* (three-sectional staff). They use momentum to cause damage to an opponent and can be effective offensive weapons in skilled hands. Multi-element weapons have good range characteristics and can be very challenging to block yet must be moving in order to cause damage hence may become difficult to control after an initial strike. In unskilled hands, they can become as much a danger to the wielder as they do to the opponent. Depending upon which weapon you choose they can be effectively used in short to mid or even long range.

Projectile Weapons

Projectile weapons include anything sent through the air with force, including hot coffee, rocks, balls, bottles, arrows, darts, certain spears, and bullets. Depending upon the type of projectile employed, these weapons can be effectively used anywhere in close to extreme range. Major subcategories include liquids, thrown objects, bows, and firearms. Chemical sprays, fire extinguishers, and other liquids can be used offensively or defensively as well. Certain liquids such as chemical irritants are even designed specifically for self-defense purposes, distracting or disabling an assailant by affecting the eyes and mucous membranes.

Modern firearms can generally be classified as handguns, rifles, or shotguns. Most handguns are readily concealable and maneuverable, hence practical for self-defense, especially on the street. Rifles are primarily used for military, sporting, and hunting purposes, too unwieldy for many self-defense applications since a majority of gunfights take place at fairly close range. Shotguns as well as handguns are popular for home defense.

Unusual Weapons

Almost anything can be used as a weapon, including bodily fluids, animals, vehicles, and explosives. Blood-borne pathogens such as HIV/AIDS, Hepatitis C, and TB can be used as weapons through syringes, rape scenarios, spittle, or open wounds. In some areas, you are more likely to be attacked by a dog than you are to be attacked by a person. These attacks can be just as dangerous as any other type of weapon. Quick thinking and use of impromptu counter-weapons can save your life from an animal attack just as it can from people. Vehicles can cause significant damage to a human being, especially when moving with any significant speed. Be cautious about pursuing a person in a vehicle if you are on foot.

No matter how well trained a martial artist you are; you simply cannot fight a bomb (or a bullet) with your hands or feet and expect to survive unscathed. The best defense is awareness of your environment as well as awareness of timing. Awareness of environment includes listening to your intuition and being aware of what is going on around you. Awareness of timing has to do with the time of day during which attacks are most likely to occur. When environment and timing converge, your level of alertness should be at its highest.

Conclusion

"Violence is the last refuge of the incompetent." [1]

— *Isaac Asimov*

Weapons can be found just about any time, anywhere. Here is a recent event that happened to my friend Kris Wilder, a karate instructor and judo practitioner. He relates, "Living in Seattle Washington, the car theft capital of America, I was not completely taken aback by seeing a person in my car that was, well, not me.

"My parking garage has a secure rolling steel door and a county sheriff parks his car not ten feet away but on an early Friday morning I stood there looking at a twenty-five or so year-old rifling my car. I dropped my bag and walked over to the passenger back door and opened it saying, 'What are you doing?' as calmly as if I had approached a co-worker at the office.

"The thief, shocked that I was there screamed at me, 'No, dude, No, don't do it!' as he brandished a utility tool knife in his right hand. I calmly repeated my question and he repeated his threat again.

"He then decided to make his escape by opening the door on the other side of the car. As he turned his head to look at the door handle, I moved on him by using my right hand to chop down on his arm pinning his weapon hand against his thigh. He had made a mistake, he gave up his back, as we would say in judo and I took full advantage of it by getting a *hadaka jime* (rear naked choke) with my left arm around his throat still securing his right hand and weapon so that he could not bring it into the fight.

"He started screaming and in a second the scream turned to a grunt as the choke set in. Now it was time for my mistake. Once I had control, I got cocky and with my right hand, I pulled my cell phone and started to dial 9-1-1. This error was enough for him to get his blood back and he began to struggle again. Without having his hips under control and using only one hand to apply the choke he managed to slip out of the car, dragging me with him.

"He tried to run and I slammed him into a support pillar with my shoulder. His adrenaline helped him as he bounced off the cement pillar in the neon lit garage and ran. He was apparently not aware of the two available emergency escape routes around the corner and consequently ran up the incline to the rolling steel door where I thought I could corner him.

"I jogged after him yelling out, 'I'm gonna choke you!' while he continued to scream, 'No, no, no, please, don't!' Before I could get there, he found the emergency button for the steel door and it started to open.

"As I ran to the door, he ran down the incline, switching places with me. I closed on him again and he continued to scream as we played peek-a-boo around a support column. Then he made his move and I attempted to take him off his feet with a clothes line, or *osotogari* (major outer reaping throw). The technique glanced off his forehead as he bowed underneath my arm and out the door, he squirted. I was talking to the police on my phone as I lost sight of him about a block and a half a way.

"Being choked has been and is a common experience for me and other martial artists. We know how to fight from the position and we know when we are in trouble. To the unskilled person choking is life threatening at the onset with all the fear and that would go along with it. This fear fueled the speed and impetus he needed to escape.[2]

"You know, on reflection nothing in my car was worth risking the possibility of opening the door and meeting a bullet or a blade in the stomach. If I had truly been thinking, and I mean really using my head, I would have ducked between two cars and called 9-1-1 then simply observed the arrest."

There are several important lessons in this story, lessons that closely align with my nine rules to live by:

Rule number one is, "Don't get hit." While he admittedly should have called the police and avoided this encounter entirely, one of the things Kris did most effectively during the fight was not get hit. He adeptly used his opponent's moment of distraction to take the weapon out of play. The thief also used this rule to great advantage too, running, dodging around a column, and otherwise keeping away from Kris. This is an excellent example of how hard it is to capture someone who is bound and determined to escape. Despite the fact that Kris is a lightning fast, highly experienced martial artist, he could not successfully secure his adversary. If awareness and avoidance fail, evasion and escape become critical aspects of remaining safe.

Pain is your friend. Although he would never have gotten himself into this situation in the first place if he were a law-abiding citizen, this is one more thing the car thief did right. While we martial arts types are used to being choked, this guy undoubtedly thought he was going to die. He nearly passed out at least once during the struggle. It is both scary and painful to grapple with a 225-pound martial artist, yet the thief used his fear and adrenaline to spur himself to action rather than giving up the fight. While I certainly do not condone his actions, you can take a valuable lesson from the car thief. No matter how much it hurts, you can still escape if you try hard enough.

Weapons are ubiquitous. While a Leatherman tool would not be most people's first choice of weapons, almost all their models contain one or more blades that can be locked open. They are well made, nicely tempered, and come from the factory very sharp. Consequently, they can be quite dangerous. The car thief is but one of the millions of people who carry around some form of deadly weapon. This is another example of how you can run into an armed assailant just about anywhere. As Kris pointed out, he never should have opened the door to confront a potentially armed thief in the first place yet he did manage to disable his opponent's weapon before he could be cut by it.

Always assume they are armed. In this particular case, Kris did not see the weapon until it was deployed. Fortunately, the bad guy only brandished it but a slightly different scenario may have ended badly for either or both of them. I imagine that the thief either used his pocket tool to break into the vehicle or was about to use it to steal the stereo or start the engine. Either way, it was already in his hand when Kris confronted him. Assuming that your assailant is unarmed is very hazardous, something you should never do. Always believe your attacker is armed until you can prove beyond a shadow of doubt otherwise.

Bad guys cheat to win; so should you. The car thief pulled a weapon to give himself an advantage. Kris countered with superior martial training to disable the weapon and psychological warfare to keep his opponent off balance and afraid. No trick is too underhanded in an armed encounter. Cheating to win is fundamental. Armed assaults place you in survival mode. Unlike a tournament, there are no rules on the street.

Understand how weapons work. A few weeks before this incident, we devoted a *dojo* session to knife combat, practicing techniques similar to what Kris employed during his encounter with the car thief. He was able to utilize the benefit of many years of training and recent practice to safely control his attacker and disable the weapon without getting hurt. He told me afterward that he was able to react with great clarity and purpose because he was confident about what he was doing. There was no significant adrenal dump or noteworthy level of fear getting in the way of his actions because he was familiar with the weapon and how to keep himself safe from it. Knowing how weapons work is an important part of being prepared to defend yourself from an armed assailant.

Expect the unexpected. Let's face it, how often do you find someone sitting in your car inside a locked security garage at 6:15 in the morning? Furthermore, people who break into cars are frequently are not armed, so the car thief's weapon came as a further surprise. Likewise, most violent encounters are unexpected. After all, if you see it coming you can avoid the situation altogether. Your opponent's tactics will attempt to take advantage of the element of surprise to defeat you. Flexibility on your part, therefore, is key to your survival.

Yell for help. Both parties followed this rule. Kris dialed 9-1-1 while the thief screamed for help. While there was no one around to overhear the ruckus that early in the morning, it was a reasonable tactic in both cases. Frankly, the car thief did an excellent job of impersonating a victim. Had someone stumbled late upon the scene, Kris would almost certainly have been mistaken for the aggressor. In retrospect he should have shouted something about his attacker's knife and certainly should not have yelled, "I'm gonna choke you," no matter how fun that must have been at the time. Creating witnesses is important in any encounter, even if you are pretty sure that no one else is present.

Check for bleeding. Fortunately, neither person was seriously injured in this encounter. Kris gets points not only for not being cut but also for attempting to subdue his attacker in a non-violent manner.* Check yourself over after every fight. If you have been cut you may not know it at the time.

This was but one of the thousands of violent encounters that take place every day, one that probably will not even make the statistics despite the fact that it was reported to the police, because no one was hurt. It is but one more example that every martial practitioner should be both mentally and physically prepared to deal with an armed assault at any time, especially when they themselves are unarmed. If your interest in martial arts is driven by a desire to keep yourself safe, you must learn about weapons in order to do so. Further, your exposure must be comprehensive enough to account for the plethora of pointy objects, blunt instruments, and unfriendly projectiles that may someday be used against you.

---

*He's a more experienced *karateka* (*yodan*) than *judoka* (*shodan*). He could just as easily have punched the car thief into next week.

Endnotes

Preface

1. Marc "Animal" MacYoung teaches experience-based self-defense to police, military, civilians, and martial artists around the world. A former bouncer, street fighter, and all around dangerous guy, his practical, real-world self-defense advice is available at www.nononsenseselfdefense.com.
2. Jeff Cooper, founder of the International Practical Shooting Confederation (IPSC), is an icon of modern pistol craft who has taught defensive handgun courses all over the world. He served with distinction as a Lt. Col. in the U.S. Marines during World War II and Korea, is a member of the NRA Board of Directors, and editor-at-large for *Guns & Ammo* magazine. In addition to his considerable expertise in firearms, he is also a history professor, philosopher, adventurer and author.

Introduction

1. Isaac Bashevis Singer (1904 – 1991), a famous Jewish author born in Poland who immigrated to the United States. He won the Nobel Prize for Literature in 1978.
2. Imi Lichtenfeld (1910 – 1998). Sde-Or is Imi's family name translated into Hebrew (he adopted this name, which means "light field," in the 1960s). Krav Maga translates as "contact combat." Mr. Sde-Or was the first chief physical fitness and Krav Maga instructor at the Israeli Defense Force School of Combat Fitness where he trained elite military and police units. While he originally developed Krav Maga as a military art, he modified it later for civilian use upon completing his active duty enlistment. Krav Maga has gained wide popularity today beyond the borders of Israel partly due to its applicability in defending against weapon attacks.
3. Kelly Worden is the first American *Datu* and Senior Blademaster of modern arnis.

Chapter 1

1. Ani DiFranco is a singer, songwriter, and guitarist. Over the years, Ani has recorded duets with both John Gorka and Jackie Chan, swapped album appearances with Prince and Maceo Parker, produced recordings by Dan Bern and Janis Ian, and performed orchestral versions of her compositions with the Buffalo Philharmonic orchestra.
2. Craig Perkins, BJS Statistician, from his report, Bureau of Justice Statistics Special Report: *Weapon Use and Violent Crime*. U.S. Department of Justice December, 2003.
3. Massad Ayoob is director of the Lethal Force Institute, an organization which trains 800 to 1,200 personnel per year in the judicious use of deadly force, armed and unarmed combat, threat management for police, and advanced officer survival in four countries. A retired police lieutenant, firearm, weapon, and unarmed combat expert, his books, articles, and classes teach law enforcement professionals and civilians realistic, street-worthy self-defense techniques. He appears selectively as a court accepted expert witness in the areas of dynamics of violent encounters, weapons, self defense, police training, and survival/threat management tactics and principles.
4. Riyad us-Saliheyn Martyrs' Brigade is a group dedicated to the creation of an independent Islamic republic in Chechnya and other primarily Muslim parts of Russia such as Dagestan, Kabardino-Balkaria, and Tatari.
5. Secular/political groups include organizations such as the Revolutionary Armed Forces of Colombia (FARC), the National Democratic Front of Bodoland (in India), the Communist Party of Nepal, the United People's Front (Nepal), the New People's Army (Communist Party of the Philippines), or the Chechen separatist movement (in Russia).
6. Marc MacYoung (see endnote 1 in the preface).
7. On January 15, 2002, the FAA published new standards to protect cockpits from intrusion, fire, axes, knife blades, small-arms fire, and fragmentation devices (e.g., grenades). The rule required U.S. and foreign operators providing passenger service in U.S. airspace to install hardened doors.

8. Ted Bundy was executed via electrocution on January 24, 1989 for killing two women in Florida and was implicated in dozens of other killings in the 1970s.

9. BTK stands for bind-torture-kill. Ten murders in the State of Kansas are attributed to the BTK killer, the first of which occurred in 1974. In the years that followed, the serial killer taunted the authorities here with grisly letters, clues, poems, photographs and phone calls. Rader pled guilty to all ten murders on June 27, 2005, graphically describing his crimes in court. He received ten consecutive life sentences for his crimes.

10. Lt. Col. David Grossman is an expert in the psychological costs of war, the root causes of violent crime, and the process of healing the victims of violence in war and peace. A West Point psychology and Military Science professor and a retired Army Ranger, he combined his experiences to form a new field of scientific endeavor which he has termed "killology."

11. Traditionally used by police officers around the turn of the century, blackjacks and other blunt weapons have given way to more modern batons. The original blackjacks were typically a leather-wrapped lead weight attached to the end of a short flexible shaft or affixed with a coil spring to a solid handle. Another way to build this weapon is to fill a sock or denim sack full of pennies or ball bearings and reinforce it with tape. This version is sometimes called a sand sock. Yet another version is a padlock placed inside of a sock. Blackjacks are not legal in many jurisdictions.

12. When attached to a rifle. Un-mounted, bayonets would be more accurately classified as knives.

13. IEDs (improvised explosive devices) are nothing new; *kayaku-jutsu* (pyrotechnic arts) date back to the early 1600s when ninja used these apparatus for assassinations in feudal Japan.

14. There are also some techniques that you can do physically but do not have the emotional wherewithal to perform on another human being (e.g., eye gouge). It is important to know what you are prepared to do before things get ugly. See combat mindset in Chapter 5 for more information.

15. Jack Feldman, Ph.D. is a professor of psychology at Georgia Institute of Technology, a Fellow of the American Psychological Association, and a Charter Fellow of the American Psychological Society. His research focuses on processes of human judgment and decision-making, both theoretical and applied.

16. Tom Givens is an author and firearms instructor who has trained law enforcement officers at the local, state, and federal level; foreign government agents; and military personnel including members of the 20th Special Forces Group.

17. Tom Givens (see endnote 16).

18. Case in point: When deputies arrested Justin Breakspear, 19, on May 19, 2005 for a breaking-and-entering incident in Middlesex County (Massachusetts), they found two sawed-off shotguns and a .380-caliber pistol in the basement where he had been hiding. The shotguns were illegal while the handgun had previously been reported stolen during the theft for which the suspect had been arrested. Breakspear denied owning the weapons, yet when he was photographed during the booking process officers discovered a large tattoo of a handgun, complete with serial number, on his hip. The tattooed weapon's serial number matched the number of the stolen handgun collected during the search.

19. Law enforcement professionals, security personnel, judges, and certain elected officials may have legal authority to demand compliance from others. Similarly, military officers or civilian managers have hierarchical authority over their subordinates due to the structure of the organization they work for, hence an ability to command compliance.

20. Tom Givens (see endnote 16).

21. While the Tueller Drill was focused on officers' reaction time in drawing a handgun and firing one to two aimed shots, the average person needs a similar amount of time to observe a threat, come to grips with the fact that the danger is real, and begin to react regardless of whether or not they are carrying a weapon. Surprise attacks eat up vital reaction time while the mind processes the threat even if you respond using empty hand techniques or a makeshift device that is already in your hand, either of which circumvent the need to draw and deploy a counter weapon. Consequently it is critical to maintain sufficient distance between yourself and a potential adversary to give yourself time to react.

22. Methods for preventing an adversary from disarming you, using your weapon against you, or otherwise keeping you from bringing your gun into play when it is needed.

23. While Tasers come with 15, 21 or 25 foot (effective range) cartridges, the 21 and 25 foot models are only sold to law enforcement, military and aviation security agencies. While civilian models have a

maximum effective range of 15 feet, they can be discharged at nearly any distance less than that. They work best at ranges where the probes have an opportunity to spread out a bit in flight, however.

24. When used for thrusting at full extension (e.g., spear) or performing other techniques that are best accomplished with a grip near the end of the shaft (e.g., overhand strike with a pole ax or *naginata*).

25. AED stands for Automated External Defibrillator. While Cardio Pulmonary Resuscitation (CPR) can keep life-giving blood and oxygen circulating after a heart attack, it cannot restart a victim's heart. An AED, on the other hand, frequently can. As prices drop they are becoming more and more ubiquitous. Most first aid classes now teach students how to use these devices in additional to traditional CPR procedures.

26. Massad Ayoob (see endnote 3 in Chapter 1)

Chapter 2

1. Buddha.
2. Massad Ayoob (see endnote 3 in Chapter 1)
3. While the rules are limited, they are generally sufficient to ensure that no one is killed or permanently maimed as a result of the competition. For example, joint kicks, eye gouges, and throat strikes are not allowed in these venues.
4. Loren Christensen is a prolific author and retired police officer with over thirty years of military and civilian law enforcement experience. A highly proficient fighter with more than 40 years of martial arts experience, he holds a 7th *dan* black belt in karate, 2nd *dan* in jujitsu, and 1st *dan* in arnis. Loren's web site is www.lwcbooks.com.
5. Marc MacYoung (see endnote 1 in the Preface).
6. Dave Lowry regularly writes articles and columns for several popular martial arts magazines and Web sites. A highly skilled and knowledgeable martial artist, he is the author of *Autumn Lightning: The Education of an American Samurai, Sword & Brush, Persimmon Wind, Moving Toward Stillness, Traditions,* and *Clouds in the West* among other excellent books.
7. From the movie, *Monty Python and the Holy Grail,* a 1974 Arthurian spoof hysterically written and performed by Graham Chapman, John Cleese, Terry Gilliam, Eric Idle, Terry Jones, and Michael Palin and released by Python (Monty) Pictures, Ltd. This song is also featured in the 2005 Tony Award-winning musical *Spamalot* (book by Eric Idle, music and lyrics by John Du Prez and Eric Idle).
8. If you are running from organized crime, law enforcement, a hired hit man, or a bounty hunter, on the other hand, you're in a lot of trouble because professionals won't give up once you are out of their sight. They also typically have access to advanced technology to track your movements and ultimately ascertain wherever you might decide to hide.
9. Christopher Caile is the founder and editor-in-chief of FightingArts.com. He has been a student of the martial arts for over 40 years, holds a 6th *dan* black belt in *Seido* karate, and has experience in judo, aikido, *Diato Ryu,* boxing and several Chinese fighting arts.
10. Mary F. Shafer, Dryden Flight Research Center, NASA.

Chapter 3

1. Dwight David Eisenhower (1890 – 1969), 34th President of the United States. During WWII he successfully commanded the Allied Forces landing in North Africa in 1942 and later in 1944 was the Supreme Commander of Allied troops invading France on D-Day.
2. Klaus, Patsy, BJS Statistician, from her report *Bureau of Justice Statistics National Crime Victimization Survey: Carjacking, 1993 – 2002.* U.S. Department of Justice, July, 2004.
3. From the American Banker's Association consumer connection web site (www.aba.com).
4. Davidson, Thomas N, from his book *To Preserve Life: Hostage-Crisis Management.* Indianapolis, IN: Crisis Incident Management Agency (CIMACOM), 2002.
5. RCW 26.50.010:
    (1) "Domestic violence" means: (a) physical harm, bodily injury, assault, or the infliction of fear of imminent physical harm, bodily injury or assault, between family or household members; (b) sexual

assault of one family or household member by another; or (c) stalking as defined in RCW 9A.46.110 of one family or household member by another family or household member.

(2) "Family or household members" means spouses, former spouses, persons who have a child in common regardless of whether they have been married or have lived together at any time, adult persons related by blood or marriage, adult persons who are presently residing together or who have resided together in the past, persons sixteen years of age or older who are presently residing together or who have resided together in the past and who have or have had a dating relationship, persons sixteen years of age or older with whom a person sixteen years of age or older has or has had a dating relationship, and persons who have a biological or legal parent-child relationship, including stepparents and stepchildren and grandparents and grandchildren.

(3) "Dating relationship" means a social relationship of a romantic nature. Factors that the court may consider in making this determination include: (a) the length of time the relationship has existed; (b) the nature of the relationship; and (c) the frequency of interaction between the parties.

6. The Public Safety Partnership is a service of King County (Washington) Metro Transit. It got its start with a grant from the Federal Transit Administration and has since received support from Local 587 of the Amalgamated Transit Union, neighborhood groups and the King County Sheriff.

7. Though a DHL A300 did sustain some damage to its left wing from a ground-launched missile in Baghdad, Iraq in 2003, there were no onboard injuries and the plane was quickly returned to service without substantial repairs so this was not counted as a successful hostile incident.

8. Suicide bombings have occurred in many countries throughout the world including Afghanistan, Algeria, Argentina, China, Colombia, Croatia, Egypt, England, India, Indonesia, Iraq, Israel, Kenya, Kuwait, Lebanon, Morocco, Pakistan, Panama, the Philippines, Qatar, Russia, Saudi Arabia, Sri Lanka, Tanzania, Tunisia, Turkey, Uzbekistan, and Yemen. While the events on 9/11 in the United States were technically a suicide attack, in this section I'm referring to someone who detonates on an explosive charge they are either wearing or carrying on their person as opposed to blowing-up or crashing a vehicle they are driving or flying.

9. The Rape, Abuse & Incest National Network (RAINN) is the nation's largest anti-sexual assault organization. Their web site address is www.rainn.org. RAINN created and operates the National Sexual Assault Hotline at 1-800-656-HOPE. RAINN also publicizes the hotline's free, confidential services; educates the public about sexual assault; and leads national efforts to improve services to victims and ensure that rapists are brought to justice.

10. Lt. Col. David Grossman (see endnote 10 in Chapter 1).

11. According to the Bureau of Justice Statistics there was an average of 1,744,300 workplace victimizations per annum between the years 1993 and 1999, just over 33,544 per week. The vast majority of those victimizations were simple assaults (75.2%). More serious aggravated assaults accounted for 18.6% of the total victimizations, while the remainder were a mix of robbery (4.0%), rape/sexual assault (2.1%), and homicide (0.1%). Given the general downward trend in overall violence since that time the current 18,000 figure quoted above seems about right. It is, nevertheless, a shockingly huge number.

12. Francis Quarles (1592 – 1644), English poet.

Chapter 4

1. The last words uttered by actress Nicole duFresne immediately before being shot to death during a robbery attempt by Rudy Fleming, a 19 year-old with a stolen gun, on January 27, 2005.

2. The Cuban Missile Crisis was a tense confrontation between the United States and the Soviet Union over the USSR's deployment of nuclear missiles in Cuba, just off the Florida shoreline of the United States. The crisis began on October 14, 1962 and lasted for 38 days until November 20, 1962. It is regarded by many historians as the moment when the Cold War came closest to becoming an all-out nuclear war, one that very likely could have destroyed much if not all of humanity.

3. Mark Twain (1835 – 1910). Humorist, short story author, and novelist, his most famous books were, *Tom Sawyer* 1876, *Huckleberry Finn* 1884, and *A Connecticut Yankee in King Arthur's Court* 1889.

4. Napoleon Bonaparte (1769 – 1821). Born on the island of Corsica, Napoleon rose from obscurity to become Napoleon I, Empereur des Français (Emperor of the French) using a combination of military and political ruthlessness.

5. From Joseph Swetnam's 1617 treatise *The Schoole of the Noble and Worthy Science of Defence.*

6. George J Thompson, from his book *Verbal Judo: the Gentle Art of Persuasion.* New York, NY: William Morrow and Company, 1993.

7. Sun Tzu (544 – 496 B.C.), Chinese general who helped the King Ho-Lu capture the city of Ying, bringing about the fall of the Ch'u state in 506 B.C. His collection of essays, *The Art of War,* is one of the best known and most quoted military treatises in the world.

Chapter 5

1. George Orwell (1903 – 1950), pen name used by British author and journalist Eric Arthur Blair. Orwell is probably best remembered for two of his novels, *Animal Farm* and *Nineteen Eighty-Four.*

2. W. Hock Hochheim, from his article, 12 Combat Commandments from the School of Hard Knocks. *Black Belt Magazine,* August, 2003.

3. Alfred Hitchcock (1899 – 1980), award-winning British film director who specialized in suspense thrillers. His most famous films included *Shadow of a Doubt, Spellbound, Rear Window, Vertigo,* and *Dial M for Murder.*

4. Ayn Rand (1905 – 1982), born Alissa "Alice" Zinovievna Rosenbaum. She was a popular and controversial American novelist and philosopher. Her most famous novels were *The Fountainhead* and *Atlas Shrugged.* Her philosophy of Objectivism emphasizes the concepts of individualism, egoism, "rational self-interest," and capitalism. She believed that every person must choose his/her values and actions by reason, that every individual has a right to exist for his or her own sake (neither sacrificing self to others nor others to self), and that no one has the right to seek values from others by physical force or impose ideas on others by physical force.

5. Born in Ireland, Burke (1729 – 1797) was an influential member of the British Parliament.

6. Luke 22:36.

7. Col. David H. Hackworth (1930 – 2005). Col. Hackworth saw action in WWII, Korea, and Vietnam. He was put in for the Medal of Honor three times; the last application is currently under review at the Pentagon. He was twice awarded the Army's second highest honor for valor, the Distinguished Service Cross, along with 10 Silver Stars and eight Bronze Stars. When asked about his many awards, he always said he was proudest of his eight Purple Hearts (a military decoration awarded to those wounded or killed in battle) and his Combat Infantryman's Badge (presented to soldiers in the grade of Colonel and below who participate in active ground combat while assigned as a member of an infantry or special forces unit).

8. Though psychological stress after trauma was documented as early as 1900 B.C., the condition of PTSD is a fairly modern discovery so this may partially be due to improved record-keeping.

9. Autogenics is a relaxation technique developed by doctors Johannes Schultz and Wolfgang Luthe in 1932 which has been used successfully in treating PTSD patients. It parallels techniques found in yoga or meditation, relaxing the body, lowering the heart rate, and controlling breathing.

10. Captain John Parker (1729 – 1775), commander of the seventy colonial minutemen (militia) that met more than seven hundred British troops who were sent to seize the guns, ammunition, and other supplies at Concord (under the command of General Thomas Gage) and fired the "shot heard 'round the world" on April 19, 1775. This event is commonly regarded as the beginning of the American Revolution.

11. Seneca (5 B.C. – 65 A.D.), Roman dramatist, philosopher, and politician.

12. Catherine "Kitty" Genovese (1935 – 1964) was stabbed and slowly bled to death near her home in the Kew Gardens section of Queens, New York, while 38 witnesses saw the attack or heard her subsequent please for help and did nothing to call the authorities or otherwise assist her in any way. An investigation of the inaction of her neighbors lead to identification of the psychological phenomenon that became known as the "bystander effect."

13. Chinua Achebe (1930 –), Nigerian writer, one of Africa's most internationally acclaimed authors and considered by many to be the father of modern African literature. His works include *Things Fall Apart, No Longer at Ease, Beware, Soul Brother, Christmas in Biafra, Morning Yet on Creation Day,* and *Home and Exile.* A paraplegic as the result of a 1990 automobile accident, Achebe currently lives in the United States where he teaches at Bard College (in New York).

Chapter 6

1. John Ronald Reuel Tolkien (1892 – 1973) was an Oxford University professor and a scholar of the English language specializing in Old and Middle English. He wrote a number of stories and books, including critically acclaimed epic fantasies *The Hobbit* and *The Lord of the Rings.*
2. United States Senator Larry Craig (R-Idaho); Congressional Testimony, June 6, 2000.
3. Loren Christensen (see endnote 4 for Chapter 2.)
4. Michael Jerome Johnson has studied martial arts for 35 years and has been a fight director for prestigious companies such as The Shakespeare Theatre, Arena Stage, The Lady Cavaliers, Double Helix Theatre, NAATCO/Fluid Motion, Round House Theatre, Folger Shakespeare Theatre, The Shakespeare Project, Theatre at Lime Kiln, Woolly Mammoth Theatre Company, Ford's Theatre, Delaware Theatre Company, and The Kennedy Center. He has taught at several schools, including, McDaniel College, Georgetown University, American University, Catholic University, National Conservatory of Dramatic Arts, University of Maryland's Opera Studio, and his alma mater, North Carolina School of the Arts. Mr. Johnson is also a professional actor. He has performed at various regional theatres, on tour, on television, and in feature films. He was also a stunt double for the television show, "A Man Called Hawk."
5. George S. Patton (1885 – 1945), United States Army general. Remembered for his fierce determination and ability to lead soldiers, he is widely regarded as one of the most successful field commanders of any army in any war. He commanded the Seventh Army during the invasion of Sicily and later the Third Army in France. Patton and his troops dashed across Europe after the battle of Normandy, exploiting German weaknesses with great success. By the end of WWII, the Third Army had liberated 81,522 square miles of territory. He was also known for carrying ivory-handled pistols.
6. Loren Christensen (See endnote 4 in Chapter 2.)
7. Loren Christensen (See endnote 4 in Chapter 2.)
8. Marc MacYoung (See endnote 1 in the Preface.).
9. Friedrich Nietzsche (1844 – 1900), German philosopher. The comic book character Superman is sometimes credited as originating from Nietzsche's concept of the Ubermensch or at least as a popularization thereof. His famous works include *The Birth of Tragedy, Beyond Good and Evil, The Twilight of the Idols, The Antichrist,* and *The Will to Power.*

Chapter 7

1. From the Federal Bureau of Investigation Web site (www.fbi.gov).
2. Marc MacYoung (See endnote 1 in the Preface.).
3. Massad Ayoob (see endnote 3 in Chapter 1)
4. Darren Laur is a full time police officer with the Victoria Police Department and the head instructor of Personal Protection Systems Inc. He has trained extensively in a variety of combat forms and specializes in reality based application and instruction.
5. Darren Laur (See previous endnote.).
6. Lloyd De Jongh is a South African martial artist who studies self-defense and criminal methods, from surprise assaults, muggings, fighting methodology, weapons use, and psychological tactics.
7. Michael Janich has taught knife fighting and self-defense techniques to Special Forces soldiers, law enforcement personnel, and civilian martial artists for many years. He has written nine books on knife fighting and other martial arts topics.
8. Loren Christensen (See endnote 4 for Chapter 2).

9. Anthony Greenbank from his book, *The Book of Survival: The Original Guide to Staying Alive in the City, the Suburbs, and the Wild Lands Beyond.*
10. Massad Ayoob (See endnote 3 in Chapter 1.).

Chapter 8

1. Massad Ayoob (See endnote 3 in Chapter 1.).
2. American Red Cross (www.redcross.org).
3. For example, if a knife blade has severed an artery it may still prevent serious hemorrhaging while it remains in place. Because the imbedded object provides pressure inside the wound it acts as a hemostat to minimize bleeding.
4. Loren Christensen (See endnote 4 for Chapter 2.)
5. Such as the 1983 study by Arye Rattner whose Ohio State University doctoral dissertation, *Convicting the Innocent: Where Justice Goes Wrong*, demonstrated that 0.5% of people arrested and charged with felony crimes in the United States annually were wrongly convicted. Eyewitness misidentification was the cause of 52.3% of those erroneous convictions.
6. Miranda v. Arizona, 384 U.S. 436. Ernesto Miranda was arrested for robbery, kidnapping, and rape in 1963. He was subsequently interrogated by police and confessed to his crimes. Prosecutors offered only his confession as evidence during his trial where he was convicted. The Supreme Court later ruled in 1966 that Miranda was intimidated by the interrogation neither understanding his right to not incriminate himself, nor his right to have counsel present during the interrogation. On the basis of that finding, the court overturned his conviction. He was later convicted in a new trial where witnesses testified against him and other evidence was presented, serving 11 years for his crimes. This Supreme Court ruling forms the basis of the "Miranda Rights" that all suspects must be read prior to interrogation by law enforcement. Police are only required to Mirandize an individual whom they intend to subject to custodial interrogation. While arrests can occur without questioning and without the Miranda warning, the warning must be given prior to any formal interrogation.
7. Laurie Shertz is a criminal defense attorney who has been practicing law in the states of Washington and Oregon since 1995. She holds a Juris Doctorate from the Seattle University School of Law and an undergraduate degree from the University of Washington. She has worked both as a prosecuting attorney and as a defense attorney focusing exclusively on criminal cases. She is in private practice in Portland, Oregon. Her web site is www.lshertzlaw.com.
8. The phrase double jeopardy stems from the Fifth Amendment which states, "…nor shall any person be subject for the same offence to be twice put in jeopardy of life or limb." This clause is intended to limit prosecutorial abuse stemming from repeated prosecution for the same offense as a means of harassment or governmental oppression after a person has already been tried for a crime.
9. In a well publicized example, Erik and Lyle Menendez were convicted of murdering their parents Jose and Kitty in 1989 despite an argument that they killed their parents in order to escape a lifetime of parental abuse. They were sentenced to life in prison on July 2, 1996.
10. Robert Frost (1874 – 1963), Pulitzer Prize winning poet. One of America's most popular and widely-read poets, he was also an advisor to presidents Eisenhower and Kennedy.
11. In many instances, except for serious felonies, there will be a recognizance process or interview where jail administration will decide whether or not you can be released on your own recognizance. Your conduct during booking can make or break your case.
12. Peremptory pleas typically include the plea of *autrefois convict*, the plea of *autrefois acquit*, and the plea of pardon. *Autrefois convict* means that the defendant claims to have been previously convicted for the same offense and that hence cannot be tried for it again. *Autrefois acquit* means the defendant claims to have been previously acquitted of the same offense, on substantially the same evidence, and that hence cannot be tried again. Pardon is where a defendant claims to have been pardoned for an offense, and hence cannot be tried for it.
13. Information sufficient to warrant a prudent person's belief that the suspect has actually committed a crime.

14. Specifically the Sixth Amendment states, "In all criminal prosecutions, the accused shall enjoy the right to a speedy and public trial, by an impartial jury of the state and district wherein the crime shall have been committed."

15. Literally, "speak the truth," a process by which prospective jurors are questioned about their backgrounds and potential biases before being invited to sit on a jury.

16. This may not happen immediately. Defendants are often returned to jail until all the paperwork is processed and then released.

17. John Entine is an investigative journalist, scholar-in-residence at Miami University (Ohio), and adjunct fellow with the American Enterprise Institute.

18. Richard Dooling is a fiction writer, essayist, and attorney. His books include *Critical Care, White Man's Grave, Brain Storm,* and *Bet Your Life.*

Chapter 9

1. Marc MacYoung (See endnote 1 in the Preface.)

2. Massad Ayoob (See endnote 3 in Chapter 1.)

3. Massad Ayoob (See endnote 3 in Chapter 1.)

4. Most concealable ballistic vests are designed to stop a bullet or a knife slash but not a hard stab from an ice pick or a narrow blade. Corrections officers and others who encounter knives on a regular basis sometimes wear special vests designed for that purpose (though they are rather expensive and not always available due to budget restrictions and other factors).

5. This poem is haiku in form, with Norse edda influence. Robin Ashley Smith is an educator, historian, tournament swordsman, and writer living in Seattle. For more information about Mr. Smith, see www.Ben-Franklin.org.

6. During the genocide that occurred between 1990 and 1994 a total of 1,074,017 people—approximately one-seventh of the total population of Rwanda—were murdered, with Tutsis accounting for 94 percent of the victims. These figures come from a February 2002 Rwandan government census report. The vast majority were hacked to death with inexpensive machetes.

7. Not something I'd recommend you do "at home." I subjected the $129 blade to that much abuse during an experiment designed to test how well-built it was (it passed with flying colors, by the way). Normally I'd use a hatchet or machete which was designed for that type of work.

8. Massad Ayoob (See endnote 3 in Chapter 1.)

9. Some jurisdictions differentiate between dangerous weapons and deadly weapons in their statutes. Nevertheless, for the purposes of this discussion anything dangerous can also be deadly if you end up on the wrong end of the weapon.

10. Marc MacYoung (See endnote 1 in the Preface.)

11. Sid Campbell is a martial artist, author, actor, stuntman, and fight choreographer. He was named California's most outstanding Okinawan-style instructor in 1974 at the Golden Fist Awards and named to *Who's Who in the Martial Arts* in 1975.

12. Charlton Heston (1923 –), actor, writer, producer, and director. He has won numerous awards for his work including Oscars for Best Actor in *Ben-Hur* (1959) and the 'Jean Hersolt Humanitarian Award' (1977). Heston was elected President of the Screen Actors Guild six times, President of the National Rifle Association (NRA) twice, and President of the American Film Institute once.

13. The power of a pepper spray is rated both by a percentage content of OC and a Scoville heat rating (SHU). The latter characteristic is most important in determining effectiveness. When looking for a pepper spray to buy, you will want to choose a spray with the highest SHU you can find as well as a high OC content (~ 10%). Typically 1.5 to 2 million SHUs is available for civilians and up to 5.3 million SHUs for police.

14. It takes far too long to chamber a round during a violent encounter in my opinion to carry a weapon without a full magazine and a round in the chamber on the street. You must, however, select a gun that is designed for safe carry with a round in the chamber before doing it that way. Some of the less expensive models are dubious in terms of safety. They may inadvertently discharge a round if struck forcefully or dropped, for example.

15. Any bullet can over-penetrate. Even pre-fragmented rounds do not always work as advertised.

16. For example, while magazines from .40 S&W caliber and 9mm Parabellum pistols can frequently be placed into the same gun, only one with the proper bullet can actually be chambered and fired. It would be bad to discover that you have loaded the wrong magazine in the middle of a gunfight.

17. If you need to remove a jammed rim fire round (e.g., 22 caliber) do not pry on the edges, use a cleaning rod to push the round backward via the barrel. These bullets are ignited by pressure on the edge of the rim. Center fire rounds, on the other hand, can usually be pried loose without fear of accidental discharge though you must continue to point the weapon in a safe direction while you are doing it.

18. Unless you are forced to do so because of a tactical situation, do not hold a pistol sideways. It looks good in the movies but increases your odds of a stovepipe failure on the street. Stove piping is when an expended cartridge is not properly extracted, jamming the weapon. Further, properly extracted brass may be more likely to fly into your face when the weapon is held incorrectly. Hot brass is very painful and potentially damaging if it hits you in the face or eye.

19. I recommend firing no less than a thousand rounds of cheap target ammo and a box of good self-defense rounds on the range before trusting a gun on the street. Even quality firearms take a few hundred rounds to break in properly. Furthermore, without adequate training and familiarity with the weapon you can become a danger to yourself or others on the street regardless of whether or not a failure takes place.

20. IPSC was founded at the International Pistol Conference held in Columbia, Missouri, in May 1976. Gun fighting legend Col. Jeff Cooper invited 40 people from around the world to attend the conference in order to determine the nature and future of practical marksmanship. The promotion of accuracy, power, and speed along with the development of procedures and rules for safe gun handling were their prime objectives. The organization's motto *Diligentia, Vis, Celeritas* (accuracy, power, and speed) was introduced to reflect this objective. IPSC is promoted in more than sixty countries from Argentina to Zimbabwe today.

21. Never cross your thumb behind the slide. If your off-hand thumb is struck by the slide it will not only hurt your hand but very likely cause your weapon to jam as well.

22. What works on the target range will not always work on the street so there is no guarantee that you will be able to do this successfully during a real gunfight; there's simply too much going on. Nevertheless, what you do in training will heavily influence what you will be able to do under stress (diminished level of effectiveness). Consequently, the more prepared you are ahead of time the more likely you will be able to survive in a violent encounter.

23. Certain large-bore calibers are frowned upon at some ranges because they can damage the facilities or increase maintenance costs.

24. John Farnam is one of the nation's top firearms instructors. As president of Defense Training International he has personally trained thousands of federal, state and local law enforcement personnel as well as civilians, in the tactical use of handguns, rifles, and shotguns. He has written several excellent books on shooting techniques including, *The Farnam Method of Defensive Handgunning, The Farnam Method of Defensive Shotgun and Rifle Shooting,* and *The Street Smart Gun Book.*

25. Ballistic gelatin closely simulates the density and viscosity of human and animal muscle tissue, and is used as a standardized target for testing firearms and ammunition. Unfortunately, a bullet's performance in gelatin does not always reflect actual penetration and expansion in humans or animals. As a bullet passes through layers of clothing or other barriers its ballistic properties are affected too. Consequently, ballistic gelatin tests are not always accurate predictors of real-life stopping power.

26. Contestants fire at standard bowling pins placed upright on a table. Rules vary but they generally must be knocked completely off the table in order to score. You typically shoot 6 tables of 5 pins consecutively per round. In most competitions I've entered all large bore guns were grouped together so there was a distinct advantage to .45 ACP over .9mm where contestants had equal skill levels.

27. Be wary of surplus submachine gun rounds which, while very cheap, can damage your firing pin. The primers on Egyptian surplus ammo, for example, are different than those designed for use in handguns and may not only blunt the firing pin but also do not always ignite every time you pull the trigger.

28. See endnote 23 in Chapter 1.

29. Major Eugene Sockut is the Chief of Marksmanship and Snipers with the Israeli Army. An American-born Jew who immigrated to Israel, he has been an advisor and consultant to the Israeli Military, Prison Service, Police, and Judicial System. Since 1971, he has published a variety of training manuals, books, and videos on arms and survival, receiving world-wide acclaim for his works.

30. An extremely toxic type of rat poison that affects the nervous system. A single dose of bromethalin is generally all that is needed to cause death unlike other rat poisons such as diphacinone and warfarin, which are anticoagulants (blood thinners) that work over time.

31. O-Isopropyl methylphosphonofluoridate, a highly toxic nerve agent which has been outlawed by the UN since 1993. Probably most famous from the March 20, 1995 Tokyo subway gas attack perpetrated by the Aum Shinrikyo cult.

32. Gavin DeBecker is a nationally recognized expert on the prediction and management of violence. His work has earned him several honors including two appointments to the President's Advisory Board at the U.S. Department of Justice and two appointments to the Governor's Advisory Board at the California Department of Mental Health. His consulting firm advises government agencies, universities, police departments, corporations, and media figures on the assessment of threats and hazards. His book, *The Gift of Fear*, spent four months on the New York Times Bestseller List, and is now published in thirteen languages.

33. Hironori Otsuka (1892 – 1982), founder of the *Wado-Ryu* (way of peace). In 1966, Otsuka Sensei received the *kun go to*, (Fifth Order of Merit of the Sacred Treasure) from the Emperor of Japan, who also bestowed upon him the *Soko Kyokujitsu Sho* medal for his contributions to the development and promotion of karate. In 1972, he received the *shodai karate-do meijin judan* or (First Generation Karate-do Master of the Tenth *Dan*), and was designated the head of all martial arts systems within the All Japan Karate-do Federation.

Conclusion

1. Isaac Asimov (1920 – 1992), Russian-born American author and biochemist. He is best known as an award-winning science fiction novelist, and scholar. His most famous works include *Foundation, Foundation and Empire, Second Foundation, The Gods Themselves*, and *I, Robot. The Oxford English Dictionary* credits his science fiction for introducing the words positronic, psychohistory, and robotics into the English language.

2. On May 11, 2005, about a week prior to this incident, another would-be car thief named Edward Zanassi was accidentally choked to death by the vehicle owner and his roommate who tried to restrain Zanassi. During the struggle, he reportedly bit the car owner's finger, so the roommate put him in a chokehold to make him release the bite. The Pierce County Prosecutor pronounced that the homicide was "justifiable and/or excusable as a matter of law" and did not file any charges in that case. I would not be surprised if this car thief heard about the other's demise since it was well covered in newspaper and television broadcasts and that the news added to his terror in this situation.

Glossary

Romaji (Romanization) note—I have primarily used the Hebon-Shiki (Hepburn) method of translating Japanese writing into the English alphabet and determining how best to spell the words (though accent marks have been excluded), as it is generally considered the most useful insofar as pronunciation is concerned. I have italicized foreign terms such that they can be readily differentiated from their English counterparts (e.g., *dan* meaning black belt rank versus Dan, the male familiar name for Daniel). As the Japanese and Chinese languages do not use capitalization, I have only capitalized those words that would be used as proper nouns in English.

Japanese is a challenging language for many English speakers to pronounce correctly. A few hints—for the most part, short vowels sound just like their English counterparts (e.g., **a** as in father, **e** as in pen). Long vowels are essentially double-length (e.g., **o** as in <u>oi</u>l, in the word *oyo*). The **u** is nearly silent, except where it is an initial syllable (e.g., *uke*). Vowel combination **e** + **i** sounds like d<u>ay</u> (e.g., *bugeisha*), **a** + **i** sounds like al<u>i</u>ve (e.g., *bunkai*), **o** + **u** sounds like fl<u>oa</u>t (e.g., tou), and **a** + **e** sounds like l<u>ie</u> (*kamae*). The consonant r is pronounced with the tip of the tongue, midway between **l** and **r** (e.g., *daruma*). Consonant combination **ts** is pronounced like ca<u>ts</u>, almost a **z** (e.g., *tsuki*).

Although there are a few words here from other languages such as Latin or German, the vast majority of words listed in this glossary come from Japanese.

Glossary of Terms

autrefois convict   plea of previous conviction

autrefois acquit   plea of previous acquittal

balisong   butterfly knife, a folding pocketknife with two handles that counter-rotate around a tang such that, when closed, the blade is concealed within grooves in the handles

borang   Filipino shortsword

bo   fighting staff, typically about six feet in length

bokken   legendary swordsman Miyamoto Musashi killed several fully armed samurai with only a wood *bokken*, demonstrating the inherent deadliness of this simple device, a wooden sword built to imitate a *katana* in size which is used in the practice of *iaido, aikido, kendo,* and other sword arts; literally "wooden sword"

budo   martial arts or ways

budoka   martial artist

buke   nobility in feudal Japan

bunkai   fighting applications found in *kata*

chudan   mid-level (chest)

chudan uke   chest block

coup d'grace   final or finishing blow; irrevocable

daimyo   warlord; literally "great name"

daisho   set of two swords carried by the samurai warriors in feudal Japan, a *katana* (long sword) and *wakizashi* (short sword)

dan   black belt rank

dao   Chinese broadsword

dojo   school or training hall; literally a "place to learn the way"

ericfine   Celtic term for blood money paid to the relatives of a man murdered or slain in ritual combat

fudoshin   indomitable or indefatigable spirit

fukidake   blowgun

gedan   downward level; below the waist

gladius   Roman shortsword

glowczyzna   Slavic term for blood money paid to the relatives of a man murdered or slain in ritual combat

Goju Ryu   an Okinawan form of karate developed by Chojun Miyagi Sensei

gross messer   literally "big knife," a large single-edged Germanic sword typically wielded two handed

gyaku tsuki   reverse punch; if one leg is in front of the other, the arm throwing the punch is on the side of the back hip

ha   cutting edge of a Japanese blade (e.g., *katana*, *wakizashi*)

hamon   temper line of a Japanese blade (e.g., *katana*, *wakizashi*) where the *ha* and *mune* meet

heiko dachi   natural stance, feet parallel

hiki uke   pulling/grasping open-hand block

iaido   a Japanese sword art

jian   Chinese straight sword (tai chi sword)

jodan   upper level (head)

judoka   judo practitioners

jutte   a truncheon used by law enforcement officers in Edo period Japan

kama   sickle

kamae   ready position

karambit   a curved knife indigenous to the Indonesian archipelago and some areas of the Philippines

karate   a (primarily) Japanese or Okinawan martial art which emphasizes weaponless or empty-hand striking techniques (e.g., punching/kicking)

karate ni sente nashi   "there is no first strike in karate," a saying made famous by Gichin Funakoshi, the founder of *Shotokan* Karate

karateka   karate practitioners

katana　*samurai* long sword

kata　a pattern of movements containing a series of logical and practical offensive and defensive techniques

kayaku-jutsu　*Shinobi* (ninja) pyrotechnic arts of feudal Japan

kiai　spirit shout, a loud yell

kissaki　tip of a *katana*

kobudo　a Japanese or Okinawan martial art featuring a variety of weapons forms derived from common agricultural tools

kubaton　invented by Takayuki Kubata, a cylindrical rod about five to six inches long and half an inch in diameter used for self-defense

kusarigama　weighted chain and sickle

kuwa　hoe adapted as a *kobudo* weapon

kwan dao　Chinese halberd

kyu　colored belt rank

kyudo　literally, "the way of the bow;" traditional Japanese archery

long *sax*　Norse shortsword

mae geri　front kick

manriki kusari　weighted chain flail

marote kamae　ready position, typically *sanchin dachi* (hourglass stance) with double *chudan uke* (chest block); the starting position for many traditional *kata*

masubi dachi　attention stance

mo gem　invented by Jim Morrell, a cylindrical rod about eight inches long and an inch in diameter used for self-defense

monouchi　blade portion of a *sai*

mune　back (unsharpened) edge of a Japanese blade (e.g., *katana*, *wakizashi*)

naginata　*samurai* glaive; a long curved blade on pole shaft

nakinshuto uchi　inside sword hand strike

naname　angle, or angled strike/block

neko ashi dachi　cat stance

neko te　*Shinobi* cat claw, metal claws affixed to the finger tips

nolo contendere　no contest (plea), literally "I do not wish to argue"

nuki　thrust, long strike

nukibo　staff thrust

nukite　finger thrust

nunchaku　rice flail; a *kobudo* weapon made from two sticks tied or chained together at one end

nunti bo　hooked spear (gaffe hook); a type of *sai* affixed to a long pole shaft

osae uke　press block

pila   Roman javelin

ronin   literally "wave man;" a masterless *samurai*

sai   a *kobudo* weapon, its basic form is that of an unsharpened dagger with forward curving projections rather than a traditional cross-guard

saifa kata   a *Goju Ryu* karate form meaning "smash and tear"

sam-jit-gwun   three-sectional staff (Chinese for *sansetsu kon bo*)

samurai   feudal Japanese warrior, literally "those who serve"

sanchin dachi   hourglass stance

sansetsu kon bo   three-sectional staff

saya   scabbard

scramasax   Norse long bladed knife similar to a modern bowie knife

sen sen no-sen   preemptively cutting off an attack before the opponent can translate the mental desire to strike to the physical movements necessary to carry out that desire

shinai   a straight bamboo practice sword used in *kendo*

shodan   first degree black belt

shozenkutsu dachi   short- or half-front stance

shuko   tiger claw

shuriken   throwing star

sjambok   a traditional South African hide whip about three to five feet in length

skean dhu   Scottish stocking knife

sotoshuto uchi   outside sword-hand strike

spatha   Roman cavalry sword

sumo   a wrestling art dating back to the Edo period of feudal Japan

suruchin   weighted chain weapon

sweihander   German greatsword

tachi   Japanese sword typically used by cavalry; as opposed to the traditional manner of wearing the *katana*, the *tachi* was worn hung from the belt with the cutting-edge down

Tagálog   main Filipino dialect

tanto   Japanese single-edged fighting knife.

tetsui uchi   hammerfist strike

tonfa   grist mill handle adapted into a *kobudo* weapon; similar to a modern side-handle police baton

tsuba   cross guard

tsuka   handle

tsukagashira   butt end of a *sai*, a striking surface

tsuki   strike or short thrust

uchi   strike

ueku   oar adapted into a *kobudo* weapon

uke   to block or receive an attack

uraken uchi   backfist strike

uraken uke   wrist block

voir dire   literally "speak the truth," a process of vetting potential jurors

wakizashi   *samurai* short sword

wergild   "man price," Norse term for blood money paid to the relatives of a man murdered or slain in ritual combat

yari   Japanese spear

yawara stick   a cylindrical rod about six inches long and an inch in diameter used for self-defense

yodan   fourth degree black belt

yumi   a longbow used in the practice of *kyudo* (Japanese archery).

yoko   sideways (horizontal)

yoku   upswept tines (cross guard) of a *sai*

zanshin   "continuing mind," a state of enhanced awareness that should exist before, during, and right after battle

zenkutsu dachi   front, forward stance

zweihander   German medieval two-handed sword

Bibliography

Books

American Red Cross. *First Aid Fast*. San Bruno, CA: The American National Red Cross, 2002.

Applegate, Rex. *Kill or Get Killed*. Boulder, CO: Paladin Enterprises, Inc., 1976.

Arsenault, Al and Joseph Faulise. *Chin Na in Ground Fighting*. Boston, MA: YMAA Publication Center, 2003.

Ayoob, Massad. *In the Gravest Extreme: The Role of the Firearm in Personal Protection*. Concord NH: Police Bookshelf, 1980.

Ayoob, Massad. *The Truth About Self-Protection*. New York, NY: Bantam Books (Police Bookshelf), 1983.

Bittenbinder, J. J. *Tough Target: A Street-Smart Guide to Staying Safe*. Philadelphia, PA: Running Press, 1997.

Campbell, Bruce. *Exotic Weapons of the Ninja*. New York, NY: Kensington Publishing Corp., 1994.

Christensen, Loren and Dr. Alexis Artwohl. *Deadly Force Encounters: What Cops Need To Know To Mentally And Physically Prepare For And Survive A Gunfight*. Boulder, CO: Paladin Enterprises, Inc., 1997.

Christensen, Loren. *Far Beyond Defensive Tactics: Advanced Concepts, Techniques, Drills, and Tricks for Cops on the Street*. Boulder, CO: Paladin Enterprises, Inc., 1998.

Christensen, Loren. *How to Live Safely in a Dangerous World*. El Dorado, AR: The Delta Group, Ltd., 1996.

Christensen, Loren. *Solo Training 2: The Martial Artist's Guide to Building the Core for Stronger, Faster, and More Effective Grappling, Kicking and Punching*. Wethersfield, CT: Turtle Press, 2005.

Christensen, Loren. *Surviving Workplace Violence: What to Do Before a Violent Incident, What to Do When the Violence Explodes*. Boulder, CO: Paladin Enterprises, Inc., 2005.

Cooper, Jeff. *Principles of Personal Defense*. Boulder, CO: Paladin Enterprises, Inc., 1989.

Covey, Stephen R. *The 7 Habits of Highly Effective People*. New York, NY: Simon and Schuster, 1989.

Davidson, Thomas N. *To Preserve Life: Hostage-Crisis Management*. Indianapolis, IN: Crisis Incident Management Agency (CIMACOM), 2002.

DeBecker, Gavin. *The Gift of Fear: Survival Signals That Protect Us From Violence*. New York, NY: Dell Publishing, 1998.

Evangelista, Nick. *The Encyclopedia of the Sword*. Westport, CT: Greenwood Press, 1995.

Gil, Itay and Dan Baron. *The Citizen's Guide to Stopping Suicide Attackers: Secrets of an Israeli Counterterrorist*. Boulder, CO: Paladin Enterprises, Inc., 2004.

Greenbank, Anthony. *The Book of Survival: The Original Guide to Staying Alive in the City, the Suburbs, and the Wild Lands Beyond*. (revised edition). Long Island City, NY: Hatherleigh Press, 2001.

Grossman, Dave and Loren Christensen. *On Combat: The Psychology and Physiology of Deadly Conflict in War and Peace*. Belleville, IL: PPCT Research Publications, 2004.

Gruzanski, Charles. *Ninja Weapons: Chain and Shuriken*. Rutland, VT: Charles E. Tuttle Company, Inc., 1967.

Janich, Michael D. *Knife Fighting: A Practical Course*. Boulder, CO: Paladin Enterprises, Inc., 1993.

(Lichtenfeld) Sde-Or, Imi and Eyal Yanilov. *Krav Maga: How to Defend Yourself against Armed Assault*. Tel Aviv, Israel: Dekel Publishing House, 2001.

Loftus, Elizabeth and Katherine Ketcham. *Witness for the Defense: the Accused, the Eyewitness, and the Expert Who Puts Memory on Trial*. New York, NY: St. Martin's Press, 1991.

MacYoung, Marc. *A Professional's Guide to Ending Violence Quickly*. Boulder, CO: Paladin Enterprises, Inc., 1993.

MacYoung, Marc. *Pool Cues, Beer Bottles, & Baseball Bats: Animal's Guide to Improvised Weapons for Self-Defense and Survival*. Boulder, CO: Paladin Enterprises, Inc., 1990.

MacYoung, Marc. Street E & E: *Evading, Escaping, and Other Ways to Save Your Ass When Things Get Ugly*. Boulder, CO: Paladin Enterprises, Inc., 1993.

Nance, Malcolm. *The Terrorist Recognition Handbook: A Manual for Predicting and Identifying Terrorist Activities*. Guilford, CT: The Lyons Press, 2003.

Orlando, Bob. *Indonesian Fighting Fundamentals: The Brutal Arts of the Archipelago*. Boulder, CO: Paladin Enterprises, Inc., 1996.

Pentecost, Don. *Put 'Em Down, Take 'Em Out!: Knife Fighting Techniques From Folsom Prison*. Boulder, CO: Paladin Enterprises, Inc., 1988.

Quinn, Peyton. *Bouncer's Guide to Barroom Brawling: Dealing with the Sucker Puncher, Streetfighter, and Ambusher.* Boulder, CO: Paladin Enterprises, Inc., 1990.

Quinn, Peyton. *Real Fighting: Adrenaline Stress Conditioning through Scenario-Based Training.* Boulder, CO: Paladin Enterprises, Inc., 1996.

Siddle, Bruce K. *Sharpening the Warrior's Edge: The Psychology and Science of Training.* Millstadt, IL: PPCT Research Publications, Inc., 1995.

Sockut, Eugene. *Secrets of Street Survival – Israeli Style: Staying Alive in a Civilian War Zone.* Boulder, CO: Paladin Enterprises, Inc., 1995.

Stanford, Andy. *Surgical Speed Shooting: How to Achieve High-Speed Marksmanship in a Gunfight.* Boulder, CO: Paladin Enterprises, Inc., 2001.

Suarez, Gabe. *Tactical Pistol Marksmanship: How to Improve Your Combat Shooting Skills.* Boulder, CO: Paladin Enterprises, Inc., 2001.

Suarez, Gabe. *The Combative Perspective: The Thinking Man's Guide to Self-Defense.* Boulder, CO: Paladin Enterprises, Inc., 2003.

Thompson, George J. *Verbal Judo: the Gentle Art of Persuasion.* New York, NY: William Morrow and Company, 1993.

Wilson, William E. *Arte of Defence: An Introduction to the Use of the Rapier.* Highland Village, TX: Chivalry Bookshelf, 2002.

Windsor, Guy. *The Swordsman's Companion: A Manual for Training with the Medieval Longsword.* Highland Village, TX: Chivalry Bookshelf, 2004.

Yang, Jwing-Ming and Jeffrey Bolt. *Northern Shaolin Sword.* Boston, MA: YMAA Publication Center, 1998.

Zabinski, Grzegorz and Bartlomiej Walczak. *Codex Wallerstein: A Medieval Fighting Book from the Fifteenth Century on the Longsword, Falchion, Dagger, and Wrestling.* Boulder, CO: Paladin Enterprises, Inc., 2002.

Articles

Ayoob, Massad. Duty Loads: Today's Best. *Guns Magazine*, March, 2002.

Ayoob, Massad. The Ayoob Files – One Gun, No Hands: The Marcus Young Incident. *American Handgunner*, Sept-Oct, 2004.

Ayoob, Massad. The Ayoob Files – Wrong Weapon: the Der/Kifer Incident. *American Handgunner*, Sept-Oct, 2003.

Ayoob, Massad. Lethal Force: Explaining the Deadly Force Decision: Justifiable Homicide. *Shooting Industry*, August, 1991.

Ayoob, Massad. Lethal Force: Explaining the Deadly Force Decision: Self-Defense in a Nutshell. *Shooting Industry*, March, 1992.

Ayoob, Massad. Lethal Force: The Dangers of Being a Firearms Expert. *Shooting Industry*, January, 1994.

Bitran, Eli. Defense Against a Straight Stab. Fightingarts.com.

Boeing Commercial Airplanes, Airline Safety Engineering. *Statistical Summary of Commercial Jet Airplane Accidents: World Wide Operations 1959 – 2003.* The Boeing Company, May 2004.

Caile, Christopher. Shot at Point Blank Range: Lessons from The Street. Fightingarts.com.

Caile, Christopher. Fighting Back At 40,000 Feet: Part 1 – Responding to Airborne Terrorists. Fightingarts.com.

Caile, Christopher. Fighting Back At 40,000 Feet: Part 2 – Group Principles, Individual Strategies. Fightingarts.com.

Caile, Christopher. Fighting Back At 40,000 Feet: Part 3 – Weapons, Shields and Artillery. Fightingarts.com.

Caile, Christopher. Defeating s Knife to the Neck. Fightingarts.com.

De Jongh, Lloyd. The Reality of Edged Weapon Attacks. Fightingarts.com.

Duhart, Detis T. Bureau of Justice Statistics Special Report: Violence in the Workplace 1993 – 99. U.S. Department of Justice, December 2001.

Federal Bureau of Investigation. Law Enforcement Officers Killed and Assaulted: 2003. U.S. Department of Justice, November, 2004.

Feldman, Jack M. Training for Situation Awareness: What? How? Teddytactical.com.

Feldman, Jack M. Unconscious Competence: What is it? How can we train for it? Teddytactical.com

Fox, Alan James. Bureau of Justice Statistics Crime Data Brief: Homicide Trends in the United States: 2002 Update. U.S. Department of Justice, November, 2004.

Givens, Tom. Controlling Fear and Making Sound Decisions Under Stress. Teddytactical.com.

Givens, Tom. Intelligence Gathering for Personal Safety. Teddytactical.com

Givens, Tom. States of Awareness, the Cooper Color Codes. Teddytactical.com.

Givens, Tom. Visualization, or Mental Imagery. Teddytactical.com.

Greenfeld, Lawrence. Bureau of Justice Statistics Selected Findings: Weapons Offenses and Offenders. U.S. Department of Justice, November, 1995.

Hart, Timothy C. Bureau of Justice Statistics Special Report: Violent Victimization of College Students. U.S. Department of Justice, September, 2003.

Hays, Tom. Actress' Slaying Teach Hard Lesson in What Not to do When Mugged. *Seattle Post Intelligencer*, February 3rd, 2005.

Henry, Tom. Job Shootings Aren't So Rare, Local Firms Told—Expert: Jeep Case Like Others. Toledoblade.com. February 25th, 2005.

Klaus, Patsy. Bureau of Justice Statistics National Crime Victimization Survey: Carjacking, 1993 – 2002. U.S. Department of Justice, July, 2004.

Laur, Darren. Edged Weapon Tactics and Counter Tactics. Lwcbooks.com.

Laur, Darren. Street 101. Lwcbooks.com

Laur, Darren. The Anatomy Of Fear and How It Relates To Survival Skills Training. Lwcbooks.com.

Perkins, Craig. Bureau of Justice Statistics Special Report: Weapon Use and Violent Crime. U.S. Department of Justice December, 2003.

Rennison, Callie M. Bureau of Justice Statistics National Crime Victimization Survey: Criminal Victimization 2000 – Changes 199-2000 with Trends 1993-2000. U.S. Department of Justice, June, 2001.

Roos, Gene. Defending Against an Ice Pick Stab. Fightingarts.com.

Roos, Gene. Defending Against an Ice Pick Stab #2. Fightingarts.com.

Truscott, Ted. Six Martial Arts Myths about Knife Defenses. Lwcbooks.com.

Web Sites

American Tactical Shooting Association web site (www.teddytactical.com).

Association of Renaissance Martial Arts web site (www.thehaca.com).

Fighting Arts web site (www.fightingarts.com).

Iain Abernethy's web site (www.iainabernethy.com).

Killology Research Group web site (www.killology.com).

Lenny Magill's concealment clothing and holster outlet (www.masterofconcealment.com)

Loren Christensen's web site (www.lwcbooks.com).

Marc "Animal" MacYoung's web site (www.nononsenseselfdefense.com).

National Counterterrorism Center Worldwide Incidents Tracking System (http://tkb.org/NCTCAdvancedSearch.jsp)

Seattle Post Intelligencer web site (www.seattlepi.nwsource.com)

Transportation Security Administration web site (www.tsa.gov).

Yahoo news (http://story.news.yahoo.com).

Videos

Bittenbinder, J. J. *Street Smarts: How to Avoid Being a Victim with Detective J. J. Bittenbinder.* Video Publishing House, Inc., 1992.

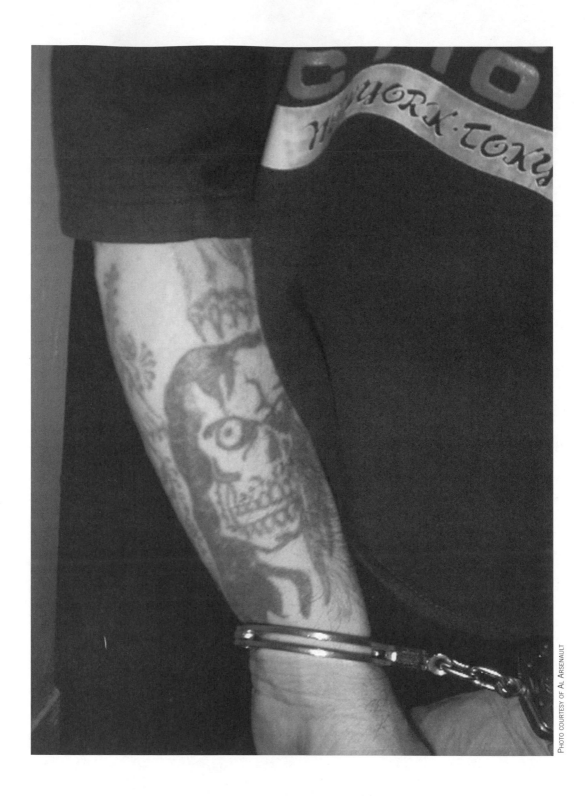

Index

About the Author

Lawrence A. Kane is the author of *Martial Arts Instruction—Applying Educational Theory and Communication Techniques in the Dojo* (YMAA Publication Center, 2004) and co-author of *The Way of Kata—A Comprehensive Guide for Deciphering Martial Applications* (YMAA Publication Center, 2005). Over the last 30 or so years, he has participated in a broad range of martial arts, from traditional Asian sports such as judo, *arnis, kobudo,* and karate to recreating medieval European combat with real armor and rattan (wood) weapons. He has taught medieval weapons forms since 1994 and *Goju Ryu* karate 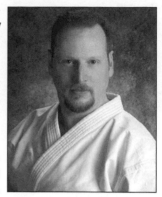 since 2002. He has also completed seminars in modern gun safety, marksmanship, handgun retention and knife combat techniques, and he has participated in slow-fire pistol and pin shooting competitions.

Since 1985, Lawrence has supervised employees who provide security and over-see fan safety during college and professional football games at a Pac-10 stadium. This part-time job has given him a unique opportunity to appreciate violence in a myriad of forms. Along with his crew, he has witnessed, interceded in, and stopped or prevented hundreds of fights, experiencing all manner of aggressive behaviors as well as the escalation process that invariably precedes them. He has also worked closely with the campus police and state patrol officers who are assigned to the sta-dium and has had ample opportunities to examine their crowd control tactics and procedures.

To pay the bills he does IT sourcing strategy and benchmarking work for an aero-space company in Seattle where he gets to play with billions of dollars of other peo-ple's money and make really important decisions. Lawrence lives in Seattle, Washington with his wife Julie and his son Joey. He can be contacted via e-mail at lakane@ix.netcom.com.

BOOKS FROM YMAA

VIDEOS FROM YMAA

more products available from...

YMAA Publication Center, Inc. 楊氏東方文化出版中心

4354 Washington Street Roslindale, MA 02131
1-800-669-8892 • ymaa@aol.com • www.ymaa.com

VIDEOS FROM YMAA (CONTINUED)

DEFEND YOURSELF 1 — UNARMED	T010/343
DEFEND YOURSELF 2 — KNIFE	T011/351
EMEI BAGUAZHANG 1	T017/280
EMEI BAGUAZHANG 2	T018/299
EMEI BAGUAZHANG 3	T019/302
EIGHT SIMPLE QIGONG EXERCISES FOR HEALTH 2ND ED.	T005/54X
ESSENCE OF TAIJI QIGONG	T006/238
MUGAI RYU	T050/467
NORTHERN SHAOLIN SWORD — SAN CAI JIAN & ITS APPLICATIONS	T035/051
NORTHERN SHAOLIN SWORD — KUN WU JIAN & ITS APPLICATIONS	T036/06X
NORTHERN SHAOLIN SWORD — QI MEN JIAN & ITS APPLICATIONS	T037/078
QIGONG: 15 MINUTES TO HEALTH	T042/140
SCIENTIFIC FOUNDATION OF CHINESE QIGONG — LECTURE	T029/590
SHAOLIN KUNG FU BASIC TRAINING — 1	T057/0045
SHAOLIN KUNG FU BASIC TRAINING — 2	T058/0053
SHAOLIN LONG FIST KUNG FU — TWELVE TAN TUI	T043/159
SHAOLIN LONG FIST KUNG FU — LIEN BU CHUAN	T002/19X
SHAOLIN LONG FIST KUNG FU — GUNG LI CHUAN	T003/203
SHAOLIN LONG FIST KUNG FU — YI LU MEI FU & ER LU MAI FU	T014/256
SHAOLIN LONG FIST KUNG FU — SHI ZI TANG	T015/264
SHAOLIN LONG FIST KUNG FU — XIAO HU YAN	T025/604
SHAOLIN WHITE CRANE GONG FU — BASIC TRAINING 1	T046/440
SHAOLIN WHITE CRANE GONG FU — BASIC TRAINING 2	T049/459
SHAOLIN WHITE CRANE GONG FU — BASIC TRAINING 3	T074/0185
SIMPLIFIED TAI CHI CHUAN — 24 & 48	T021/329
SUN STYLE TAIJIQUAN	T022/469
TAI CHI CHUAN & APPLICATIONS — 24 & 48	T024/485
TAI CHI FIGHTING SET	T078/0363
TAIJI BALL QIGONG — 1	T054/475
TAIJI BALL QIGONG — 2	T057/483
TAIJI BALL QIGONG — 3	T062/0096
TAIJI BALL QIGONG — 4	T063/010X
TAIJI CHIN NA	T016/408
TAIJI CHIN NA IN DEPTH — 1	T070/0282
TAIJI CHIN NA IN DEPTH — 2	T071/0290
TAIJI CHIN NA IN DEPTH — 3	T072/0304
TAIJI CHIN NA IN DEPTH — 4	T073/0312
TAIJI PUSHING HANDS — 1	T055/505
TAIJI PUSHING HANDS — 2	T058/513
TAIJI PUSHING HANDS — 3	T064/0134
TAIJI PUSHING HANDS — 4	T065/0142
TAIJI SABER	T053/491
TAIJI & SHAOLIN STAFF — FUNDAMENTAL TRAINING — 1	T061/0088
TAIJI & SHAOLIN STAFF — FUNDAMENTAL TRAINING — 2	T076/0347
TAIJI SWORD, CLASSICAL YANG STYLE	T031/817
TAIJI WRESTLING — 1	T079/0371
TAIJI WRESTLING — 2	T080/038X
TAIJI YIN & YANG SYMBOL STICKING HANDS–YANG TAIJI TRAINING	T056/580
TAIJI YIN & YANG SYMBOL STICKING HANDS–YIN TAIJI TRAINING	T067/0177
TAIJIQUAN, CLASSICAL YANG STYLE	T030/752
WHITE CRANE HARD QIGONG	T026/612
WHITE CRANE SOFT QIGONG	T027/620
WILD GOOSE QIGONG	T032/949
WU STYLE TAIJIQUAN	T023/477
XINGYIQUAN — 12 ANIMAL FORM	T020/310
YANG STYLE TAI CHI CHUAN AND ITS APPLICATIONS	T001/181

DVDS FROM YMAA

ANALYSIS OF SHAOLIN CHIN NA	D0231
BAGUAZHANG 1,2, & 3 —EMEI BAGUAZHANG	D0649
CHIN NA IN DEPTH COURSES 1 — 4	D602
CHIN NA IN DEPTH COURSES 5 — 8	D610
CHIN NA IN DEPTH COURSES 9 — 12	D629
EIGHT SIMPLE QIGONG EXERCISES FOR HEALTH	D0037
THE ESSENCE OF TAIJI QIGONG	D0215
QIGONG MASSAGE—FUNDAMENTAL TECHNIQUES FOR HEALTH AND RELAXATION	D0592
SHAOLIN KUNG FU FUNDAMENTAL TRAINING 1&2	D0436
SHAOLIN LONG FIST KUNG FU — BASIC SEQUENCES	D661
SHAOLIN WHITE CRANE GONG FU BASIC TRAINING 1&2	D599
SIMPLIFIED TAI CHI CHUAN	D0630
SUNRISE TAI CHI	D0274
TAI CHI FIGHTING SET—TWO PERSON MATCHING SET	D0657
TAIJI BALL QIGONG COURSES 1&2—16 CIRCLING AND 16 ROTATING PATTERNS	D0517
TAIJI PUSHING HANDS 1&2—YANG STYLE SINGLE AND DOUBLE PUSHING HANDS	D0495
TAIJIQUAN CLASSICAL YANG STYLE	D645
TAIJI SWORD, CLASSICAL YANG STYLE	D0452
WHITE CRANE HARD & SOFT QIGONG	D637

more products available from...
YMAA Publication Center, Inc. 楊氏東方文化出版中心
4354 Washington Street Roslindale, MA 02131
1-800-669-8892 • ymaa@aol.com • www.ymaa.com

YMAA
PUBLICATION CENTER